*"Estrogen's Storm Season* provides perimenopausal women (and their healthcare providers) with brilliant insights and practical solutions to help them weather the rigors of this important life stage."

—CHRISTIANE NORTHRUP, MD, author of *Mother-Daughter Wisdom, The Wisdom of Menopause,* and *Women's Bodies, Women's Wisdom*

"Dr. Prior is a caring and cautious clinician, and at the same time a most innovative researcher. She wrestles with the questions that too many doctors ignore, and has saved a substantial number of women from—for example—unnecessary hysterectomies. How does she do this? You must read and study this highly informative book to see. To those of you who experience extremely heavy bleeds—your search to overcome them gently begins right here."

—BARBARA SEAMAN, author of *The Greatest Experiment Ever Performed on Women: Exploding the Estrogen Myth* and Co-founder of the National Women's Health Network

"It has been fifteen years since I bravely followed Dr. Prior's lead where other clinicians feared to tread and started treating my perimenopausal patients with progesterone. What a boon her wisdom, research and evidence has provided for patient care and self knowledge. Since we can't all sit down with her, these eight stories have something for all of us, into and out of menopause, past or present."

—JEAN MARMOREO, MD, CCFP, family physician, specialist in mid-life medicine, author of *The Middle Ages: Women in Midlife,* and columnist for the *Globe and Mail* newspaper

"Dr. Jerilynn Prior has a long history of fine scholarly work on the role of progesterone in relation to health and well-being during the transition to menopause and beyond. As a scholar and clinician she has published her provocative views in the biomedical literature; these are often controversial in spite of their scientific underpinning. In this book she engages the reader in her clinical focus as she works with women to help them solve menopausal issues that have resisted classical medical approaches. For women who have problems with their menopausal experience, she may well serve as a last resort. Here women may find a unique approach to bring relief. Dr. Prior's focus is on the medical exceptions; those women whose problems with bleeding and other hormonally invoked changes do not respond to "standard practices."

—WINNIFRED B. CUTLER, PhD, President and Founder of
Athena Institute for Women's Wellness, Inc.

"Prior teaches the essential facts of perimenopause through stories instead of cold medical diagrams and jargon. In so doing, she proves that complicated medical facts and debates may resonate more with women if they are embedded first in women's actual lives. *Estrogen's Storm Season* is an engaging and thoughtful account of the various struggles some women may experience with perimenopause."

—KATHLEEN O'GRADY, Research Associate, Simone de Beauvoir
Institute, Concordia University, Director of Communications
for the Canadian Women's Health Network, Past editor of
"A Friend Indeed," the newsletter for women in menopause
and midlife (Women's Health Clinic) and Co-author of
*Sweet Secrets: Stories of Menstruation*

# ESTROGEN'S STORM SEASON

# ESTROGEN'S STORM SEASON

## DR. JERILYNN PRIOR

*stories of perimenopause*

Library and Archives Canada Cataloguing in Publication
Prior, Jerilynn C., 1943-

Estrogen's Storm Season: Stories of Perimenopause / Jerilynn Prior.

Includes bibliographical references.
ISBN 0-9738275-0-5

1. Perimenopause--Popular works.
I. Centre for Menstrual Cycle and Ovulation Research.
II. Title.

RG188.P74 2005          618.1'75          C2005-903185-9


Edited by Suzanne Bastedo
Cover and book design by Fiona Raven


Photograph on page 20 reproduced with kind permission of Rachel Ada Prior.

Quote by Ursula K. LeGuin reprinted with permission of the author and The Virginia Kidd Agency, Inc.
In: *Women of the 14th Moon: writings on menopause.* Sumrall AC, Taylor D, eds. Freedom, California:
The Crossing Press, 1991.

Quote by Susan Griffin reprinted with permission of the author and Random House, Inc.
In: *A Chorus of Stones.* Griffin, Susan. New York: Random House, Inc., 1993.


First Printing July 2005
Printed in Canada by Friesens

We are committed to protecting the environment and to the responsible use of natural resources.
This book is printed on 100% ancient-forest-free paper (100% post-consumer recycled),
processed chlorine and acid free. It is printed with vegetable-based inks.

Published by

**Centre for Menstrual Cycle and Ovulation Research (CeMCOR)**
Suite 308 – 575 West 8th Avenue, Vancouver BC Canada V6Z 1C6
Tel: 604-875-5927 Fax: 604-875-5915  **www.cemcor.ubc.ca**
CeMCOR logo created by the Atelier-Pierre Ruiz

# contents

# *author's note*

This book is for the perimenopausal woman who no longer recognizes herself. It is for the woman who finds work and fun are disturbed by the changes of perimenopause. It is for the woman who can't find a clear and reasonable explanation for what she is experiencing. It is for the woman who has seen many physicians, been referred to specialists, and seems to be getting worse rather than better. If you are this woman, or someone who knows a woman like this, I wrote this book for you. My belief is that you, too, can survive estrogen's storm season—perimenopause—the years of change before, and one year after, the final menstrual flow.

Let me introduce myself. I am a professor of endocrinology with a specialty in women's hormonal health. I, personally, had a difficult perimenopause. Perimenopause seemed to go on forever—mine actually lasted over ten years! My breasts were sore, I was relentlessly hungry, and I was angry. I was angry because, as a doctor, I had learned that midlife women suffered from dropping estrogen levels. What I knew was that my estrogen levels felt sky-high! I even dreamed I was pregnant.

My university job means that I study and teach. For urgent personal as well as academic reasons, therefore, I set myself to figuring out how hormones really changed in perimenopause. In the process I read and studied the new and old scientific papers and books written about perimenopause. I came up with and published good evidence for the existence of high estrogen levels in perimenopause. And I made reasonable guesses about how estrogen levels got that way. I also found that estrogen's essential partner hormone, progesterone, was clearly often too low.

I thought that everything would change once I'd figured out the unexpected patterns of estrogen and progesterone levels in perimenopause. I thought that writing clear, scientific papers was sufficient. Medical students would learn accurate information. Doctors would know how to explain the changes of perimenopause to women who were having a rough time. Women would understand what they were experiencing and feel less out of control. Perimenopausal women would stop having surgeries without an effective trial of medical options. Doctors would stop prescribing estrogen to women in perimenopause.

My 32-page perimenopause review was published in 1998. Seven years later, the books written for women and doctors still describe dropping or low estrogen levels in perimenopause. And young women and men medical students, even at the University of British Columbia, my own university, are still not learning about the dramatic differences between perimenopause and menopause. Doctors continue—almost automatically— to prescribe estrogen to perimenopausal women. Perimenopausal women with heavy flow are still being treated with the Pill. When that extra-high estrogen therapy doesn't fix their flooding menstruation, women continue to be told that they need endometrial ablation or a hysterectomy. And all before they even know that they are in perimenopause!

As it has for centuries, medicine continues to change slowly. But I feel that new information is urgently needed to help the millions of "baby-boom" women now needlessly suffering through a difficult time in perimenopause.

This book represents my decision to convey the new information about perimenopause to more women than I can ever see as a physician. What I learned during my own perimenopause was valuable. I know it will help other women. I have learned about treatments that have been intensively and scientifically tested, and those that have not. I have listened to and learned from hundreds of perimenopausal women whom I have treated. I have learned how variable perimenopause is—no two women experience it in the same way. I have reviewed countless Daily Perimenopause Diary records kept by numerous women over many years. I can feel the excitement and confidence grow as a woman sees patterns and understands what's going on with her own health.

I decided to write this book as a series of connected stories of eight women who see Dr. Kailey Madrona, a woman endocrine specialist physician. Why stories? Because I love them. When I was born, my mother's Mom, Celia Ashmun Benthin, gave me a big book of stories. My mother, Joyce Elliot Smith, read and told me stories beginning before my first memory. I wrote this book as women's stories because all the midlife women I know are eager to hear the perimenopausal experiences of other women.

All of the stories in this book are crafted to show the variety of difficulties and problems of perimenopause and to hint at how our lives interact with our symptoms. You may see resemblances with yourself or others you know. And you may think that Dr. Kailey Madrona resembles me. She certainly knows what I know, because in this fictional plot she works with me in the Centre for Menstrual Cycle and Ovulation Research in Vancouver, British Columbia. However, Dr. Madrona is fictional and each patient she sees or treats represents no one woman I've ever seen or treated.

Don't make the mistake of thinking that this book is about the experiences of most or even all perimenopausal women. In fact, these stories describe only the 10–20 percent of perimenopausal women who, like me, have a difficult perimenopause transition. There are many women who are absent from these pages. They are the most common women in perimenopause—the women who are noticing changes, but are not greatly troubled.

Although this book is about fictional people living through hormonal and situational challenges, it is based on science. The book, therefore, contains new words and ideas that you may find a bit challenging. Each time I use what my patients call a doctor-talk word, I've explained it. You will notice that a new word is shadowed the first time I mention it. You can find all of those shadowed words, in alphabetical order, in the glossary at the end of this book.

Because my job is writing and reading scientific papers *I* need to focus on often-dry science. You don't have to. However, I assume that you are both curious and intelligent. I use this assumption also in writing for the Centre for Menstrual Cycle and Ovulation Research website (www.cemcor.ubc.ca) and in everything I present for women. I also know that some of you could care less about the whys and wherefores. So I've given you a choice. If you wish to read or at least know where the original information was published, I've put a reference number like this (1) where a reference fits in the story. You will find the reference associated with this number in the List of References at the end of the book.

$\sim$

The Centre for Menstrual Cycle and Ovulation Research is publishing this book as a way of earning funds to support its ongoing research and the CeMCOR website. Many, many thanks to Joanne R. Silver, Executive Director for CeMCOR, who has kept us on task, and to Linda Redmond, retired associate publisher and CeMCOR volunteer, for seeing that this book became real. My thanks to all of those who have shared their stories with me and listened to mine. Thanks to Matt Prior, Rachel Prior-Tsang, Linda Redmond, Joanne Silver, Lori Smithers-Ruiz and Yvette Vigna who did the tedious task of proofreading. Special thanks also to Yvette for her support, honest criticism and sense of humour.

*"The woman who is willing to make that change
must become pregnant with herself, at last."*

URSULA K. LE GUIN, 1991

*"The telling and hearing of a story is not a simple act.
The one who tells must reach down into deeper layers of the self,
reviving old feelings, reviewing the past. . . .
The one who hears takes the story in,
even to a place not visible or conscious to the mind, yet there."*

SUSAN GRIFFIN, 1992

# 1

*strangers* in perimenopause

I walk into the plain meeting room for the Division of Endocrinology and see eight women sitting around a long table. They look as different as eight women can be—tall or short, skinny or fat, fair or dark, dressed for a fashion show or for the garden. They are neither really young nor very old. One woman is talking quietly to the woman next to her. Another is holding a cell phone to her ear. A few others are leafing through some papers in front of them—I recognize a green sheet with "The ABCs of Midlife Osteoporosis Prevention" and a purple pamphlet about the Centre for Menstrual Cycle and Ovulation Research. The women look up as I come in.

My secretary, Lana, comes in just behind me. She says, "I forgot to tell you. There are pens and pencils for anyone who wants to take notes. Oh—and I just got a call from the woman we were waiting for from Dawson Creek. Bad weather, so her flight was cancelled. Everyone's here that can be, so you can start. Good luck!"

I place my folder of transparencies for the overhead projector on the table, then sit down in the empty chair at the head of the table.

"Hi, I'm Dr. Kailey Madrona," I say. "I'm a specialist in endocrinology at the University of British Columbia. I'm particularly interested in women's reproduction, especially women's periods, ovulation and perimenopause. Your family doctors have referred each of you to me because of problems that either they or I thought were related to perimenopause."

A heavy-set woman with dark straight hair interrupts. "There must be some mistake!" she blurts. I'm here because I have a problem with *menopause*. I don't even know what perimenopause is!"

Blond, graying, auburn and other brown heads nod.

"Most every one gets perimenopause and menopause mixed up," I say, laughing. "You're not alone in asking me the difference! Perimenopause means the stretch of time from when you first notice that things are changing until one year has passed since your final menstrual flow. That's when true menopause begins—when you are one year without flow. I, for one, am proud that I've both survived perimenopause and graduated into menopause!"

I notice that only a couple of women smile. I think that they must be feeling anxious. Here they are, sitting with a new doctor and with a room full of strangers.

"I invited you to this information-sharing session today for several reasons," I continue. "First, I wanted you to know that you are not alone in having midlife miseries. Many other women are also going through frustrating changes; they just may not talk about it! Secondly, I asked you to come as a group because I don't have a free appointment for several months. You are all waiting for your individual consultations with me. However, you can learn something today, and get started toward an understanding about perimenopause.

"The final reason that I started offering sessions like this is that I want to introduce you to some tools that my colleagues and I have developed. The Daily Perimenopause Diary (1), which I'll explain to you shortly, certainly made me feel more in control during my perimenopause. It can help you track what is changing in your experiences and your menstrual cycles. When Lana calls to remind you of your individual appointment with me, she will also ask you to bring any records that you have. If you keep just one month of the Diary record, or even notes about your periods on a calendar, we'll have a head start in understanding what's going on for you. When I meet with you individually, we'll go over your completed records and I'll explain what I see."

I look around at the eight upturned faces.

"Let's talk about what's ahead in this session. We'll talk together for about two hours with a few breaks. It could last longer if you have lots of questions. I'll cover the essential stuff first so if you need to leave, you can. We'll start by going around the table, giving each of you a chance to say who you are and why you are here. Then I'll explain about the hormonal changes in perimenopause. It's important for you to know how the actual changes differ from what I was taught in medical school and from what most doctors still believe. Next, I'll introduce you to the Daily Perimenopause Diary and show you how to record information for yourself. If we have time, and if anyone here is interested in becoming pregnant, I'll explain how the old-fashioned basal temperature can be used to figure out whether you have ovulated (2)."

A diminutive black-haired woman gasps, and everyone looks at her. "Sorry!" she says, looking embarrassed. "I think about baby." She pauses, struggling to find words. "I surprise you talk about baby."

"I've been thinking about babies recently, too. I feel sad . . . " another woman says. She's tall and thin and wearing an attractive iridescent green-brown shawl.

I nod. "It is very common to think about babies in perimenopause—even if you have all the children you ever wanted. Perimenopause means the end of that possibility. I've heard many perimenopausal women describe dreams in which they are pregnant. The passage from reproductive to non-reproductive selves is important—to all women and from many cultures. It's even recorded for Nisa, a !Kung woman and member of a hunter-gatherer tribe from the Kalahari desert in Africa (3)."

"Dreaming of pregnancy sounds like a bloody *nightmare!*" a thin woman with light brown hair says suddenly, her voice loud in the quiet room. "That is the last thing I want—I've got more than enough to deal with right now, thank you very much!"

I see that many women are laughing. I start speaking again.

"Let's finish what I'd like to cover with you. After we talk about basal temperature, we'll discuss some healthy habits that are especially important at this time of our lives, things we can do that help prevent osteoporosis and diabetes from developing. Finally, I've given you some homework." I grin, trying to take the possible threat out of my words, and point to the papers they have in front of them. "There will be lots of opportunities for questions. Don't be afraid to say something or ask as we go along. And take notes if you want. Lana has provided pens and pencils as well as extra paper."

I pause and look around. Some of the women look relaxed, but others still seem uptight. "An essential first part of this session is to share as little or as much as each of us feels comfortable with. Why don't I start?"

I lean back in my chair. "I'm 54 years old. I can't believe it—I don't feel as old as that still sounds to me! I grew up in Masset, a fishing village in the Queen Charlotte Islands, and, as a little girl, wanted to be a public health nurse. However, an older nurse friend of mine in university said I asked too many questions to be a good nurse! I know nurses ask many questions today, but that was in the sixties."

A heavy-set, dark-haired woman blurts, "You're darn tootin' we ask questions!"

I smile and continue. "I wasn't sure, in those days and as a woman, that I *could* become a doctor, so I majored in psychology and history. I also took all the pre-medical science and math courses I needed. After eventually getting into medical school and graduating, I received my specialty training in internal medicine and endocrinology. I've worked as a doctor in Boston, Toronto, and the Queen Charlottes as well as here at Vancouver Hospital, where I have been since 1980.

"I know that I was taught that the doctor is the boss. But I have a bit of a different idea about a doctor's job. I believe in working with each person to figure out what is right for her. Giving orders is not my idea of medicine. I'm dreadful at taking orders myself!"

Everyone smiles at this.

"I knew I was in perimenopause—one morning in the wee hours. I awoke with a migraine headache—vomiting, blurred vision and all. I'd had a migraine before, when I was 20, and five days into taking the super high-dose estrogen birth control pill from the 1960s. So I knew what a migraine felt like. I got up quietly to avoid waking my partner then sat on the cold bathroom floor vomiting."

A woman in a flannel shirt pipes up, "Doesn't it just piss you off when your honey is snoring peacefully and you're wide awake!"

Several women murmur, "You bet!" and "Nothing worse!"

"That was the beginning of my *awareness* of perimenopause. In retrospect I'd been having worsening premenstrual symptoms, and heavier flow—I just didn't twig before that dramatic migraine."

"That first migraine was in November of 1993 when I was 43. And I didn't have my final menstrual period until 2002 when I was 52."

All of the women are listening intently. "One of my proudest achievements is having survived perimenopause—they were the most difficult years of my life. Migraines punctuated most weeks, my breasts were sore all the time and swollen. I resented it as they grew from a "B" cup to a " D"!"

I note that only the tall woman with red-highlighted brown hair nods. The rest look blank or puzzled.

"My professor had studied perimenopause so I knew that high estrogen levels could produce what I was experiencing. I guess I hadn't really taken her work seriously until I was in the middle of estrogen's storm season myself!"

"Wow! I never thought of estrogen and storms before," a young-looking woman with straight blond hair interjects. "Estrogen's storm season is a great way to describe perimenopause! *Anytime* is storm season in Newfoundland, where I grew up!"

"Right, and the Charlottes too!" I say. "So I decided I had to figure out, for myself, what was going on. I borrowed a Daily Perimenopause Diary sheet from the office and began to keep my own record. Since then I've plotted many migraines. But I'm happy to say I haven't had a migraine now for six months!

"I'm interested in the history of scientific ideas especially about women. For example, why is it so difficult for doctors to accept perimenopause or its high estrogen levels? So, because I was miserable, I tried to look for the first evidence of the word 'perimenopause' being used along with a description of high estrogen levels. What I found was that a woman, with no medical training, wrote a book for ordinary women about what she called 'menopause' back in 1977. She said, 'I know for myself that my body produces an enormous amount of estrogen' (4).

"It took until the mid-1990s for a medical author to use the word 'perimenopause' for women with regular cycles. She showed that these women in their forties had high estrogen and low progesterone levels compared with premenopausal women (5). Around that same time, an Australian researcher studied women ages 45-55 and showed very high estrogen levels (6) during what he called 'the menopausal transition.' But he didn't even recognize that estrogens were high (7). He was stuck on proving that old idea that estrogen levels are dropping." I pause and look around. Seeing a couple of women nodding, I continue.

"The first review to clearly show evidence for high estrogen levels in perimenopause was by my teacher, Dr. Prior (8). She also showed, in another review, that progesterone levels were also too low in perimenopause (9). I probably wouldn't even know this—because trends in medicine are so local—if I'd stayed to work in Toronto."

"My doctor says Dr. Prior's on the fringe!" a heavy-set, dark-haired woman interrupts.

"I might have thought so too," I say. "All I know is that she's a professor, which isn't easy to achieve in a faculty of medicine. But I'll admit that I didn't take her research very seriously either, until it explained my symptoms in early perimenopause."

"I guess most doctors and women still believe that perimenopause is about dropping estrogen levels. All I know is that I'm grateful to have better information. The neurology specialist I saw for the migraines would have treated me with estrogen if I hadn't known better. I think it's the high and swinging estrogen levels that *caused* my perimenopausal migraines.

"One time," I continue," when I was still having regular periods, I flew to Halifax for a research meeting. Any of you ever flown there?" The blond woman with the Newfoundland accent nods energetically.

"It's four time zones away—I spent the whole day on airplanes. I remember being thankful that I was finishing my period. After arriving late at night at the hotel, I showered and went straight to bed. I woke a couple of hours later with doubling-up cramps and found I was flooding. I spent the rest of the night, half-asleep, running to and from the bathroom. When I fell into the closet on the way to the toilet, I realized I was dizzy with blood loss. So I made a pot of peppermint tea and dug out and ate the salty crackers and chips that I had hoarded from the flight. Then I took ibuprofen for cramps and flow. I started to feel a bit better. Still, I was pale and fatigued when I staggered to my meeting in the morning."

I look around the table. "How many of you know that ibuprofen helps with heavy flow?"

No one raises her hand.

"Well, it's important. A randomized study of women with heavy menstrual bleeding showed that drugs that block the formation of prostaglandins, non-steroidal anti-inflammatory drugs, like ibuprofen, reduce the amount of flow by a quarter as well as treating the cramps (10). Dr. Prior has posted an article about heavy bleeding on the Centre for Menstrual Cycle and Ovulation Research website." I pause and write the CeMCOR website address: www.cemcor.ubc.ca on the board. "Take a look at 'Very Heavy Menstrual Flow,'" I suggest.

"I've had that kind of unexpected mother of all periods!" says a tired-looking woman with straggly light brown hair. "The worst is that it surprises you." A couple of other women nod.

"One of the things I vowed that night in Halifax," I continue, "was that I would make sure every perimenopausal patient of mine knew what to do for heavy flow. And that, when traveling, they carried emergency treatment for flooding."

"Did you get anemic?" the slim woman with auburn hair asks.

"I probably had a low blood count," I reply, "but I guess I was too busy. I don't think I went to see my doctor or to get a test. However, because I suspected anemia from loss of blood, I did buy a years' worth of iron tablets and took one pill every day until they were gone."

"Why did you take that ibuprofen? That's what you said, isn't it? My doctor says those can make you bruise and bleed easily," a heavy-set, dark-haired woman asks.

"Yes," I nod, "ibuprofen, can cause increased bruises. But with heavy flow and cramps, ibuprofen prevents formation of prostaglandins that are made in the uterus and are causing the pain. It also brings into balance a number of hormones acting on the endometrium and therefore reduces flow.

"Although ibuprofen made it possible for me to complete my work in Halifax, I flooded my way home to Vancouver. When I arrived that next evening, I called my doctor who prescribed 15 medroxyprogesterone pills. They're a kind of progestin. I took two that same night, and one every day afterwards until I finished. It was amazing—my flow was gone by morning!"

At that moment I feel the start of a hot flush. I take off my suit jacket and turn to hang it on the back of my chair. "The worst things for me," I continue," are hot flushes and night sweats. Thank god they're not bad and don't wake me at night any more. They're particularly likely when I'm feeling stressed!"

Everyone laughs. I continue. "Not that teaching you is really stressful. Actually, I quite enjoy it. I'll miss sessions like this soon because I'm going to stop seeing new patients. Although I'll continue to follow old patients one day a week, I'm headed back to university to get a Masters in the history of medicine."

"Why do some of us get hot flushes and others get off scot free?" asks the auburn-haired woman. She looks worried.

"I don't really know," I answer. "Those of us who have more premenstrual symptoms early in perimenopause are at greater risk (11), as are those whose lives are most stressful (12). I remember complaining bitterly to my cousin Elspeth, who is my mom's age, about why I was having such a bad time with perimenopause when she, my mom and my younger sister—provided she's telling the truth—have sailed through it."

"What did your cousin say?" asks a quiet, light-haired woman. "I've wanted to ask a question like that myself!"

"Elspeth said that I was *meant* to! I was to learn about perimenopause so that I could help other women!"

We all laugh.

"On that note, let's take a short break. The washroom's down the hall and there's bottled water in the corner. Fifteen minutes?"

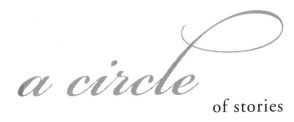

*a circle* of stories

I look around the room at the eight women. They are now chatting with each other and looking much more at ease.

"Let's resume," I say. "Now that you've heard a bit about me, it's time for each of you to share who you are and why you are here. Although each of you will have a different story, we probably share a lot of experiences."

I notice that two of the women look away. They remind me of students who don't want to be called on. I try to reassure them. "Because we don't know each other," I say, "we need to make sure everyone feels comfortable. Only say what you feel ready to share. We don't need last names. And let's remind ourselves that everything we say here is private. Agreed?" I hear murmurs of approval and see that all heads are nodding, including the two who had looked worried.

"Who wants to start?" I ask.

"I will," says a brown-haired woman on my left.

"I'm Jennifer, and what's bothering me most is feeling sick to my stomach all the time. It's worse in the morning . . . Don't laugh! I'm not pregnant. And if I were, it wouldn't be funny!" A few women who have laughed look embarrassed. "My doctor can't figure out what's causing my nausea. I've had all kinds of blood tests for liver disease, a scan for gallbladder trouble, and everything's normal. Oh, I forgot to say—I'm 38 years old and work as a counselor for differently abled kids. My periods are regular as clockwork."

"Does that sick feeling take away your appetite?" asks a stocky woman across the table. "If it does, I'll trade you!" Several women snicker.

"No!" says Jennifer. "That's what's weird. I get very hungry sometimes, even while I'm feeling sick to my stomach. And I'm gaining weight." She pauses and pats her rather slim tummy. "I'm gaining weight despite watching what I eat and feeling sick to my stomach most of the time."

Jennifer looks around the table. "That's me," she says. "Who's next?"

Abruptly the next woman down the table begins speaking. "I Beverley," she says. "I fine. Not sick. Don't get pregnant. Doctor say no more eggs." She shakes her head with a quizzical look on her face. "But my period perfect. My age, 39. That all."

"That's no fun," One of the women says. "I remember making a job out of trying to get pregnant when I was in my 20s."

Beverley smiles at the sympathetic woman and twirls an expensive-looking green pen with her thumb and first finger. It's a fascinating skill! "No fun," she says. "My mother eight children. Want Canadian grandson."

Everyone now turns toward the woman beside Beverley. I see she is doodling and her straight blond hair is falling on the paper. "Oh," she looks up suddenly, "I guess it's my turn! I'm Alison and I'm 46. I used to teach high-school math, but now I'm home with my three sons who are ages six to 13. What bothers me most are migraines. Nothing seems to help the migraine headaches or the night sweats. They both are worst before my monthlies. My migraine specialist has given up. We've tried every medicine he normally uses plus some experimental ones. He suggested estrogen treatment—I said I wanted a referral!" She nods at me, then turns to the woman beside her. "You're next!"

"My name is Eva," says the tall, trim woman. "I am—or at least I *was*—a champion master's 10-K runner. That means I run 10-kilometre races. Several times I came in first for women over 45. I'm 47 and just getting to the age that most women have stopped running. I love to run. And I was getting better. But now I can't manage to train properly. I still run at least an hour a day, but there's no way I can run uphill. I just plod. I'm not anemic and I'm taking iron. My thyroid's fine too. Nobody seems to know what to do."

"I know that Dr. Prior did studies of runners in the past," Eva continues, "so I asked for a referral to this centre. I hope you can help. What I want to know is, what the hell does difficulty training have to do with menopause?" Eva looks challengingly at me.

"I'm only a jogger," I reply, "but I experienced something like what you describe. It was early in my perimenopause. I had to walk up the small hills in my neighbourhood. Before that, I could run up easily. I couldn't figure it out either. But you'll be glad to know that my legs are much stronger now! My hunch is that interfering with exercise is one of the things that high estrogen does. Does being able to run uphill change at all with your cycle?"

Eva concentrates for a minute. "I don't think so, but it hasn't crossed my mind before."

"When we meet, be sure to bring your training log," I say. She nods.

"Who's next?" I ask.

"I'm Darlene," says the heavy-set woman beside Eva. "I'm 43 years old and bleeding to death!" She laughs and others join in. "I'm serious! When my period comes, I can't go to work. I'm a nurse in the Intensive Care Unit at Surrey Memorial Hospital. I have to stay home and stuff my crotch with towels. I can't get up without blood running down my legs. It's like what happened to Dr. Madrona in Halifax. But for me it is a week or two of every two or three weeks! I tried the Pill but it gave me migraine headaches, sore boobs and the bloats. And they didn't help the flow. I finally asked for 'Mirena.'"

Seeing the puzzled looks around the table, I interject, "That's a kind of IUD with progestin imbedded in it. It's new here. But it has been tested and used for over 20 years in Finland and for some time in Australia and Europe. It significantly decreases flow (13;14) ."

"But I got wicked cramps on it!" Darlene says. "I couldn't *stand* them." She starts again. "I took naproxen, but got gastritis! And I was still miserable most of the month."

"Naproxen is similar to ibuprofen," I explain. "They're both anti-prostaglandin medicines. Any members of that drug family can cause stomach irritation. Tell me, how are you taking them?"

Darlene sits up straight in her chair. "Yes, yes, I know!" she says. "I take them every four hours with food, and I'm still passing clots. I begged my family doctor to take out that IUD thing after one month. He wasn't happy because it spoiled the statistics for the study I was in! And now my gynecologist says I have to have the whole thing out, or fry my innards. I'm hoping you can see me before I decide to just get scooped out and be done with it!" Darlene sounds angry and frustrated. The other women are silent.

"If you really don't want a hysterectomy operation," I respond quietly, "I'll do everything I can to help you avoid it. Your gynecologist is referring to either a hysterectomy in which the uterus is removed through surgery or an endometrial ablation. Endometrial ablations involve use of heat or laser to remove the layer of the uterine lining that bleeds each month. I'll certainly put you on my cancellation list, Darlene. Before then, be sure to take at least one tablet of iron every day, otherwise you'll get a low blood count. Please give my secretary your family doctor's name and I'll phone her with some suggestions for dealing with your flow and cramps." I smile at Darlene and jot her name on a slip of paper.

The woman next to her speaks up. "Compared to what you all have been through, my story sounds like nothing!" she says. "I'm Floreena. I'm a fabric artist. I just turned 50. I'm continually having sore lumps and cysts in my breasts. I've had so many mammograms. . .and more biopsies than I can count." She stops for a minute to re-adjust her silk scarf. "I really worry at this rate that I'll get breast cancer before I hit menopause!"

The other women are leaning forward, their faces showing their concern.

"Do you think I should start Raloxifene?" Floreena asks, looking at me.

I reply slowly, measuring my words. "Raloxifene is a new kind of drug called a 'selective estrogen receptor modulator' or SERM for short. That means that it acts *like* estrogen as well as acting *against* estrogen. It is a newer cousin of tamoxifen, which was the first kind of estrogen receptor modulator drug we had. I think, if estrogen levels are high, anything acting like estrogen should be avoided during perimenopause—even though Raloxifene may prevent breast cancer in menopausal women. I would be slow to take a new drug, about which a lot is not yet known, without being part of a well-designed scientific study."

A hush settles on the room. I wonder whether, like me, everyone is thinking about those they've known with breast cancer.

"Ok, it's my turn!" A sturdy woman with short hair and a red face jumps into the silence. "I don't know what I should admit! But—I'm Carla and I think I'm going crazy! I had the bleeding all over the shop, a bit like you." She nods toward Darlene. "I also tried the Pill and it was a nightmare. They said hysterectomy was my only choice. I decided that I never wanted to use my womb anyway, so I thought, what the heck, just take it out!"

Carla leans forward in her chair. "After the surgery I was so happy to not have bleeding any more. But then I started having night sweats. My doctor put me on Premarin. Now I feel murderous most of the time, forget my phone number, am depressed, and to top it all, the night sweats aren't any better. My partner is ready to turf me."

"What do you think is going on?" I ask.

"I feel like I have PMS all the time—wretched moods out of the blue—and I just can't figure anything out anymore," Carla says, sounding exasperated.

"That reminds me of the words of a nurse clinician in a book I've read," I say. "Here it is:

'At menopause [I'd use the word, perimenopause] life can turn into one long premenstrual experience. Hormones slap you up against the doors of your unfinished business' (15)."

There is silence. The words seem to me to be slowly sucked into the consciousness of the listening women. I start speaking again. "Several studies show that women who have a hysterectomy have a more difficult time in perimenopause and see physicians about twice as often as women who haven't had surgery (16;17). Many women tell me that they feel lost after a hysterectomy. They lose their sense of connection to their bodies. Your period," I look at Carla, " for all its difficulty, at least gave you a feeling about timing—if bloating and moodiness happened, and then you got your period, you knew why."

"You're damned right I feel out of control!" Carla snorts. "The million-dollar question is, can you help?"

"If you start keeping the Daily Perimenopause Diary, you'll begin to see patterns again," I answer. "Anyone else have any ideas that would help Carla?"

"It seems to me that, if estrogen levels are already high in perimenopause, then the Premarin won't be helping much," offers Alison.

"Yeah, but Premarin's the best we've got for hot flushes!" retorts Darlene.

"You're both right," I say. "Premarin is estrogen, and estrogen's not a good idea in perimenopause. Your mood swings also tell you you're making lots of your own estrogen. However, having had a hysterectomy means that your ovaries will stop making estrogen sooner and will make lower levels of hormones for the rest of your life. That's a good-news story. Hysterectomy is associated with about a 13–26 percent lower risk for breast cancer (18). You're not alone, Carla. About 40 percent of North American women end up having a hysterectomy. However, most women having a hysterectomy are in their mid-forties and in the early phases of perimenopause when they still have regular periods (19–21). I think it's wrong that women have major surgery without ever realizing that the high estrogen and low progesterone levels of perimenopause are the reason for their heavy flow (22)."

"I'm looking forward to hearing about that danged Diary!" blurts Carla. "I'm not very good at keeping records, but I'll try. I'd like to get a handle on my bloating and mood swings. And then I may try stopping the estrogen. It's not helping my drenches at night anyway."

"You're probably on the burgundy-coloured, 0.625 mg, standard dose of

Premarin, right?" I ask. Carla nods and I continue. "Get a prescription from your doctor for the green ones that are half strength—0.3 mg. Take a look on the Centre for Menstrual Cycle and Ovulation Research website for the article titled 'Stopping Estrogen Therapy.' Print that out and show it to your doctor. It will tell you about gradually decreasing the dose for several months before stopping completely.

"Why can't I just ditch the stuff?" asks Carla.

"I think that the brain gets used to high estrogen levels," I answer. "That's true whether the high estrogen is made by our ovaries, as in perimenopause, or comes from a pill, like Premarin. When the estrogen levels suddenly drop, our brain reacts like an addict's in withdrawal. That's what hot flushes and night sweats are all about."

"That makes sense," Carla says. I notice that several of the women are looking as if they suddenly understand.

"Well, I'm last as usual," interjects the next woman, looking at the group with a tired smile. "I'm Henrietta, I'm 48, and I'm here because my doctor and I are arguing about whether I need an anti-depressant. So far I've refused. As a compromise, she made me promise to see an endocrinologist." She looks toward me.

"I've survived the flooding—now my periods are skipping and farther apart. But I have hot flushes all day and night sweats all night! I just can't cope. If I don't watch out, I'll lose my job—I work as a head waitress." She stops suddenly, looking like she could cry. Several of the women who have been gazing intently now look down. Carla pats Henrietta's shoulder.

"I haven't had a full night's sleep for months," Henrietta continues. "I've refused HRT more times than I am years old. Maybe you think I'm stubborn, but I just don't want to take medicines. To my mind, most things doctors give women are nasty. They have bad side-effects. Plus they cause harmful things that aren't discovered until years later. And usually they've only been tested in men anyway!" Henrietta slumps in her chair.

"You're right to be cautious, Henrietta," I say. "And men *are* the experimental subjects on whom most medicines have been studied. However, nowadays, unless it's something like prostate cancer that women don't get, government research money, by law, must be spent equally on studies in women and men."

"That's great!" Carla bursts out and all of the women smile.

"By the way," I ask as I look around at the eight women, "what do you think about HRT?"

Floreena leans forward. "Wasn't there a big study from the States a few summers ago? And didn't it show that HRT caused breast cancer and heart attacks (23)?"

"And," Eva interjects, "some women are starting class-action lawsuits against the company that makes Premarin because it causes strokes and blood clots and heart attacks."

"But Hormone Replacement prevents hip fractures and colon cancers," Darlene retorts.

"The latest I read is that HRT doubles the risk for Alzheimer's," says Carla (24). "And all these stuffed-shirt doctors have been telling us it was so great for us. One said to me, 'No problem if you have your insides cleaned out, you'll feel great on Premarin!'"

"Yeah, but that study you're talking about from the States is only *one* study," Darlene interjects. "Millions of women have been studied showing HRT halves the risk of heart attack and keeps women healthy and attractive into old age!"

I decide to jump in. "Let's talk more about the several studies called the Women's Health Initiative," I say. "They looked at estrogen plus progestin and at estrogen alone, each compared with placebo, a pill identical in looks but without anything active in it. What's important about these studies, called WHI for short, is that all of the women who took part were menopausal and healthy and had no symptoms. The women were randomly assigned, by chance, like a roll of dice, to take either an active hormone pill or a placebo. The many studies you're talking about, Darlene, were observational, which means that women and their doctors chose who would and who wouldn't take the hormones. In those studies, it turned out that the healthier women and those who were better at taking pills and exercising were the ones who took hormones. Ones who didn't smoke, and were getting check-ups for diabetes and high blood pressure and high cholesterol levels were also more likely to be on estrogen. Some doctors thought that all of the healthy outcomes in that group were due to estrogen, when really the healthy outcomes were probably caused by the women's good health and pill-taking habits (25;26)."

I notice that Darlene looks sceptical. "We now have proof that estrogen with low-dose progestin caused harm," I continue. "The estrogen plus progestin arm of the WHI was stopped years earlier than planned, in July 2002. In March 2004, we learned that the estrogen arm of the WHI, in women who had hysterectomy, was *also* stopped about a year early because too many women were having strokes and blood clots (27). I'm extremely happy that we finally have well-designed randomized studies to tell us what I suspected!"

"So the WHI didn't tell us about perimenopause," Floreena muses quietly.

"That's true," I say. "And I agree with you about not taking 'HRT,' Henrietta. For a start, I think the idea of 'replacement' is wrong. Dr. Prior taught me to call it 'Ovarian Hormone Therapy' or OHT for short. Furthermore, there are no randomized studies showing that OHT helps hot flushes in *peri*menopausal women."

"Well, what therapies have been studied for us?" Jennifer asks.

"Not many," I answer. "Dr. Prior and I've tried for three years in a row to get funding to study therapy for heavy flow, hot flushes, and breast tenderness in perimenopausal women. The large federal granting agency in Canada has repeatedly rejected our application."

"What can do?" Beverley asks. "No Canada research money."

"Let's wait to talk about these treatment questions until we've learned a little more about perimenopause," I suggest. "We now have a good idea about how different each woman's perimenopause can be. Yet hot flushes, night sweats, worry about breast cancer and lack of sleep affect most of us who have symptoms. After just this short time together as a group, we feel more like we're neighbours than strangers."

Several of the women grin at each other.

"Ok, let's have another break—be back in 15 minutes. Lana will make a pot of tea and some decaffeinated coffee if you like. Sorry that I can't lay on snacks. But there are many coffee shops within a block of here. We'll review what we know and don't know about perimenopause when we start again."

# 3

*puzzles* of perimenopause

We're all settled around the table again. "There are three things to keep in mind while I introduce the main concepts about perimenopause," I begin. "First, as you already sense, there's a lot yet to learn. Next, from the variety of our stories, we know that each woman's experience of perimenopause is different. Finally, we represent the 10–20 percent of women who have the worst time with it. We're the *unlucky* ones! Lots of women notice a few mild changes, skip periods, and then one day realize they've been more than a year since their last flow. They suddenly know they are truly menopausal.

"When I'm giving a slide talk about perimenopause, I use a photograph to illustrate how variable the course of perimenopause is. The Yukon River delta has low foothills in the misty background. In the foreground, thousands of little streams all flow toward the sea. The paths women take in perimenopause are like dozens of leaves falling into separate small rivulets up in the foothills. Each takes a different route to the ocean.

I gather my transparencies and walk to the projector. "I'm going to use the overhead projector to show you some of the important aspects of perimenopause. We'll stay awake—and the figures will be visible—if we leave the lights up." I place a sheet on the overhead, turn the projector on, and return to stand in front of the room.

"I want to start by putting perimenopause into the bigger hormonal course of our lives. Let's begin by looking at a sketch of the life cycle of estrogen. I'm starting with estrogen because it is dominant in our culture.

As a doctor once wrote in an Okanagan newspaper, 'Estrogen's what makes a girl a girl!'

"This diagram shows the ages of women across the bottom, from birth to older age, and higher estrogen levels toward the top.

## ESTROGEN'S LIFE CYCLE IN WOMEN

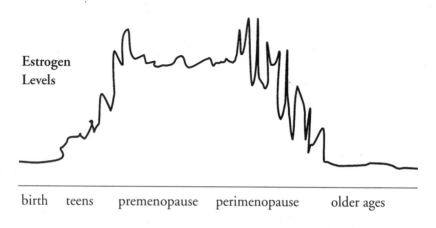

Estrogen
Levels

birth    teens    premenopause    perimenopause    older ages

"Notice that estrogen levels are low when we are newborn and children. As we grow to be nine or ten years old, our estrogen levels start to rise. At this point, pituitary hormones that direct our ovaries have already begun to increase during sleep. Hypothalamus or brain hormones boss the pituitary ones, giving their signals in bursts, like pulses. Initially pituitary hormones are only increased during sleep. Then, around the time of the first period, called menarche, estrogen levels become high (briefly, for some teens even higher than normal) and pituitary hormones develop their adult pattern of signals that are regular about 90 minutes apart—through both the day and the night."

I point to the middle of the diagram. "Next, there is a relatively flat, high plateau of estrogen from our late teens or early twenties until about our mid-forties. I've drawn estrogen as high and steady, but this is the *average* of the swings in estrogen levels that are part of the normal menstrual cycle. Sometime, in approximately the mid-thirties to the late forties, estrogen levels become chaotic and higher than normal. On average, estrogen levels are 30 percent higher—individual values can *double* the highest level normally found in the menstrual cycle (8).

"No wonder my breasts hurt!" Floreena exclaims. Sympathetic laughter ripples through the room.

"So you see that in early perimenopause," I continue, "estrogen levels not only become higher, but also start being unpredictable. They sneak up on us! Early in perimenopause when cycles are still regular, estrogen swings from higher-than-normal to normal. Later with skipped periods in perimenopause, estrogen swings from higher-than-normal to normal or low. These swings continue, even during the final year following our last period. After menopause, although the average estrogen levels are still decreasing, estrogen levels may again rise to very high levels—although this happens rarely. That's why about 5 percent of us will get a further period after we've been a full year without flow. We'll then have to re-start that final-year clock."

"What a pain!" blurts Alison. A murmur of agreement swells, with many heads nodding.

"It was!" I resume. "That happened to me. I had been proudly saying I was menopausal. I was 16 months since my last flow. Then I got a lot of period-type cramps, for weeks. And I had one migraine after another and breasts got sore again. Once my final-final period started, I felt much better! I, for one, will be happy to have low estrogen levels for the rest of my life!"

"Not me!" grumbles Darlene. "Estrogen deficiency makes you old and ugly."

Perhaps sensing conflict, women lean forward, several starting to speak.

"Yes, Darlene," I say. "You're voicing a common medical point of view. Let me ask another question," I put another overhead on the projector. "Is this seven-month-old baby girl estrogen-deficient?"

Several women look puzzled. Alison answers slowly. "Well, yes and no," she says thoughtfully. "Her estrogen levels are low, but from that last diagram, it looks like that is normal for a child."

"Then the same is true for a *menopausal* woman!" Eva asserts.

"But . . . low estrogen is bad for you," Darlene says, less strongly this time.

"Hell no!" Carla blurts. "It's normal for babies to have low estrogen!"

I decide to summarize. "The confusing thing is that low estrogen levels are perfectly normal during some parts of our life cycles. Children, both boys and girls, have low estrogen levels." I pause for a moment.

"Isn't it clear from babyhood on, who's a boy and who's a girl?" I ask.

Most of the women nod. Jennifer and Alison murmur, "Yes" and "For sure."

"If both have low estrogen levels, then estrogen is *not* what makes a girl, a girl!" I exclaim. "The same is true, I believe, about menopausal women. Here

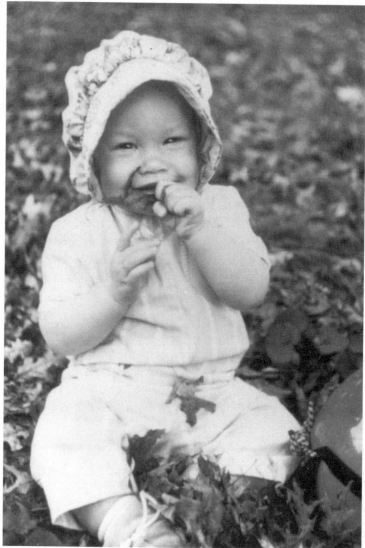

PHOTO BY BY JERILYNN C. PRIOR

Rachel Ada Prior, age 7 months.

again, low estrogen levels are normal and appropriate for that part of the life cycle. I, for one, feel vastly better since my estrogen levels became low."

Carla interrupts. "I think that idea about menopause meaning estrogen deficiency is prejudice! As well as being just plain wrong!"

Darlene looks upset. "I'm a nurse. I know that estrogen deficiency causes osteoporosis and vaginal atrophy and incontinence," she says. "Until the Women's Health Initiative, we believed that menopause caused heart disease. How can these diseases be normal?" She looks around, her chin at a challenging angle.

"Well it *is* very confusing," I say, "and doctors and scientists sometimes disagree. I've looked at the history of this idea. We've thought of 'hormone deficiency' as a disease since the 1920s and 1930s when the three main sex hormones—estrogen, progesterone and testosterone—were first discovered (28). A huge industry grew up in which 'Estrogen Replacement Therapy' was advocated for everything. We now know that the company that makes Premarin from pregnant mare's urine was very effective, not only in marketing their drug, but also in selling the *idea* of estrogen deficiency. The concept of estrogen deficiency became accepted and taught. Hundreds of non-randomized studies were designed, funded, performed, and published to confirm this idea. It took years before scientists realized that there had been no randomized, placebo-controlled trials of hormone therapy that were double blind in which the women and the scientists didn't know who was taking the real thing. Women's groups and scientists complained to drug regulators that men wouldn't be treated with drugs that hadn't been studied with randomized controlled trials showing they were effective and safe. Others said that the observational studies were misleading because healthier women who participated took estrogen. It was only in the last ten years that the National Institutes of Health in the USA designed and funded the Women's Health Initiative studies that we discussed earlier (23;27).

I look around to be sure I'm holding their interest. Eyes are riveted on me. "During the almost two years before the Estrogen arm of the WHI study was discontinued because it caused harm, many doctors tried to blame the low dose progestin or medroxyprogesterone. The WHI has since been criticized for everything under the sun. But a number of randomized controlled trials from several countries all show the same negative results from estrogen treatment (29). I, for one, was very disappointed that the idea of 'menopause as estrogen deficiency' didn't change as we got new and strong scientific evidence. I can only guess the reason is that human beings like the comfort of holding on to old ideas."

"Let's move on, or we won't get to perimenopause!" I say. The women are listening intently. I look at the serious faces, deciding to lighten things a little. "Dr. Susan Love, the popular author of *Doctor Susan Love's Menopause and Hormone Book*, declared, 'If estrogen deficiency's a disease, all men have it!'(30)." My hands are on my hips, my voice brash. Everyone laughs, except for Darlene who still looks disgruntled.

"When I was in perimenopause," I continue, "one of the other things I guessed about hormones was that the brain and pituitary control system must be out of kilter. For example, when I was younger, I occasionally had sore breasts and premenstrual symptoms. I learned these would get better if I exercised more and avoided sweets. So when I started having the same symptoms in perimenopause, I knew what to do—I increased my exercise and skipped candy. To my shock, it didn't help! Around the same time, I learned from Dr. Prior that the feedback system, or the thermostat, for controlling the ovary was wacky because of lower levels of a kind of brake-like hormone called inhibin. This is a small hormone that is made by cells surrounding the eggs in the ovary. Inhibin B levels appear to decrease early in perimenopause."

"I never heard of inhibin before," Darlene protests.

"I hadn't either," I reply. "It looks like lower levels of Inhibin B allow the pituitary's follicle stimulating hormone or FSH levels to go up a bit. FSH then pushes the ovary to make more estrogen. The increasing estrogen levels, without enough inhibin, are no longer able to keep FSH levels low like they did during the premenopausal years (8)."

I move to the overhead and switch to a new transparency. This one shows a diagram of the normal menstrual cycle.

"Speaking of estrogen," I start again as I walk back to the front of the room, "where is it made?"

Several voices chorus, "The ovary!"

"You're right," I say.

"And some from fat cells," Eva adds.

"Yes, especially after menopause," I say, looking at Eva, "when the low levels of estrogen from fat become quite important. But when we are menstruating, most of our estrogen comes from the ovary."

I look around the room. "Is estrogen made by the *whole* ovary, like thyroid hormone is made by the whole thyroid gland?" I ask. No one answers.

"The answer is no," I say. "Each menstrual cycle's estrogen comes from a single pinhead-sized group of cells called a follicle. These are the cells that belong with and make a circle around a particular egg. We're born with about a million of those follicles and their eggs. Until puberty and the high pituitary signals during sleep, those cells release almost no estrogen. Instead, a few each week start the process of growing and then, for reasons we don't understand, become permanently inactive. That means we have about 100,000 eggs left at our first period and about 1,000 left at perimenopause. The process of follicle growth and then inactivity seems to speed up in women's late thirties (31). I think that's at least partly why estrogen levels become higher in perimenopause.

"But back to my question about what makes estrogen. All of the high hormone levels during a given menstrual cycle are made by the particular set of cells surrounding one egg. Each cycle has a different follicle that's its own hormone-producer! What's amazing is that any of us ever manage to have regular menstrual cycles!"

"Some of us don't!" Carla chimes in. "Not even before I hit perimenopause!"

I nod. "We still need to learn about the normal pattern of menstrual cycle hormones because, despite the exceptions that everyone has, the pattern of hormones across the menstrual cycle gives us the 'gold standard' to indicate what is normal. And we need to know what is normal during the premenopausal years to understand the changes during perimenopause."

I pause to see whether this appears to make sense to the eight women around the table. "So, now for the next question," I begin again. "Are estrogen levels ever low during the menstrual cycle?"

"No! Menstrual cycles mean normal estrogen levels," Darlene says with conviction.

"That's generally true, Darlene," I reply, "but actually estrogen is low during flow and for the first few days of the menstrual cycle. Estrogen levels are as low during the early days of the cycle, as in a child, a menopausal woman, or a man."

A few of the women laugh. I point to the diagram on the screen. "You see that estrogen levels on this figure are drawn as a solid line. If you look during flow, here, estrogen levels are very low. Those three to six days of low estrogen levels are important to give our breasts a break from the demands of estrogen. Never, except during pregnancy, do estrogen levels stay high naturally. And

## CHANGES IN MENSTRUAL CYCLE HORMONES
### ACROSS A MENSTRUAL CYCLE

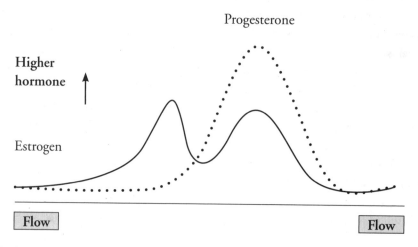

during pregnancy, high estrogen levels are counterbalanced by high progesterone levels."

"Earlier Floreena talked about cysts in her breasts," I say. "How many of you have heard of cysts in the ovary?" Most of the women nod or raise their hands. "Do you know what causes them?"

Darlene starts confidently. "I know about Polycystic Ovary Syndrome when the ovary has many cysts and the woman has trouble with things like hirsutism, acne, obesity and infertility."

"You've got a lot of medical knowledge, Darlene," I say trying to feel appreciation. "Yes, Polycystic Ovary Syndrome is a hereditary, but reversible, problem in which ovulation is rare and the ovary makes too much estrogen and androgens as well as not enough progesterone. I call it 'Anovulatory Androgen Excess' rather than naming it after cysts, because, as you will see, ovarian cysts are a normal and essential part of the menstrual cycle."

I point to the menstrual cycle diagram again. "Look at the estrogen line about Day 7," I say.

"About midway through the follicular phase, estrogen levels start to rise. What is happening inside the ovary is that several follicles have grown and are each starting to make more estrogen. The one closest to the outside of the ovary, and the biggest one, then becomes the 'boss.' It's called the dominant follicle and becomes the estrogen maker for this entire cycle. As the dominant follicle grows, a hollow appears in its centre and fills up with hormone-rich fluid. It is now a cyst. When the dominant follicle's cyst reaches the size of a Canadian loonie, or a dollar coin, it's making enough estrogen to produce the midcycle estrogen peak. That is the highest estrogen level during the cycle. At the midcycle peak, estrogen levels have increased by 220 percent from their low level during flow (32).

"That estrogen peak," I point to the diagram, "triggers a sudden spike in the pituitary hormone called Luteinizing Hormone or LH for short. That LH peak triggers the dominant follicle or largest fluid-filled cyst to burst and release its egg. That bubble-bursting process is called ovulation."

Beverley interrupts. "Can tell if ovulate?"

"Anyone know?" I ask.

"Every cycle I got this stitch in my side," Henrietta says. "Usually it only lasted a minute or two, but once I had to go to Emergency because the pain was so bad. It was on my right side, so at first they thought I had appendicitis."

"I can tell when I ovulate because I get stretchy mucus on the toilet paper when I wipe myself," Darlene declares.

"Yeah, I used to get that stretchy stuff in the middle of the month, but now it happens all over the cycle. I can even get mucus just before my period!" says Alison.

"Right! Sometimes now I get flow mixed with mucus," says Jennifer. "I swear it's like currant jelly!"

Everyone laughs. "Here we are laughing and talking about menstrual cycles like it was the weather!" Carla observes.

"What makes that stretchy mucus?" I ask. The room goes silent again. "It's made by high estrogen levels stimulating the glands of the cervix, at the mouth of the uterus," I say. "That mucus has the job of making it easy for sperm to swim upward and to make the vagina well lubricated for intercourse."

"I guess that must mean I had high estrogen levels just before my last period," says Jennifer. "I thought so—I was bloated and had really bad nausea."

"It does sound like you had very high levels, Jennifer," I agree. "And you've just figured out one of the most common perimenopausal changes—high estrogen levels before flow! Normally that stretchy mucus increases gradually from about Day 5 until the time of the midcycle estrogen peak. Around that peak it can usually stretch out about 4–7 cm—an inch or two. After that, the mucus normally disappears. Does anyone know why stretchy mucus goes away?"

"I just thought of it," says Floreena, "I'm sure mine doesn't go away."

"Your observation is telling us something about the second hormone of the menstrual cycle, progesterone," I say. "If you look just past the midcycle estrogen peak on this overhead, you'll see that progesterone, shown by a dotted line, begins to rise and increases very fast. It is progesterone's job, also by acting on the glands of the cervix, to stop production of that slippery mucus. That prevents more sperm from having easy access when the time is no longer right for fertilizing an egg."

"So, mucus all time, mean no egg?" asks Beverley. "Maybe this why no pregnancy?"

"I must not be ovulating then, either," says Floreena.

"You are both probably right, but there is another possible explanation. The effect of estrogen and progesterone on the cervical glands depends on the balance of the two hormones. So it's possible to ovulate, but have such high estrogen levels that the estrogen effect dominates. Or it is possible that estrogen levels are normal but that progesterone production is too low."

I point again at the progesterone line on the picture. "Does anyone know how much progesterone increases from its low levels during the first half of the cycle to its peak?"

"I'm just guessing," says Jennifer, "but it looks like it also rises about 200–300 percent."

"I'm sorry to confess that this diagram has different scales for each hormone," I say. "If the authors had drawn estrogen and progesterone to the same scale, the progesterone peak would reach the floor above us! Progesterone rises to its highest point—about 1,400 times higher than its baseline!"(32). That happens within a week after ovulation."

"That's huge!" says Carla.

"I never knew that!" says Darlene. "All of the stuff we studied in nursing school looked just like your diagram."

"I think inaccurate drawings are part of the reason we've always emphasized estrogen. Another reason is that laboratories report estrogen and progesterone in different units. Estrogen's unit is pmols—this is smaller, so its numbers seem higher. Progesterone's unit is nmols—1,000 times higher—it looks like it is lower because its numbers are smaller.

"What does all this have to do with perimenopause?" I ask, rhetorically. "Not only do estrogen levels get higher (5;8)," I continue, "but also progesterone levels get lower than normal in perimenopause (5;9). Again, part of the problem is faulty brain-pituitary-ovary coordination with lower Inhibin B levels. Also, the estrogen peak may be less likely to trigger an LH surge and ovulation in perimenopause (33;34)."

I remove the diagram from the overhead and replace it with a new one. "I believe that there are some common experiences we usually pass through in perimenopause," I say. "I'm showing you these phases of perimenopause because I believe knowing them will help you feel you're making progress toward menopause. We haven't properly studied the amount of time for each phase, so we've used our best guesses."

### PHASES OF PERIMENOPAUSE (9)

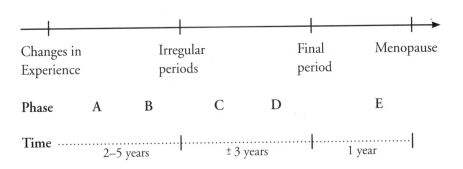

I point to the screen. "This diagram shows the timeline through perimenopause divided into five phases," I say. "Phases A and B are similar because in them menstrual cycles stay regular. Many women don't notice any changes. I did, mostly because I got difficult migraines."

"Tell me about it!" blurted Alison. "I never even heard of migraines before. They began out of the blue and have gotten continually worse."

"That's right," I reply. "Sore breasts are another high estrogen symptom early in perimenopause and before periods change." I glance at Floreena. "Or nausea," I say, looking toward Jennifer. "And some of us get heavy flow, like I did in Halifax. Others may find it puzzling that they've again started to have dysmenorrhea, menstrual cramps. The typical pattern for women who've had children is that cramps go away after the first child. For many women, the cramps return in early perimenopause, along with heavy flow."

"I have wicked cramps. I'm bleeding like stink! And I haven't heard diddly-squat yet about how to fix it," protests Darlene.

"Let her finish!" Alison says sharply. Women turn quickly. Then Alison interjects, "Can't tell I'm an old school marm, can you?" I feel the women relax into laughter.

"Yeah, sometimes I become a total bitch," Jennifer says. "I understand your impatience, Darlene. I must be still early in perimenopause, 'cause my flow hasn't skipped a beat."

"In Phase A of perimenopause" I continue, "if you were tracking your cycle lengths, you'd notice they become shorter than your usual, which, for many women, is about 28 days. Often cycles average 24–26 days apart. The follicular phase gets shorter—that's from the start of flow until mucus is most stretchy—averaging about 10 days rather than the usual 14 or so. A short follicular phase is a sure sign of high estrogen levels (35)."

"Night sweats often start," I say, "usually along with premenstrual mood changes and breast tenderness (1). Because of sleep disturbance, some women get extremely achy and tired. Some of us, early in perimenopause, are diagnosed with chronic fatigue syndrome or fibromyalgia. If we knew that our symptoms were part of perimenopause, we'd have room for hope. Instead, we're often given a diagnosis and end up going on disability, losing not only our health, but also our identities and our jobs. Finally, as I mentioned before, women with heavy bleeding end up with a hysterectomy before they know they're early in perimenopause and that flow will eventually improve.

"In Phase B of perimenopause," I continue, pointing to the next phase on the diagram, "cycles become the shortest. They may even average 21 or 22 days apart. Some cycles will be as short as two weeks apart."

"That's me!" Darlene exclaims. "Only my flow happens with barely a break."

"I had the same thing before I got disgusted and took the hysterectomy route," Carla adds.

"Yes," I say, "women that are going to have heavy flow, commonly start having it during Phase B. Although menstrual cycles remain regular, ovulation is less consistent. Lower progesterone levels combined with higher estrogen levels are the makings of heavy flow (22). During this phase, the women who, earlier, had severe premenstrual symptoms, begin to have real trouble with night sweats.

"The difficulty for perimenopausal women—and for doctors trying to help—is that a group of experts met in 2001 at a Stages of Reproductive

Aging Workshop called STRAW for short (36). These experts decided that perimenopause began when periods got variable and an FSH level on Day 3 was increased. So, all of the things that trouble us before periods become irregular are not, officially, part of perimenopause."

Several faces around the table look shocked. "I know," I say. "I couldn't believe it, either, when Dr. Prior came back from that conference and told me. She said it was a horrible experience. They didn't listen to her or believe what she said about women's experiences."

"Who the heck are those experts, anyhow?" demands Carla.

"Most of them are specialists in gynecology," I reply, "plus representatives of many medical groups and companies. I think I can partly understand. They connect irregular cycles with dropping estrogen levels. For them, that feels comfortable, because it fits with the old idea about declining estrogen levels before menopause. They haven't changed their minds in spite of several papers (5;37) and Dr. Prior's review (8) showing the significantly higher estrogen levels in perimenopause compared with premenopause. That STRAW decision means that many more of us will struggle through six or more years of misery that we, and our physicians, can't explain, before we even get to irregular cycles, and a diagnosis of perimenopause!

"Phase C of perimenopause," I continue, pointing to the diagram, "is when periods become slightly, but noticeably, irregular. As I said, most experts say perimenopause begins here, with irregular flow (36;38). I don't think so, because to say *that* would be to ignore both what we, as women, experience and the higher estrogen levels that begin when flow is still regular (5;8).

"At Phase C," I continue, "it's about four years, on average, until menopause. A random sample of about 3,000 women from Massachusetts who were part of a two-year observational study showed that it averaged four years from the start of Phase C, until menopause, the end of Phase E (38). Breast tenderness may start to improve and mood and bloating get better here (39)," I say, pointing. "Often flow is better, but the majority of women have at least one flooding menstrual flow at the start of Phase C (40). This is startling! It makes about a quarter of us see our doctors (16). Around this time, flow may start to alternate between heavy and light."

"If I can still add," Henrietta blurts, "this whole thing is almost ten years long! I don't know if I'll last!"

"Come on, don't start fearing the worst," I say. "You may be more than halfway there already. In fact, if I remember correctly, you said you were getting day and nighttime sweats every day." Henrietta nods. "That indicates to me that you are at least in Phase C," I say. "Many of us start to get daytime hot flushes in Phase B that can become more frequent in Phase C. And our night sweats start coming any old day, not just before flow. Many of us then totally get over those flushes and sweats, but for others, like me, and I guess you, Henrietta, they increase in difficulty through Phases D and E (39)."

I look over at Alison. "Your migraines will virtually go away when you reach menopause, Alison," I say. "Your migraines will start improving as soon as your hot flushes are controlled."

Alison holds her head. "It can't happen too soon!" she says.

"When you skip a whole period, you've gotten to Phase D! Night sweats and hot flushes get more intense especially during long cycles. Flow is now mostly far apart and usually not heavy. During this phase, women may just have a spot or less. But it still counts! Even though periods are far apart, breast tenderness, that had been improving, often signals that a period is coming. And estrogen levels are still sometimes very high. Premenstrual-like symptoms can occur totally without any relationship with periods. Those women whose cramps increase may find that they come any time during the cycle."

"I think I'm almost there!" Henrietta sputters. "I'm at least four months since my last period. I almost forgot . . ."

"Yep! One day you realize it's been a long time since you had a period. With any luck, you've tracked your periods on a calendar, so you can look back and start the one-year clock ticking. During that final year of perimenopause, most things that have been troublesome, except hot flushes, are better (39)."

"I can't wait," says Floreena fervently.

"However," I continue, "those women with night sweats will find they are waking with them most nights. Then, one day, you'll realize that it's been a whole 12 months since your last flow. You feel so happy and relieved that you just have to find someone to tell. In fact, it is a cause for celebration!"

"Bring on a party!" exclaims Jennifer. "If we were to share phone numbers or emails, we could let everyone here know when we reach that magical day." Then ruefully, "I'm afraid I can't imagine having a staff-room party at work about it!"

"That's a great idea," says Floreena. She takes a blank piece of paper from the table, writes down her telephone number and email address, and starts the list around the table. "I've got no one that I'd feel comfortable sharing all this with," she says, pausing. "Except for you." She looks around the table.

"That's too bad, isn't it?" I say. "Society's negative ideas about aging and menopause make it much harder for us to cope with all the changes of perimenopause (41). I feel very lucky. My kids, my partner, my workmates, and even some of my patients knew when I reached menopause. That's my hope for each of you—that menopause will mark the beginning of a new era in your life, a graduation. Now, let's take that break I promised. Would anyone besides me like some water?"

# 4

*decoding* midlife mysteries

"Ok," I say, "Now that we've re-assembled. I'd like to move on to talking about ways you can learn to track and understand perimenopausal changes.

"By now you know that perimenopause isn't something I can exorcize with a wave of my stethoscope. It is a life phase that we each must live through. However, it *is* something I can help you understand. And, I can treat some of the problems it brings. We have a tool that will help you live through perimenopause. That tool is called the Daily Perimenopause Diary (1). My colleagues and I at CeMCOR have developed and refined this Diary over many years. I've given you a paper copy today, but in the future you can download and print blank Diaries from the CeMCOR website at www.cemcor.ubc.ca.

"Slow down!" says Carla. "I'm trying to write all this."

"Don't worry," I reply. "It's on the board," I raise the screen.

"Thanks," says Carla.

"Keeping the Daily Perimenopause Diary is a bit like my looking at the flag on top of City Hall," I begin. "Seeing that the wind is from the east doesn't mean that I'll be happy when it starts to rain. But seeing the wind direction provides me with a way of predicting, and thus preparing for, a storm. Knowing that I can observe and predict the weather helps me to cope with it. The same is true of perimenopause—when I keep the Diary, I can start seeing patterns in my experiences and anticipate what's coming. Also, if I decide I'm going to try some treatment or other, I can track any changes, and decide if it's helping me or not. It gives me a kind of power. Self-knowledge makes me feel more in control, and less frustrated by the changes that I'm facing."

I see that the women are listening intently. I lower the screen again, put on a new transparency and turn the projector on before moving to the front of the table again. "This video," I pick up the purple video case sitting there, "that Dr. Prior made in 1999 is called the 'Puzzle of Perimenopause' (42). It's a 44-minute film that includes most of what we've already discussed about the hormonal changes of perimenopause, and what we're about to learn about the Diary. CeMCOR is distributing it for a donation of $35 CDN from which you'll get a $20 tax receipt—or $25 US without a tax receipt." I explain that CeMCOR's ongoing perimenopause research is funded by distribution of the video. "If you want a copy, you can see me afterwards or go to the CeMCOR website to order it."

"Is it also available in DVD?" asks Eva.

"Not yet. Stay tuned. It's in the works," I say. Several women make notes. I wait for them to finish. "Ok, back to the Diary," I continue. "I suggest that you fill in the Diary in the evening, just before you go to bed. You will need to record everything that occurred from your bedtime the night before—it becomes a goodnight ritual. If you forget one night, just skip that day. Ok?" I look around.

### Daily Perimenopause Diary

Name: _____   Month: _____   Year: _____

| Cycle Day | 1 | 2 | 3 | 4 | 5 | 6 | 7 | 8 | 9 | 10 | 11 | 12 | 13 | 14 | 15 | 16 | 17 | 18 | 19 | 20 | 21 | 22 | 23 | 24 | 25 | 26 | 27 | 28 | 29 | 30 | 31 |
|---|---|---|---|---|---|---|---|---|---|---|---|---|---|---|---|---|---|---|---|---|---|---|---|---|---|---|---|---|---|---|---|
| Date | | | | | | | | | | | | | | | | | | | | | | | | | | | | | | | |
| Tampons/pads/day | | | | | | | | | | | | | | | | | | | | | | | | | | | | | | | |

"You'll notice that the first line gives the cycle day," I continue. "Cycle Day 1 is the first day of flow. In the first three phases of perimenopause, you'll find it easier to see patterns if you start a new Diary sheet with a new period. That means that two partial months may need to be written at the top—like April-May. However, in Phase D of perimenopause, when you start skipping periods, you can keep the Diary by the month.

"The next line is for flow," I say, pointing to the screen. "It's the actual number—as nearly as you can remember—of *soaked*, normal-sized tampons or pads you've used in the previous 24-hour day. Let's practise. Say it's the first day of your period, and you soaked a pad overnight and three tampons during the day. What would you record in the flow box under Cycle Day 1?"

"Four," says Beverley.

"Right, Beverley," I nod.

"You said *regular* tampons and pads. I always need maxi-pads and super-tampons! What do I do with that?" asks Darlene with a little smirk. I feel that she is trying to catch me out.

"Good question!" I reply, keeping my voice bland. "Let me answer as I ask all of you a question: How many teaspoons of blood does a normal-sized tampon hold?"

"Maybe three," says Carla.

"Probably less, more like two," interjects Henrietta.

"You may be surprised to know this," I say, "because it looks like more when it's all spread out on a tampon. The answer is: *a soaked pad holds one teaspoon.* That's the same amount of blood that is in one of those glass tubes they use to take blood at a laboratory. Maxi-pads and super-tampons hold about twice as much, Darlene, which means you have to double the regular tampon count. So, if you use one super-tampon overnight and six regular-sized ones, what would you record?

"Two plus six makes eight," Alison blurts. "Eight," says Beverley almost at the same time.

| Record 0 = none, 1 = minimal, 2 = moderate, 3 = moderately intense, 4 = very intense | | | | | | | | | | | | | | | | | | | | | | |
|---|---|---|---|---|---|---|---|---|---|---|---|---|---|---|---|---|---|---|---|---|---|---|
| Amount flow | | | | | | | | | | | | | | | | | | | | | | |
| Cramps | | | | | | | | | | | | | | | | | | | | | | |

"That's right," I say. "You would record eight in your Day 1 box."

"Does anybody know how many soaked pads or tampons on average we use during one whole menstrual flow?" I ask.

"Maybe 30," says Carla.

"Probably ten," says Beverley.

"I think 20," asserts Darlene. "That's what I always had before I started flooding. But, Dr. Madrona, this system isn't accurate—you've no way to record clots. They plop into the toilet every time I pee!"

"I'll answer Darlene before we finish talking about usual flow," I say evenly, trying not to show my frustration. "When soaking through everything, Darlene, you'd still record the number of soaked tampons and pads on the line we're talking about. However, on the 'Amount flow' Diary line, you can make a judgment about how heavy your flow was. For clots and flooding, you'd write a '4'."

"Ok," I say, "back to what's the usual number of soaked regular-sized pads and tampons in one menstrual period. Any more guesses? So far we've heard from 10-30." I pause a moment, looking for more suggestions. "The answer is, about eight—the normal range is from two to 12 during the whole period. The absolute *too-much flow* that was learned from a population-based study is 16 soaked normal-sized pads or tampons in any one period (43). That means you would have lost about 80 ml of blood—about 2.5 ounces. We need iron in our red blood cells and we get it from food. Sixteen soaked tampons is more blood loss than the iron you eat allows your blood to replace each month (43). If you continue having 16 or more soaked tampons every cycle, you will become anemic and develop a low blood count or low hemaglobin level."

"I've soaked 20-30 tampons every six weeks since I was a kid. No wonder my blood count's so low that they won't let me donate blood!" Darlene exclaims.

"Are you taking iron?" I ask her.

"No!" she says. "No one ever said to," she adds defensively.

"Being anemic is hard on the whole system," I say. "It makes you tired, lose hair, and become at increased risk for infections. Anyone soaking 16 or more tampons during her periods needs to take one iron tablet a day. You can buy those at a drugstore without a prescription. Keep it up for a whole year." I reply a little stiffly, thinking she should know this from her nursing training.

"If you have heavy flow and find you're anemic, it means the iron stored in your bone marrow is completely gone," I continue. "When you take iron, your blood count usually becomes normal in weeks. But it takes a whole year of iron therapy for the bone marrow iron stores to return to normal."

I look around at the women taking notes. "If anyone is having heavy flow of 12 or more tampons a cycle, or any clots or flooding," I continue, "it's wise to take a daily multivitamin that has 4 or 5 mg of iron in it. That may prevent anemia."

"What if I only partly fill a tampon?" asks Alison. "I change them every time I go to the toilet—just to be clean, you know."

"That's a very good question, Alison," I answer. "If you partially soak a pad or tampon, make a guess as to what part was soaked—for example a quarter, or a half. A panty-liner, for example, would usually hold about a quarter of a tampon. If you changed tampons eight times in a 24-hour day, and each time, the tampons were half full, you'd record '4' below Cycle Day 1."

"What about spotting?" asks Eva. "I seem to spot for days and days before my flow really starts, and I sputter on for a couple of days after it should be over."

"There's also a place to record spotting on the 'Amount flow' line," I say. "That's the same line that allows record of flooding and clots. Use a '1' to mean spotting. And if you need something like a panty-liner or mini-pad, write ¼ on the tampon/pad line as well."

Seeing some worried faces, I continue. "The number of soaked tampons is the best that you can remember. Don't worry!" I exclaim. "Your best guess is good enough. You don't have to get obsessed or go marking on your hand!" Some of the women laugh. Alison pantomimes writing on her palm.

"Just do the best you can," I say. "That's plenty good enough. It's so both you and I can get a clear idea of what you're experiencing."

I point to the main section of the Diary on the screen. "Ok," I say, "although we've already started to talk about grading flow, I'd like to explain what the scoring system here is all about."

I point to the line on the Diary where it says: 0 = None, or absent, 1 = Minimal, 2 = Moderate, 3 = Moderately Intense, and 4 = Very Intense. "You'll use this same grading system for the whole top part of the Diary," I say. "It's easy to use—put a 0 if you didn't experience something that day. That '0' is probably the most important thing you'll write down! Any idea why?"

"I guess it's good if you don't have stuff like cramps," says Carla.

"Yes," I nod. "But, I also like the zeros because they tell me that you've thought about each part of the Diary. I know—when I see 0—you've thought about it and truly didn't experience whatever it is that day."

I point again to the Diary. "This line is your judgment call about flow. We already talked about spotting (a '1') and flooding or clots (a '4'). Obviously, if you didn't have flow, you'd write a '0.' If flow was normal or light, it's a '2'—if normal to heavy, it's a '3.' Any questions about that?"

"This is a pretty clever system, Dr. Madrona. How did you come up with those two different ways to record flow?" asks Eva.

"Well, that happened before my time," I reply. "I asked Dr. Prior that same question. The story goes that a young research assistant, about 20 years ago, used the daily Menstrual Cycle Diary (44) and saw, like Darlene, that just counting pads and tampons wasn't complete. It was then that this line was added to give a more accurate picture. When the Daily Perimenopause Diary (1) was developed later, we kept the same system. What's interesting is that those two lines also give me a clue about a woman's sense of what's normal. For example, if you were to write a '2' in the second line yet record seven soaked tampons on the first line, I'd know for sure that you're used to heavy flow!"

Several of the women laugh and Carla nods.

"The next line is about menstrual cramps," I say. "When Dr. Prior first adapted the original Menstrual Cycle Diary into this Daily Perimenopause Diary, she added hot flushes and night sweats but took away cramps. Very soon, from what midlife women told her, she had to add cramps back! Anyone know why?"

The room is quiet—several faces are looking puzzled. "Cramps can be severe in teenagers. After having a child, cramps often go away. That's why Dr. Prior took cramps off. However, in perimenopause, cramps may come back with a vengeance. And after Phase C, cramps may occur any old time of the cycle!"

"That's true," says Alison thoughtfully. "One month, when my migraines were really bad, I kept thinking my period would start. Almost all that month I was having that dull, way-down pelvic ache of cramps."

| Breast Sore: Front | | | | | | | | | | | | | | | | | | | | | | | | | | | | | |
| Breast Sore: Side | | | | | | | | | | | | | | | | | | | | | | | | | | | | | |
| Fluid Retention | | | | | | | | | | | | | | | | | | | | | | | | | | | | | |

I move on, pointing at the next lines on the Diary. "These two lines about breast soreness are especially for you and me, Floreena!" I say. "But I'll show you what they tell us about hormone action in perimenopause. The first line gives breast soreness, or tenderness, in the front of the breast. That is most reliable sign we have of high estrogen levels! If it's as bad as a '4,' it hurts even to take off your bra at night! When it's a '1,' you wouldn't realize that your nipple was sore unless you brushed against something.

"Because breast tenderness is such an important sign," I continue. "I want you to actually test for it. To do this, push the palm of your hand straight back and firmly into the front of your breast. Come on, try it!" I demonstrate.

"Ow! That hurts!" exclaims Jennifer. "You thought high estrogen was causing my nausea. There's the proof, right?"

"True, Jennifer! The check for breast soreness is to apply the same pressure on your thigh. If your breast is more sore, you'd need to record at least a '1.'"

Most of the women are pressing their breasts and then their thighs and murmuring among themselves. I notice that neither Eva nor Beverley is checking. Both look uncomfortable.

"I hardly dare touch," Floreena says. "I know they're sore as a boil!"

"Why do you have a second line for breast soreness, Dr. Madrona?" asks Eva.

"Great question!" I say. "The reason is that different areas of the breast seem to respond differently to high estrogen or to progesterone. The area of the breast that is particularly responsive to progesterone is way high up under the armpit in what is called the axillary tail of the breast. The whole breast can be sore from just estrogen. However, if the whole breast is *not* sore, but the armpit part of the breast is tender, it means that progesterone is present. Interestingly, I think for 'tail-of-the-breast' soreness both estrogen and progesterone levels are needed. For example, I'm still taking progesterone to treat night sweats and migraines, and I'm not sore at all," I say, pushing my fingers into my breasts near my armpit. "In summary, high side-of-the-breast tenderness in menstruating women means ovulation."

"Has that been proven? Or are you and Dr. Prior making wild claims again!" demands Darlene.

"That's a fair question," I say, struggling to sound reasonable. "Over and over I've seen that breast sign correlate with ovulatory results on the quantitative basal temperature (2). Dr. Prior has published that the absence of this high side-of-the-breast tenderness predicts low progesterone levels (45). Anyone have more questions?" I pause.

"I want you to practise checking your breasts for ovulation." I demonstrate by pushing the backs of my hands onto each armpit with my elbows sticking out. "Try it!" I encourage. "I know that we're taught that good little girls don't touch themselves! However, it's important that we know and own our own bodies."

This time most of the women copy me. "I call it the 'Chicken-Tonight-Sign'!" I say, playing the clown as I flap my sticking-out elbows and dancing about. Everyone laughs.

"Hurts!" says Beverley. She sounds surprised and a bit excited. "Does mean ovulate?"

"Only if the rest of your breast *isn't* sore, Beverley," I reply. Beverley touches the front of her breast and frowns.

"So, Beverley, that means high estrogen levels—it looks like your breasts are sore both in the front and up under your arm," I say. "There's likely no ovulation this cycle. Ok! Enough of breasts!

"The next line is about fluid retention," I continue, pointing to the Diary. "This is also influenced by estrogen. Here a '1' means waking once to urinate at night or puffy fingers in the morning."

"You mean, like I'm up peeing all night?" Carla exclaims. "I never used to."

"That's what I do, too," says Jennifer. "On the days with the worst nausea, my eyes and fingers are swollen in the morning!"

"That would be a 2 or 3, Jennifer. With ovarian hyperstimulation," I explain, "a complication of an infertility treatment, so much water is retained, it's an emergency! Gynecologists inject pituitary hormones to stimulate follicles to grow and ovulate. Estrogen levels sometimes become extremely high. When that happens, women will retain fluid in their bellies and may even go into heart failure. Most of the time, we don't notice swelling. We just have to urinate a few hours after we fall asleep.

| Hot flushes - day | | | | | | | | | | | | | | | | | | | | | | | | |
|---|---|---|---|---|---|---|---|---|---|---|---|---|---|---|---|---|---|---|---|---|---|---|---|---|
| # of flushes - day | | | | | | | | | | | | | | | | | | | | | | | | |
| Hot flushes - night | | | | | | | | | | | | | | | | | | | | | | | | |
| # of flushes - night | | | | | | | | | | | | | | | | | | | | | | | | |

Some of you know all about night sweats and a few know about hot flushes." I glance at Henrietta. "But others of you haven't experienced them. . .yet. I say 'yet' because most of us will have a few. Basically hot flushes mean a sudden feeling of heat with or without dampness that lasts for a few seconds to many minutes. Thankfully only about 10 or 15 percent of us will have severe hot flushes and night sweats.

"The next four lines," I continue, "describe day and night hot flushes. The first two lines are about daytime flushes and the second two are about night sweats during sleep. The first line labeled 'Hot flushes—day'" I point to the screen, "is your best judgment of how intense your hot flushes are. A '1' means a mild feeling of heat that you might not notice if you were really busy. An intensity of '2,' like the hot flush I had earlier, makes you fan yourself or take off clothing. It may only cause a little clammy feeling or a hot feeling without sweat. A '3' is something you will find hard to ignore. It makes you take off clothing, go to a window or fan yourself. At this score, at least half of your body is sweating. A '4' is a tropical rainstorm!" There is laughter. "You are hot and dripping!" I continue. "At that level, you take off clothes, fan yourself *and* go to a window. You can easily become dehydrated—you need to drink two extra litres of fluid a day."

"That's me!" exclaims Henrietta.

"The second line under daytime hot flushes," I continue, after nodding at Henrietta, "is the actual number of hot flushes you had during one whole day—from the time you awoke in the morning until you went to sleep at night. Again, as with tampon counts, you don't have to be exact—although some days I could remember precisely what I was doing at each flush!"

"Will I actually flush, I mean, turn red?" asks Floreena.

"No," I reply. "Most of the time, someone else can't see a hot flush in our faces. If there is any change it is often looking pale or peaked. The veins in our hands do get bigger and our fingers become warm. Flush is just part of a phrase that has come to describe this experience."

"Why don't you call them *flashes*?" Darlene asks. "That's the right name!"

"Most of the English-speaking world calls them 'flushes,'" I reply. "But in the USA they are usually called 'flashes.' Either term is ok."

All of a sudden Carla puts her hands on her hips and announces in a loud voice: "I don't have hot flashes, I have power surges!" We all laugh and clap.

"That's cool! Ahh, I mean *hot*!" exclaims Alison. "That expression makes hot flushes sound like something strong and exciting, not miserable!"

"Yes," I agree. "And speaking of power surges reminds me of what makes hot flushes so difficult—they come with a sudden sense of anxiety or anger, our hearts racing for no reason, and feelings of I-can't-sit-still restlessness. The rush of adrenalin and other brain hormones that are part of a hot flush cause those unpleasant experiences. In fact, the closest thing to a hot flush is what an addict goes through when quitting heroin. The same brain hormones surge when we have a hot flush."

"You know, I can tell when I'm about to get one," exclaims Henrietta. "It's like knowing your milk is going to let down when you're nursing." Alison and Jennifer nod. "I usually feel kind of dizzy or sick to my stomach, then I feel the heat creeping up my body—I just want to scream! Especially when I'm at work and some jerk complains his eggs aren't fried the way he asked!" Several women nod sympathetically.

"You're right, Henrietta," I say. "Some hot flushes do have an aura that tells us they're coming. I think those drug-withdrawal hormones cause that feeling. An aura will only happen for me when I'm stressed. The other day my colleague was yelling at his secretary. All of a sudden I had a weird feeling—I knew I was going to get a flush!"

"I think I've had flushes, but instead of getting hot, I get frozen!" says Eva. "Is that possible, Dr. Madrona?"

"Cold flushes are similar to hot flushes," I say. "Some women—especially those who have less insulation and are thin—are more likely to experience a coldness feeling as a flush has passed. After more intense hot flushes, our temperatures drop because moisture evaporates from our damp skin. You can get a wet-dog-shaking kind of sudden chill. Occasionally the flush feels like a cold shiver all by itself."

"Are we going to talk about treatment?" Henrietta interjects. "I can't take this any more!" I notice that Henrietta's face is drawn, and she is taking off her vest. She begins to sip from her big blue water bottle.

"Yes we'll talk treatment, and soon, Henrietta," I reply. "Hot flushes and night sweats are the most unpleasant experience that *well* women ever have. Severe night sweats require urgent treatment. You can't be healthy if your sleep is continuously interrupted. The only greater perimenopausal urgency is heavy bleeding. Henrietta, after we're done with this group session, ask Lana to put you on the list for a cancellation appointment. And also ask your family doctor to phone me. I'll discuss treatment that you could start before I see you."

"I don't want estrogen or anti-depressants!" Henrietta protests.

"I remember, Henrietta," I say. "I'm going to suggest natural progesterone taken at night." I pause, "However, no treatment in the world will completely take away hot flushes and night sweats *if we are very stressed*. I suggest two things you can start now that will make your hot flushes and night sweats better. First learn, and regularly practise, yoga breathing, deep and slow (46). And second, begin or increase your exercise—it can be anything active like walking, bicycling, dancing, aerobics, kick-boxing, Tai Chi—something you like (47)." Henrietta and several other women make notes.

"Which brings us to night sweats," I say pointing to the line of the Diary that says Hot flushes—night. "These occur during the time we are sleeping. A night sweat scored '1' will usually not waken us. Occasionally I'll get up to go to the washroom and realize my neck is damp. Because it didn't wake me up, I'll record a '1.' Night sweats that are a '2' or stronger wake us up! Even if we don't need to change our nightclothes or bed linens, we often have trouble going back to sleep because of surging brain hormones. A woman who has severe night sweats several times a night often gives up trying to sleep with her partner. A patient of mine complained bitterly: 'I can't cuddle, without a puddle!'"

A chuckle spreads through the small room. "What can we do to make them better—open the bedroom windows when it's frosty, and turn on a fan?" asks Carla.

"One of my patients with bad night sweats said she goes to bed in her all-or-nothings with one bath towel under her and one over her. Each time she has a night sweat, she replaces the wet towels with dry ones."

"What about when I'm on night shift and I sleep during the day?" asks Darlene.

"What do you think?" I ask in return.

"I think I would record the flashes during the daytime when I am sleeping, as 'Night sweats' and the ones during the night when I am working, as 'Daytime hot flashes,'" she answers.

"You got it!" I say, and everyone laughs.

| Mucous Secretion | | | | | | | | | | | | | | | | | | | | | | | | |
|---|---|---|---|---|---|---|---|---|---|---|---|---|---|---|---|---|---|---|---|---|---|---|---|---|
| Constipation | | | | | | | | | | | | | | | | | | | | | | | | |
| Headache | | | | | | | | | | | | | | | | | | | | | | | | |
| Sleep Problems | | | | | | | | | | | | | | | | | | | | | | | | |

I point again to the screen. "The next line on the Diary is for that stretchy vaginal mucus we discussed earlier. Here a '1' would be some shiny stuff on the toilet paper. And anything you could stretch out to 4–5 cm—an inch or two—would be a '4.'"

"What about vaginal discharge that isn't stretchy? How do I record that?" asks Alison.

"Thanks for asking, Alison," I reply. "What we care about is the stretchy characteristic of the mucus. That sign, like sore breasts, reflects high estrogen levels. So, record a 0 for any vaginal discharge that isn't stretchy."

"I just remembered—I used to keep that kind of record," says Jennifer. "I was trying to time my first pregnancy. A woman who used to be a nurse gathered a bunch of us who were interested. We met at the women's centre in Quesnel, where I grew up. I was like what's-her-name in the movie and book called *Fried Green Tomatoes*. I couldn't get the hang of looking in my vagina!"

"We did that in the outports of Newfoundland, too!" Alison chimes in.

"I never learn monthlies in Hong Kong," says Beverley.

"I also heard about that temperature and mucus method, not in medical school, but from some non-medical friends in Boston," I say. "I guess things that help women understand what's going on just spread from woman to woman."

I look at Beverley. "I'll bet old grandmothers in rural China knew lots of things about women's cycles," I say. "Maybe you just didn't hear about it, Beverley, growing up as you did in a big, westernized city."

I turn back to the Diary on the screen. "The next line is constipation. It's in the Diary, not because it differs in perimenopause, or because it is related to menstrual cycles—just because it's common for women in this culture. But I've noticed I tend to get constipated when I'm stressed or depressed."

"The next line is for headaches," I say, beginning to feel the pressure of time. "Headache is something that some of us have rarely, and others have severely and often. These can be tension-type headaches"—here I rub my temples—"or sinus, or because you were in bright sun without a hat or sunglasses. Whatever kind it is, score it as you would any other experience."

"How do I record my migraines?" asks Alison.

"If you have a migraine," I reply, "score the headache on the 0-4 scale, but also put a dot in the box with that number. That tells you, and me, that it was a migraine headache."

"I always get a tension-type headache just before my period—sometimes it turns into what I think is a migraine," says Eva.

"You can tell when it's a migraine because your head is throbbing, everything is too bright, you feel sick to your stomach, and you just want to crawl into a dark hole," Alison explains.

"Sounds like they're migraines. Thank goodness they don't come every period, nor do they appear at any other time of my cycle!" says Eva.

"Let's look at the line for sleep," I say, pointing to the screen. "How many of you regularly had problems with sleep when you were younger?"

"I had trouble falling asleep before an exam," Darlene says, contributing more easily now. "Most nurses have trouble because we work shifts. But I wouldn't say I usually did."

"Most of my life," says Henrietta, "I'd spend the first hours of the night just lying there, worrying. I've always been high strung. But now it's different. I fall asleep instantly—I'm dead tired. Lord knows I've got enough to worry about! Then I jolt awake with my first night sweat about two hours later. After that, I usually can't fall asleep again."

"Well, I've always been a good sleeper," Carla adds, "but now I do the same as Henrietta—I fall asleep and sleep hard for four hours, then I'm awake. Once I wake up, I know exactly what time it will be, so I fuss with myself about whether or not I'll check the clock!" Sympathetic giggles swirl around the table. "It's always at 3:13!" she continues. "Every night! And I try not to watch the clock but it's at least an hour before I fall into a restless sleep again."

"Those middle-of-the-night wakening problems you're describing are very typical of perimenopause," I say. "I used to think night sweats that women couldn't remember wakened them in the middle of the night. But from listening, and from my own experience, I know that perimenopausal sleep problems occur without any night sweats at all. This line of the Daily Perimenopause Diary is for sleep problems of any kind."

I stretch my neck a bit, feeling a tightness increasing. It got stiff when I was practising in a recorder trio last night. "Speaking of sleep," I say, "we're nearing the end of our session together. Now we're reaching some lines on the Diary that are more difficult. They relate to how we *feel*. Most of us, as women, were raised to know when our mom was having a bad day, or if our co-worker feels anxious. We know these things without a word being spoken. We've been trained to perceive other people's body language and feelings—unfortunately, often without being aware of, or acknowledging, our own. The next three lines are for feelings of frustration, depression and anxiety.

| Feeling Frustrated | | | | | | | | | | | | | | | | | | | | | | | | | | | | |
|---|---|---|---|---|---|---|---|---|---|---|---|---|---|---|---|---|---|---|---|---|---|---|---|---|---|---|---|---|
| Feeling Depressed | | | | | | | | | | | | | | | | | | | | | | | | | | | | |
| Feeling Anxious | | | | | | | | | | | | | | | | | | | | | | | | | | | | |

"You know what frustrated means. Initially Dr. Prior put 'Angry' on that line. But in the 1980s, at least, women just wouldn't admit to anger!"

"I don't have a problem with being angry!" Carla fairly shouts. "I just wish I didn't feel that way the whole g-d time!"

"It looks like you'll have lots of '3s' and '4s' for that line in your Diary, Carla," I say. "That reminds me of one of the best early randomized studies of estrogen treatment. It was by gynecologists who clearly believed that estrogen was the bees' knees. They were studying sleep and night sweats in menopausal women. Half the women got the pill form of estrogen and the other half got placebos. The estrogen-treated women had a 90 percent improvement in their night sweats and about a 50 percent improvement in sleep. The authors also recorded results of some emotional tests each woman did before and after treatment. They wrote that the women on estrogen had an unexplained 'increase in internally directed hostility' (48). That's doctor-talk for if-you-don't-show-your anger-you-become-depressed. Anger or depression increased for the women on estrogen, even though they otherwise felt and slept better."

There is utter silence in the room. Some women are looking down at their papers.

I point to the next line of the Diary. "That brings us to the next line, called Feeling Depressed. That doesn't mean you need a psychiatrist, or are clamoring for the newest anti-depressant drug. It can simply mean you feel a little blue or sad. Remember that you don't have to have a *reason*—you feel the way you feel! I, personally, find it hard to admit I'm feeling sad. I'll realize I'm a bit blue only when I've finished filling out the lower part of the Diary. I'll have recorded decreased energy and lower self-worth—those commonly mean that I'm feeling sad. Many a time I've written a '0' on the Feeling Depressed line, then I've changed it to a '1' or even a '2.'" I take a deep breath. "By the way, it's ok to change something on the spot. Just don't do any revising later!"

I tap my finger on the line following. "The final line of this section of the Diary is called Feeling Anxious. That's easy for most of us to understand—especially when we see it in others. For example, one time I had a woman sitting in front of me practically vibrating, wringing her icy cold hands and declaring, 'I'm not anxious—I've got nothing to be anxious about!'"

Everyone laughs. "Well, that completes the first part of the Diary," I say. "Anyone have any questions before we go on to the next section? It's easier and shorter, by the way."

"How do I record if I can't tell if I'm feeling angry or depressed or anxious, if they're all mixed up?" Carla asks. She looks utterly earnest. A couple of women giggle.

"I'm glad you asked that!" says Floreena.

"I'd guess you'd have to record a '2' or more for each, Carla," I reply. "These feelings can become a tangled mass! I remember reading that Marjorie Nichols, a loud-mouthed, controversial political reporter from the 1970s and 1980s in Ottawa, wrote: 'Anger is, of course, the tattletale of fear' (49)."

"The bottom Diary section is about *change*. Therefore," I say, pointing to the screen after moving the transpareny up on the overhead projector, "it has a different scoring system. This system centres around 'U' for what feels usual or normal for you. Like the rest of this Diary, there are no rights or wrongs. Just put down your best call. Dr. Prior told me she switched from the numbering system in the top part of the Diary because she didn't want to see zeros for breast size!" There is a general, embarrassed laugh.

Record  M = much less, L = a little less, U = usual, Y = a little increased, Z = much increased

| Appetite | | | | | | | | | | | | | | | | | | | | | | | | | | | |
|---|---|---|---|---|---|---|---|---|---|---|---|---|---|---|---|---|---|---|---|---|---|---|---|---|---|---|---|
| Breast Size | | | | | | | | | | | | | | | | | | | | | | | | | | | |
| Interest In Sex | | | | | | | | | | | | | | | | | | | | | | | | | | | |

"So," I continue, "the scale uses higher alphabet letters like Y and Z meaning 'increased a little' and 'increased a lot' and lower letters like L and M meaning 'a little decreased' or 'a lot decreased' from your *usual* experience. Any questions?"

The women are silent, but look absorbed. "Ok, the first line is Appetite. Ask yourself as you fill this in: Has there been any change today in my usual appetite?"

"I'd have to make that a 'Z' every time!" exclaims Eva. "I'm peeved to be hungry when I know I shouldn't be. I just can't stop myself from eating."

"Me too!" interrupts Carla. "My *teeth* feel hungry!"

"I just go from the cupboard to the fridge, then back again—I can't find anything that will satisfy me," complains Darlene. "Then I give in. I eat a candy bar and have a cigarette even though I've promised myself I won't."

"I know what you mean," I say. "And I think that kind of hunger is from higher insulin levels in perimenopause. When I was in early perimenopause, I got obsessed with my weight for the first time in my life. I was always slipping off to weigh myself—after I'd been to the washroom first, of course!"

Eva laughs.

"It's really weird," says Jennifer, "even though I'm vomiting, I still feel hungry. The only time I felt like that before was when I was pregnant."

"Well I'm just the opposite," says Henrietta. "I could care less if I never ate again. Maybe it's because I'm throwing greasy food at ghastly people all day. What puzzles me is why I'm not losing any weight."

"There is an almost supernatural resistance to weight loss in perimenopause," I say. "If any of you want to lose weight, it makes more sense, right now, to prevent *gain*. Then, when you have graduated into menopause, you can think about becoming more trim. I rationalize my weight gain as a natural protection against bone loss."

I smile, but a few of the women look worried or disgruntled. I try to lighten the mood.

"There's an old British saying: 'If tha' doesn't widen, tha' wizen!'" I say. "That translates, in plain English, into: If you don't gain weight in midlife, you become an elderly potato chip!"

All of the women laugh—but now, Eva's sitting on the edge of her chair. "But, I *can't* gain weight and be any good as a runner!" she exclaims. "I hate the way my clothes fit. I swear I'll get gangrene of the waist before I'll buy bigger work suits!"

"You're not alone in being distressed by weight gain," I say, " but to prevent wrinkles, it is probably wise to gain some weight at perimenopause. Besides, I don't think anyone can avoid a gain of about 2–5 kg—that's about 5 or 10 pounds. Let's add a French saying to the British one: 'Mind your face, not your hips!'"

I notice that Floreena rubs her face thoughtfully. "Whether it's increased or decreased, the change from *your sense* of what's usual for you is what matters," I continue. "This next line is Breast Size. In perimenopause, I moaned as my breasts just kept getting bigger and bigger. I remember one night, as I was doing my Diary, my then-teenaged daughter came into my bedroom and was watching me. 'Mo-om,' she said, sounding incredulous, 'How can your breasts be bigger than usual *all* of the time?'"

Laughter carried me to the next line of the Diary. "Interest in Sex is the next thing that may change in perimenopause. I think it's normal to have a decreased interest in sex during the perimenopausal years. 'Go away, honey! You're too hot,' or 'I have a headache,' or 'I'll be awake half the night listening to you snore!'" I frown, and mime pushing away a partner. "We can't explain this decreased sex interest by low estrogen or even decreasing testosterone (50). I think it's because we have way too many changes in our bodies and feelings to have any energy left over for sex. Sexual interest doesn't seem to be 'hard-wired' into us the way it is into guys. I think for most of us, sex is like icing, something that's delicious, but that we can live without."

"*Does* it get better?" Floreena asks, looking worried.

"It does," I answer firmly. "Most of the women I've listened to over the years say so. That is, provided you have a partner that you care about, and who is understanding. By the way, the only time I've heard that sex is great in perimenopause is when you find a new partner. Then, perimenopause or no, you're in that shimmering-can't-think-of-anything-else phase of a new relationship!"

"How do I record that if I've got no partner and am not having sex?" asks Jennifer.

"Thanks for reminding me," I reply. "Sexual *interest* is different from sexual *activity*. We can be quite interested, and even pleasure ourselves, despite no partner. Although some single women in past studies have left that line blank," I admit, "because they simply didn't feel comfortable acknowledging any sexual interest."

I look around. "The next Diary line is Feeling of Energy," I continue. "That means the get-up-and-go to do the things you want to do. Some days, for no reason, I just feel listless. I think those days are great for just vegging."

| Feeling Of Energy | | | | | | | | | | | | | | | | | | | | | | | | | |
|---|---|---|---|---|---|---|---|---|---|---|---|---|---|---|---|---|---|---|---|---|---|---|---|---|---|
| Feeling Of Self-Worth | | | | | | | | | | | | | | | | | | | | | | | | | |
| Outside Stresses | | | | | | | | | | | | | | | | | | | | | | | | | |

At this, many heads nod in agreement. "If only I could," mumbles Henrietta.

"I just call in sick. It's a Mental Health Day!" Darlene states, looking around.

"I heard that at any one time, one-third of all of the teachers and nurses in this country are off work," I add. "Think about it! What's the average age of most women in nursing and teaching today? It's about our age. That's why I think understanding and treating perimenopause is so important, not just for our own well-being, but also for the economy and for our society.

"Ok, enough of my soap box! The next line is called Feeling of Self-Worth. That refers to liking ourselves, feeling today as though we are a good partner, mother, worker, or whatever we consider ourselves to be. However, there are days when I just don't feel good about myself. So I would record an 'L' or 'M.'"

"'L' or 'M' would be my usual response, too," Henrietta says ruefully.

I smile in sympathy. "You'll feel better when you get a good night's sleep!" I declare.

"The final line of the Diary is called Outside Stresses." I say. "Here, I'd like you to be objective about what stuff's coming at you. Pretend that you're Tinkerbell—you know, Peter Pan's little flying friend—sitting on your shoulder and watching what you have to deal with in a day—the kids' clothes, the sick parent, the unbalanced chequebook, the boss who ignores your good work. You get the picture. On this line, record what's happening in the rest of your life." I look around to be sure the women are getting it.

"This much I know!" I declare. "No one can be well who, for weeks at a time, records 'Ys' and 'Zs' for Outside Stresses!"

"Some days I just wish I could give myself 'time out,'" exclaims Jennifer. "The way I *make* my acting-up kids chill!"

"Yes," I say, "we all need time-outs. Whether or not we *think* we can, most of us are able to either decrease the stresses in our lives or decrease our reactions to those stresses. We don't have to volunteer to drive this or that kid to hockey. We don't have to serve on the Christmas-party committee at work. We can actually say no. We can also decide to ask for what we need. That's a hard lesson for most of us, as women, to learn. We've succeeded so far, only by proving ourselves again and again. In many cases, we've had to be better or work harder than most guys. But, I'm convinced that we women who have a hard time during perimenopause will get sick or go nuts if we don't take time for ourselves when we are in this phase."

"I've begun to realize that," says Alison thoughtfully. "I'm trying to raise my boys to be responsible citizens. Not men who expect 'mom' or 'wife' to do everything. It isn't easy, but when I'm having a migraine, the boys *have* to help out. And maybe they'll grow up to be better around the house than their dad."

A few women nod in agreement. "Well," I say, "that's the last line on the Diary except for this one for recording your first morning temperature. Beverley, you and anyone else who wants to learn about recording and analyzing your basal temperature can look on the CeMCOR website for instructions. Briefly, you take all the temperatures in one cycle, calculate the average, and consider that the luteal phase begins when your temperature goes above and stays above that average. If you need to, ask Lana to print you a copy of the basal temperature instructions.

"The final bit of the Diary has a place for a word or two of comments. This has become a kind of journal for me. I'll write down 'Aunt Matilda visited—still crotchety' or stuff like that."

Everyone laughs. I look at the clock on the wall.

"And—we've run out of time," I announce. Some women glance at their watches.

"I've got to feed my parking meter in five minutes!" Henrietta jumps up and starts to put her things together. "I can't afford another ticket!"

"Five minutes is more than enough time to finish," I say. "There's not much left to cover. I'll just ask each of you to take home and read the handouts I've given you: 'The ABC's of Osteoporosis Prevention for Midlife Women' and 'Perimenopause—the Ovary's Grand Finale.' Both of these are also on the CeMCOR website. Some of you who are interested in figuring out where you are in perimenopause may want to read the new handbook, *Transitions through the Perimenopausal Years,* that Dr. Prior and some Victoria colleagues just published (51). Again, information about ordering *Transitions* is on the CeMCOR website. I've already given each of you the information about ordering the *Puzzle of Perimenopause* video. If any of you want one now, I'll get it for you." I look up to see Eva's hand raised.

"Finally," I say, "I've had a good time today. You're a lively group. I'm already feeling sad that you may be my last perimenopause group. I'm not accepting any new referrals because I'm going back to university. Thank you all for coming and participating today."

"Thanks to *you,* Dr. Madrona," says Carla, and all the women clap. Women start talking among themselves. I leave the room to get a video for Eva. When I return a minute later, Henrietta, looking tense, is headed out the door.

"Wait," Alison says. "I'd like to get together again. We've had fun here. May I take the list of names and contacts we made? I'd like to meet again soon? Any objections?"

"Fine with me," Carla says. The rest nod.

"Me too," says Jennifer.

"It's hard for me to come from the Valley," says Floreena, "but I'd like to."

"Yes, for sure I'll come from Victoria," says Carla. "I'll take the bus—that way we could go for a beer afterwards!"

"Does Friday afternoon work?" asks Jennifer.

"I got time off to come to see the doctor, but I couldn't just for a meeting," says Darlene.

"Why don't we make it a late Saturday afternoon, instead," suggests Alison. "That Saturday their dad will just have to take care of the boys' soccer games and piano lessons. And I bet we could use my church's basement. There's free parking. Anyway, I'll get back to all of you and we'll see. I've found it very helpful to know others were going through midlife miseries besides me."

The women mill out through the door.

"'Bye, Dr. Madrona!" Eva says. "See you at my appointment. I'm looking forward to it even more."

"'Bye, everyone," I say. "I'll look forward to seeing each of you again. Safe travels!"

The door closes behind them. I start picking up the overhead transparencies, feeling both exhilarated and tired.

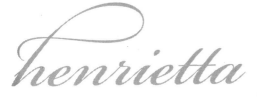

nightmare night sweats

"I'm glad you had a cancellation! And so happy I could find someone to take my shift!" Henrietta is out of breath and looks as though she's been rushing.

"It is good to see you again!" I say, taking her hand. "Are you ready to start?" She hands me a pile of Daily Perimenopause Diary records.

We reach my examination room-office, which is decorated only with a Norway calendar and a large framed Women's Day print from a few years back. It is a small space equipped with a desk, a scale and an exam table. We settle ourselves in our respective chairs.

Henrietta glances around, sips water from the bottle in her hand and takes a deep, slow breath. Then she nods.

"Good for you," I say, observing how she has calmed herself.

"What you mentioned about yoga breathing is really helping, Dr. Madrona," she says. "I didn't realize how uptight I've been. . . I was getting furious every time I woke at night. I was cursing that I was getting menopausal—I mean *peri*menopausal. My getting upset was making my night sweats even worse!"

"You've already learned the most important thing about hot flushes, Henrietta!" I exclaim. "Let's take a look at your Diary records first." I spread out her Daily Perimenopause Diary sheets on the desk.

"Good records, Henrietta!"

"Thanks," Henrietta says. We both shift positions so that we can look at her Diary together.

"Looks to me as though your hot flushes *are* improving," I say. "Good for you! Oh, you've marked an 'M' down here at the bottom. What does that mean?"

"I wrote 'M' for meditation—I put a check for each time I meditate 10 minutes or more," Henrietta says. She thinks a moment. "Yes, I guess the daytime flushes are better. The night-time ones, though, are still getting me down. I was a basket case when I came to that group session. You see, my mom is sick.

### HENRIETTA'S MARCH DIARY

Name: **Henrietta**     Month: **March**   Year: **2004**

| Cycle Day | 1 | 2 | 3 | 4 | 5 | 6 | 7 | 8 | 9 | 10 | 11 | 12 | 13 | 14 | 15 | 16 | 17 | 18 | 19 | 20 | 21 | 22 | 23 | 24 | 25 | 26 | 27 | 28 | 29 | 30 | 31 |
|---|---|---|---|---|---|---|---|---|---|---|---|---|---|---|---|---|---|---|---|---|---|---|---|---|---|---|---|---|---|---|---|
| Date | | | | | | 6 | | | | | | | | | | | | | | | | | | | | | | | | | |
| Tampons/pads/day | | | | | | | | | | | | | | | | | | | | | | | | | | | | | | | |

Record 0 = none, 1 = minimal, 2 = moderate, 3 = moderately intense, 4 = very intense

| | | | | | | | | | | | | | | | | | | | | | | | | | | | | | | | |
|---|---|---|---|---|---|---|---|---|---|---|---|---|---|---|---|---|---|---|---|---|---|---|---|---|---|---|---|---|---|---|---|
| Amount flow | | | | | | | | | | | | | | | | | | | | | | | | | | | | | | | |
| Cramps | no flow | 0 | 0 | 0 | 0 | 0 | 0 | 0 | 0 | 0 | 0 | 1 | 1 | 0 | 0 | 0 | 0 | 0 | 0 | 0 | 0 | 0 | 0 |
| Breast Sore: Side | 1 | 0 | 0 | 0 | 0 | 0 | 0 | 0 | 0 | 0 | 0 | 1 | 2 | 1 | 1 | 1 | 0 | 0 | 0 | 0 | 0 | 0 | 0 |
| Breast Sore: Front | 2 | 3 | 1 | 2 | 0 | 0 | 0 | 0 | 0 | 0 | 1 | 0 | 3 | 3 | 1 | 1 | 0 | 0 | 0 | 0 | 0 | 0 | 0 |
| Fluid Retention | 2 | 2 | 1 | 2 | 1 | 0 | 1 | 1 | 1 | 0 | 1 | 0 | 0 | 1 | 1 | 1 | 1 | 1 | 1 | 1 | 1 | 1 | 1 |
| Hot flushes - day | 3 | 2 | 3 | 2 | 3 | 3 | 3 | 2 | 2 | 3 | 2 | 2 | 2 | 1 | 2 | 1 | 2 | 1 | 2 | 1 | 1 | 1 | 0 |
| # of flushes - day | 6 | 3 | 5 | 2 | 2 | 7 | 5 | 4 | 5 | 6 | 4 | 2 | 3 | 2 | 2 | 3 | 1 | 2 | 3 | 2 | 3 | 2 | 3 | 2 | 1 | 0 |
| Hot flushes - night | 3 | 2 | 4 | 2 | 2 | 3 | 3 | 3 | 3 | 2 | 2 | 3 | 4 | 3 | 2 | 2 | 3 | 2 | 2 | 3 | 2 | 3 | 2 | 3 | 2 | 2 |
| # of flushes - night | 4 | 3 | 2 | 2 | 3 | 5 | 2 | 3 | 4 | 3 | 3 | 4 | 5 | 6 | 3 | 2 | 1 | 1 | 2 | 3 | 2 | 3 | 3 | 4 | 3 | 2 |
| Mucous Secretion | 0 | 0 | 0 | 0 | 1 | 0 | 0 | 0 | 1 | 2 | 0 | 0 | 0 | 1 | 0 | 0 | 0 | 0 | 0 | 0 | 0 | 0 | 0 | 0 |
| Constipation | 0 | 0 | 0 | 0 | 0 | 0 | 0 | 0 | 0 | 0 | 0 | 0 | 0 | 1 | 0 | 0 | 0 | 0 | 0 | 0 | 0 | 0 | 0 |
| Headache | 2 | 1 | 0 | 0 | 2 | 3 | 0 | 0 | 1 | 0 | 0 | 0 | 2 | 2 | 0 | 1 | 0 | 0 | 2 | 0 | 0 | 0 | 0 | 1 | 1 | 2 |
| Sleep Problems | 4 | 3 | 3 | 2 | 2 | 4 | 2 | 3 | 3 | 2 | 2 | 3 | 4 | 3 | 2 | 3 | 2 | 2 | 2 | 3 | 4 | 2 | 3 | 2 | 3 | 2 |
| Feeling Frustrated | 2 | 3 | 2 | 1 | 2 | 2 | 0 | 2 | 2 | 1 | 3 | 2 | 2 | 2 | 1 | 2 | 0 | 0 | 1 | 0 | 2 | 2 | 1 | 0 | 1 | 1 |
| Feeling Depressed | 2 | 3 | 3 | 1 | 0 | 2 | 4 | 2 | 1 | 1 | 0 | 0 | 1 | 0 | 0 | 1 | 0 | 0 | 0 | 1 | 0 | 1 | 0 | 0 | 0 | 0 |
| Feeling Anxious | 1 | 0 | 1 | 2 | 1 | 2 | 1 | 3 | 2 | 1 | 1 | 0 | 0 | 1 | 1 | 0 | 0 | 0 | 0 | 0 | 1 | 0 | 0 | 0 | 0 |

Record M = much less, L = a little less, U = usual, Y = a little increased, Z = much increased

| | | | | | | | | | | | | | | | | | | | | | | | | | | | | | | | |
|---|---|---|---|---|---|---|---|---|---|---|---|---|---|---|---|---|---|---|---|---|---|---|---|---|---|---|---|---|---|---|---|
| Appetite | L | M | L | L | L | U | L | M | L | L | M | M | L | U | U | L | U | U | U | L | L | U | U | U | U |
| Breast Size | U | L | U | U | L | U | U | U | L | L | U | L | U | U | Y | Y | Y | U | U | U | U | U | U | U | U |
| Interest In Sex | basically zip | | | | | | | | | | | | | | | | | | | | | | | |
| Feeling Of Energy | L | L | M | L | L | M | M | L | L | U | L | U | L | L | M | M | L | L | U | U | U | U | U |
| Feeling Of Self-Worth | L | L | U | U | L | U | L | U | L | L | U | U | U | Y | L | U | U | U | Y | U | U | U | U | U |
| Outside Stresses | Y | Z | Z | Y | Y | Y | Y | U | U | U | Y | Y | Y | Z | Y | Y | Y | Z | U | U | U | U | Y | Y | Y | U | Y |
| ~~Basal Temperature~~ M✓ = 10 min | 0 | 0 | 0 | 0 | 0 | 0 | 0 | ✓ | ✓ | ✓ | ✓ | ✓ | ✓ | ✓ | ✓ | ✓ | ✓ | ✓ | ✓ | ✓ | ✓ | ✓ | ✓ | ✓ | ✓ | ✓ |
| Comments (Temperature Taken Late, Feeling Sick, Poor Sleep, Etc.) | | | | | | | | | | | | | | | | | | | | | | | | | | | | | | | |

I work as a waitress about 50 hours a week to make ends meet, commuting into the city from Surrey by bus because I can't afford a car. I spend all my free time going to see my mom, who can be very demanding. She lives on her own in North Vancouver, which is hard to get to from here!" She takes a breath.

"Then my son and his three-year-old moved back in with me after a kind of separation—his wife had to take a job in Cranbrook. They couldn't afford to keep two places, and he couldn't risk losing his mechanic's job here. I would have been ok with that, but pretty soon my son was acting like I would be so happy to take care of him and my grandson, and cook and clean and entertain. Well, I wasn't! And I didn't have the gumption to tell him so."

Henrietta pauses and I listen, feeling drawn into her story. "Once I'd been doing some meditation—I suddenly saw that I needed to take better care of myself or I wouldn't be able to help anybody. I asked John—that's my son—to make the evening meals, to do his own and his son's laundry and all of the shopping—in short, I asked him to share the tasks. He's also contributing to the rent. And he takes turns with me in visiting Mom—he lets me drive his car when I have to go to see her after a day shift. So, what was a disaster is turning out to be good, now that I've learned to ask for what I need."

"And started meditating" I add. "It's no wonder your hot flushes and night sweats were difficult. You're dealing with a whole bunch of big life stresses."

Henrietta takes another long, deep breath, and a sip of water.

"I guess another part of it is that my mom went through menopause when I was a teenager. She has bipolar affective disease. She had a terrible time—was hospitalized for months before they realized why she was so crazy. I've always known I'd have a tough time with meno . . . *peri*menopause, and I was angry that it came so soon and when I've got so much on my plate."

"It isn't fair, is it?" I say, feeling sadness prickle my eyes. "But, as you have proved to yourself, you can help things get better. And the good news is that perimenopause eventually ends. Meanwhile, it's my job to help you live through this." I pause, taking my own deep, yoga-breath.

"My first job is to understand you better. You're 48, aren't you?" I say as I write it on the form in front of me. "That's just about the average age for periods to start becoming irregular. When did you first skip a period?"

"Last year. I missed it in December. Since then I've only had a couple, which is a relief, although my periods were never difficult. I was basically paying no attention until I started waking two or three times a night and having to change my sheets. When I complained to my doctor, he said I was depressed.

That set me off! I am not like my mom! After that, I didn't trust him. And I refused to take everything he prescribed!"

"Bipolar affective disease *does* tend to run in families," I say, "but it doesn't sound as though you have it. It seems more likely to me that you're perfectly sane. A combination of disturbed sleep and financial, family and work stresses is getting you down. That's plenty to make anyone a bit depressed."

"If blue means not having fun anymore, then my doctor's partly right. I felt like I had nothing to look forward to. Each morning I wondered if I could make it through the day. But I feel so much better now that I understand I'm not the only one. And you've taught me something I can *do* for myself."

"Have you ever had a spell of depression before?" I ask.

"Yeah, when Dad left us. I was ten. I missed him because I was his 'special big girl.' He left to take a job in Quebec and then just didn't come home again. Mom got depressed and would holler at us and then go off and cry. I had to be a little mom for the two younger ones. It was a hard time—I used to hide in the library before and after school."

I reach over and touch her hand.

"The librarian, Miss Wang," Henrietta continues, "saw how rough things were and made me her little friend. She would invite me over for tea on Saturdays. When I was away, Mom had to cope with Sissy and Teddy. And gradually I came to realize that it wasn't my fault that Dad had left."

"So you have *two* risks for perimenopausal depression," I say. "First, depression is more common in perimenopausal women who've ever been depressed before (52). Secondly, depression is more common in those who are having trouble making ends meet (12;53)."

I jot down her history.

"What exercise do you regularly do?" I ask.

"Before I had to move to Surrey for cheaper rent, I used to do this long walk on the dyke in Richmond after work and at least once on a weekend. But now I'm only walking from my house to the bus and back again—that takes about 20 minutes a day. Of course, when I'm working I'm running all day. I know I need to exercise, so I've started doing some long walks—the restaurant where I work is downtown, so I walk to Stanley Park and have a good brisk walk a couple of times a week."

"Good for you," I say. "The walking will help a lot. Lack of exercise is another of those risk factors for depression in perimenopause (54). Several studies have also shown that exercise makes depression better" (55;56).

"I like walking," says Henrietta. "It's usually the only time I really have to myself."

"What supplements or herbs are you taking?" I ask.

"I use sage tea for the flushes—I learned that from a friend who works at a health-food store. I take chamomile tea before I go to bed and in the night if I can't sleep. I'm taking oil of evening primrose capsules three times a day, Remifemin three times a day, dong quai twice a day, and black cohosh morning and evening. And I have at least two soy-based foods a day—soymilk or tofu."

"You're taking all of those for treatment of hot flushes and night sweats, aren't you?" At her nod, I continue, "The best studied of these is black cohosh—it is packaged as the commercial product called Remifemin. Randomized placebo-controlled trials show that Remifemin causes some improvement in hot flushes. Don Quai is an estrogen-like herb—no good studies show that it is effective for hot flushes. Soy foods contain phytoestrogens, natural plant hormones that act like estrogen, and are often recommended for hot flushes. Only about half of the dozens of randomized placebo-controlled studies show soy helps hot flushes and it's not much more effective than placebos (57). Garden sage has recently been recommended for hot flushes but has not yet been scientifically studied. Oil of evening primrose is a plant-derived oil that has been touted for premenstrual symptoms but has never been scientifically tested.

"You're trying everything that may help, aren't you?" I say cautiously, feeling unwilling to put doubts in her mind about things that she finds useful. "However, I would be careful of oil of evening primrose and dong quai because they may act like estrogen and might make your underlying risk for flushes worse. Also, black cohosh and Remifemin are really the same. So you could skip one—you don't want an overdose."

"And I take Vitamin E," Henrietta adds. "I increased to 400 IU a day. I also take a special vitamin supplement in three capsules a day and 1,000 mg of calcium citrate with magnesium at bedtime."

"All of those are probably helping you right now, Henrietta. Keep a record on your Diary of what you are taking. Before you run out of each one, taper it down while recording and see whether you notice any changes. If you see no change, you can stop it. That also will allow you to save some money."

"That'd be good," Henrietta says, "because I spend about a hundred dollars a month on those supplements alone, and I really can't afford it!"

"Ok," I say, "besides skipping periods, the night sweats and the hot flushes, have you noticed any other changes with perimenopause?"

"I didn't think I had," she replies, "but when you were describing shorter cycles, breast tenderness and increased cramps in that group meeting, I realized I'd experienced those and just taken no notice. The thing I didn't get was weight gain. I've lost weight in the last few years. I eat really well, when I eat. But sometimes I'm just too stressed."

"Have you ever been seriously ill, injured, hospitalized, or broken a bone or had surgery?" I ask.

"I had my tonsils out when I was a kid. And I guess I was really small at birth because my mom was a smoker. They wondered if I'd live. And in my mid-twenties I had whiplash from being rear-ended. I've noticed that my neck is bothering me, especially when I've had a bad night and am feeling like I can't cope. Otherwise I've been well."

I look up from writing in my chart and watch Henrietta's always-moving hands.

"Are there any illnesses besides bipolar affective disease that may run in your family?" I ask.

"My mom developed hypothyroidism, an under-active thyroid, in the last few years, but the doctor said that was from her medication. She had a blood clot when she went on hormone replacement therapy for osteoporosis. She has lots of crushed vertebra in her back. There's osteoporosis in my family for sure. My grandma broke her wrist and got very short as she got older. My dad's family I don't know that well. I think it was a heart attack that killed his father when I was little."

"Do you think you're at risk for osteoporosis?" I ask.

"Yes, because of Mom, and Grandma, although I've never smoked and I've been careful to exercise. I'm allergic to milk, so I've been supplementing calcium for many years."

"You have at least two big risks for osteoporosis," I say gently, "besides your family history and low food calcium. One risk is your low weight and weight loss and the other risk is that you are in the phase of perimenopause during which *everyone* loses bone. Would you like me to order a bone mineral density test now so that we can see where you stand?"

"How would you treat me if I had osteoporosis, Dr. Madrona?" asks Henrietta, frowning. "I don't want medicines."

"There is real benefit from higher amounts of calcium, and vitamin D, good exercise and a healthy weight gain, Henrietta," I say. "And, I think, from improving sleep and night sweats so you have lower cortisol levels. But if those supplements and lifestyle things are not sufficient, I may recommend a non-hormonal medicine that slows bone loss. Remember, if I recommend a medication you don't feel comfortable taking, you make the final choice to take it or not."

"Ok, I'd like a bone density," Henrietta says. "By the way, I forgot—I broke my ankle when I fell a few years ago."

"Were you running or jumping when you had that ankle fracture?" I ask.

"No, I was walking and just didn't see a small step-down. I twisted my ankle as I fell."

"That means that you already have osteoporosis, Henrietta," I say softly, but firmly. "A normal, strong bone would not break with that little force."

Henrietta sits up straight in her chair. "Don't give me any more diseases! Perimenopause is enough to cope with right now!"

"I'm not *giving* you diseases, Henrietta," I say. "I have a responsibility to tell you the truth. Osteoporosis is something that we can work on together. Perimenopause is indeed enough, and it's not a disease at all, just a phase of life you'll out grow. Once you are sleeping through the night, everything will look brighter (58)."

Henrietta relaxes slowly into her chair.

"Besides milk, are you allergic to anything or to any medicines?" I ask.

"I am allergic to cigarette smoke. That's why I'm so glad I work in Vancouver where the bylaws prohibit smoking in restaurants. Oh—and I got hives from tetracycline for an infected gum when I was teenager."

"Ok," I say. "Let's run through what you've eaten in the last day, starting with breakfast this morning."

"I had a whole wheat and nut bagel with tofu cheese that I ate on the bus as I went to work and a banana and a ground-grain kind of fake coffee at my break. At a later break, I ate the carrot sticks and apple I brought with me."

"That sounds good," I say. "How about for lunch and dinner yesterday?"

"At lunch," Henrietta pauses, "I can't remember. . .but I had supper with my mom. She had fixed scalloped potatoes and wild salmon steaks and"—she makes a wry face—"overcooked broccoli. Oh, now I remember. I had lunch on the run—clam chowder from work, organic corn chips with homemade fresh salsa, and a handful of peanuts as I left work to go to Mom's."

"Did you have anything besides chamomile tea before bed?" I ask.

"No, I was tired. I didn't even have my tea. I just took my calcium, sat on my bed, did my breathing, and went to sleep."

"You do eat healthily, Henrietta," I say. "But I don't think anything you ate yesterday, except your mom's food, had any of the essential oils. Could you add some olive or other natural oil to each meal?"

"Yes, I'll try doing that. Maybe flaxseed oil capsules."

"That's like adding another supplement, Henrietta," I say. "I was thinking you could make some salad dressing with olive oil or sauté food in oil. How often do you skip a meal, or have a tiny one, like that soup yesterday?"

"More than I'd like," she says. "I guess I'll have to make my lunch and take it to work. I think I'll start taking my breaks together with lunch so I can both eat my lunch and do some walking."

"Do you drink any coffee, tea or colas, or use alcohol?" I ask.

"I used to drink eight or ten cups of coffee a day and thought it was keeping me going. But I started getting heartburn, feeling shaky, and having headaches both at the end of the day and before my first morning coffee. So I quit about nine years ago."

I nod.

"I used to have a social drink or wine with dinner," she continued. "It became a habit when I was married. But I don't like how I feel with it, and I'm a cheap drunk, so I just avoid alcohol totally now."

"Do you use any recreational drugs?" I ask.

"I smoked pot when I was a teenager and during my marriage. But I don't like marijuana smoke any more than cigarette smoke. And when I bake with it I never know when the effects will start, so I just leave it alone now."

"Do you regularly check your breasts?" I ask.

"Yes. Except I forgot last month . . ."

"Now that your periods aren't regular, you can use the twelfth day of every month," I say.

"The twelfth? Oh, that's my birthdate! Ok, that'll be easy to remember."

"Have you had a mammogram?" I ask.

"No, I read about the controversy and don't believe that testing while you're in your forties is useful because the breasts are too dense. I'll have one when I'm 50—then I'll have one every couple of years after that. I know that I don't have any risk factors. My period came late at 15 and I had my first child when I was 21."

"How were your periods after they finally started?" I ask.

"I skipped a lot when I first got them, then I got to be regular. I tried the birth control pill when I first had a steady boyfriend, but it made me sick. So

I went to Planned Parenthood and learned how to use a diaphragm and jelly, which I've always used since. Not that I need it nowadays!" She laughs.

"How many times have you been pregnant?" I ask.

"Three. I had a miscarriage after my son—the one who lives with me—and then had a second son who is now going to Queens' and studying architecture," she says with pride.

"How are your bowels?" I ask.

"I used to be constipated—I was for most of my life. Now I almost have diarrhea every morning. It's lucky I have to get up so early for my shift, or I think it would wake me. I think it's the vitamin E."

"Oh, I'll bet it's the magnesium in your calcium pills, Henrietta," I say. "You remember milk of magnesia—it's magnesium making what I call 'intestinal hurry.' Even though the health-food stores are very insistent, the studies they quote are in rats whose diets are low in magnesium. Good human evidence shows that we who have healthy bowels don't need magnesium to absorb calcium (59). Anyway, your diet is full of whole foods so I think you're getting enough magnesium. Try buying some calcium tablets without magnesium and see if that makes any difference in your morning diarrhea."

"Ok," says Henrietta, "I'll do that. Calcium without extras is usually cheaper anyway."

"Are there any things bothering you that we haven't talked about?" I ask.

"What is bothering me most, even with my yoga and meditation, is the night sweats. I use your trick of the big towel under and over me. When I wake with a sweat, I just replace the two towels with dry ones and try to get back to sleep. But I still feel hyper, and even though I do my breathing and try to relax, I often can't fall asleep again. And I'm still wakening, as you can see from my Diary, at least three times at night."

"I know that natural progesterone will make that better, Henrietta," I say. "But we'll talk about a plan of action once I've examined you. Ok?"

~

After I've examined Henrietta, we settle into our own chairs again. I pass Henrietta's Diary records back to her. "Here are your original diaries, Henrietta. While you were changing clothes, I made a copy for your chart. If you have a fax available, you could keep in touch by sending me your Diary each month as you finish it. Then I'll know whether things are improving or you need some help."

"I'd prefer to try everything myself first, Dr. Madrona," says Henrietta firmly.

"Ok, Henrietta, you may certainly try. Let's summarize. You are basically a very healthy woman except that you are too thin. Your BMI, body mass index, a way of putting the height and weight together, is 19.2, which is just within the normal range for a teenager, but too low for a woman in her forties who's at risk for bone loss."

"How much *should* I weigh?" she asks.

"Let's see," I say. You now weigh 52 kg and are 164 cm tall. Ideally you would increase to 60 kg, which would make your BMI just over 22. Do you think you can do that?"

"I'm not sure—I've only ever weighed that much when I was pregnant. If you think that would be good for my bones, I'll try."

"Great!" I say, smiling. "You are now in Phase D of perimenopause. Remember the timeline we discussed? You have one or two years until your final menstrual period and a year from that until you graduate into menopause."

"Yes, I remember," she says. "I thought I might still be in Phase C."

"You're farther along than that because you've skipped whole periods, and are not just irregular. Irregularity is the characteristic of Phase C," I say.

I notice that Henrietta is taking notes as I talk.

"Your blood pressure was fine at 136 over 72," I say. "Your pulse is a bit too fast at 84. But as you learn to use your meditation skills wherever you are, that will slow—it will also improve as you increase your exercise. Your breasts are generally soft, except for those nodular areas I showed you. They're not a worry because they match from side to side. Since they are lumps you remember feeling before and they haven't changed, we won't worry. I worry when a woman doesn't check her breasts and so has no idea whether something was there before or not."

Looking at my notes, I say, "The rest of your examination was perfect except that you have very skinny arms and your hands are freezing."

"I know! I've had cold hands all my life. What do skinny arms and frozen fingers mean besides that I haven't been lifting bar bells?"

"To me they say that you are under a lot of stress. When we're stressed our bodies make higher than normal levels of cortisol and that makes us burn muscle for fuel. We also make too much cortisol when we don't have enough calories to meet our bodies' needs. Both reasons cause low muscle, especially in the arms. And, it's warm in here. So your cold hands are not simply because you are thin or the environment is cold, but also because the stress hormones called catecholamines . . . "

"Like adrenalin?" asks Henrietta.

"Yes, adrenalin and noradrenalin are made in higher amounts with stress. One of their jobs is to make sure that our heart and lungs have enough blood so that, if we needed to, we could run or fight. To do that, they take blood from the hands and feet, causing them to be cold."

"Oh," says Henrietta.

"As you meditate," I add, "you can practise warming up your hands."

Henrietta smiles. "So there's something more *I* can do!" she says.

"Right," I agree. "And we've already talked about your weight and set a goal to work toward. That will help with your bones as well as giving you a buffer for when you have to skip meals."

"You're right that I should be heavier," she says. "I didn't like losing weight, but I can gain some now by taking my own lunch, by adding some good fats to what I eat, and by not skipping meals."

"You've got it!" I say. "The other thing is osteoporosis. I'll order a bone density of your lower back and hips. It could be done the same day you come to see me in a few months. That would save you an extra trip into town. Or you could come on a Saturday. They have started doing them on Saturdays here at the hospital."

"I'd prefer to make one trip," she says, "although I've started reading on the bus and don't feel travel is as big a waste of time as I did when I drove."

"Good," I say. "And there are a couple of things besides gaining some weight and starting more regular exercise that will also help your bones. Do you use the Internet? Good. Please go to the Centre for Menstrual Cycle and Ovulation Research website at www.cemcor.ubc.ca and look under perimenopause for the 'ABCs of Osteoporosis Prevention in Midlife Women.' Remember that I mentioned it in our group session? It explains that healthy bones are a 'whole meal deal.' Healthy bones in midlife involve reducing stress, having regular ovulation or taking progesterone to increase bone formation, getting to and maintaining normal weight and doing good exercise as well as taking calcium and vitamin D.

"I'll also order a urine test," I continue, writing out the laboratory form. "We'll do that test every six months for the next several years. It is a measure of bone loss. Collect this urine for your first test after you have been doing everything we've discussed for about two or three months. You want to collect *all* the urine you make in the middle of the night and the first urine in the morning. The test is called deoxypyridinoline or D-pyr for short because that's the name of a cross-linked protein that comes from bone. We all lose some bone normally, so the normal range for this D-pyr protein in the morning urine is 3–7.4. But if you are losing too much bone despite gaining some weight and taking enough calcium and vitamin D, I'd like you to consider further treatment."

"I don't want to take medicines unless I absolutely have to, Dr. Madrona."

"I know, Henrietta. As I said earlier, you will always have that choice. I just want you to know that *everyone* loses bone in Phase D of perimenopause. You are different than the average woman because your bone mineral density is likely already low and you've already had a low-trauma fracture. Plus, you are likely to lose bone more rapidly than average because of your family history of osteoporosis.

"You also need to get a total of 2,000 mg a day of elemental calcium," I say. "At Henrietta's puzzled look, I explain that "elemental" means the weight of just the calcium without the other things like carbonate or citrate with which it is always paired.

"The total elemental calcium can come from both food and supplements, but needs to be spread across the day. The most calcium that will be effectively used at any one time is 600 mg."

"I know that a cup of soymilk has 300 mg of calcium," says Henrietta, "and my diarrhea pills!"—she laughs—"that's what I'll call my calcium/magnesium pills!—have 250 mg in each. I could take two rather than four at bedtime, and have one at breakfast and one at lunch. Plus I could have a glass of soymilk at supper as well as at bed." She does some figuring in her notebook. "That will give me 1,600 mg a day. Is that enough?"

"That is nearly perfect, Henrietta, except I'd like you to add one more high-calcium food or tablet because only about 200 mg is absorbed from each cup of soymilk. A healthy diet with vegetables and nuts has about 300 mg of calcium in it counting all of the small amounts from various foods.

"I'd also like to see you getting 1,400 IU of Vitamin D each day. You are probably getting 400 IU from your multivitamin now—take a look at the label. If you were to add a single 1,000-unit Vitamin D pill each day, you'd have exactly what you need. And each pill only costs about eight cents a day."

"Can I take cod liver oil pills instead?" asks Henrietta.

"Yes, if you prefer, but I find I often taste that fishy oil all day!" I make a face. "The maximum amount of vitamin D from the usual cod liver oil pill is only 200 IU. Each cod liver oil pill also contains 5,000 IU of vitamin A. Since the maximum amount of vitamin A you should get is between 3,000 and 10,000 IU a day, you would get 'way too much from the five capsules you'd need to take to get 1,000 IU of vitamin D. And they would cost more than a single vitamin D pill."

"Thanks for telling me about vitamin A. I guess a natural source is not always better, eh?"

"Right, Henrietta. Oh—also, when you run out of your brand-name vitamins, you could try replacing them with generic multivitamins that cost about two cents each. You can also replace that expensive calcium citrate with cheaper calcium carbonate. Evidence says that carbonate and citrate are nearly equally effective"(60).

"Any questions?" I ask. "No? We're almost finished. You will definitely improve your sleep with continued meditation and more walking. You might also try taking an old-fashioned antihistamine—the kind that makes you drowsy—at bedtime."

I shake Henrietta's hand—now slightly warmer—and walk out of the room with her.

"Remember to do a urine test about two weeks before I see you next time. That will tell us whether what you are doing is sufficient to prevent bone loss. We'll send in the requisition for your bone density test. Lana will coordinate everything for you."

"Here's Henrietta, Lana" I say. "I'd like to see her again in about three months and have a bone density done that same day, just before I see her."

"Thanks, Dr. Madrona," says Henrietta.

"Take care, Henrietta," I say. "You're doing a great job."

A couple of months later, Lana tells me that a distraught Henrietta is on the phone.

"Yes, I'll speak with her," I say to Lana. "Please put her through while you round up her file and that last Diary she faxed."

I pick up my phone. "Hello, Henrietta."

"Oh, Dr. Madrona, thank you so much for talking to me. I'm just having a hard time. I can't sleep, I ache all over,"—she starts to sob—"and I can't cope anymore!"

"Slow down, now," I say. "Tell me what's changed since I last saw you. I've got your Diary from May and it's looking better. At least the daytime flushes seem less."

I can hear Henrietta blow out a big breath. "The big thing is that Mom got manic, was smoking all night, then fell asleep. Now she's in the hospital with burns. And the house is bad. . . " Henrietta begins to sob again.

"I'm sorry, Henrietta. Is your mom going to be ok?"

"She's lucky, she burned only one arm and her side. She's ok. They're talking about sending her home in a few days. But where can she go? Her house needs fixing, the insurance agent is phoning, the social worker at the hospital is calling and calling me. I'm aching all over, and my whiplash is horrible. I can't sleep. . . ." Her voice trails off.

"What do you think would help, Henrietta?" I ask.

"I think I need to start that natural progesterone you mentioned in the group session. I tried the progesterone cream from the health-food store, even a triple dose, but it doesn't seem to help. If Prometrium is supposed to help sleep as well as hot flushes, I'll take it!"

"I'll be happy to phone that prescription to your pharmacy, Henrietta," I reply. "I'll prescribe Prometrium in 100 mg capsules. Each looks like a beige-coloured salmon egg—you need three at bedtime every night. Take them just as you are on your way to bed, or you may feel dizzy. Also, the first night or so after you take them, you may feel groggy in the morning. It's your body's way of trying to catch up on dream-sleep. Give me your pharmacy's phone number. And," I pause, "Henrietta, I know things are rough right now. But you need to start doing that yoga breathing and meditation again. Your sore neck and aching all over are just because you haven't been sleeping. They'll get better soon," I say, consciously being reassuring and positive.

About a month after her desperate phone call, Henrietta arrives for her follow-up appointment.

"Hi, Henrietta!" I say. "Lana tells me you seem much better. Tell me what's happening."

"I'm lots better!" she pulls out her June Diary and shows me that the hot flushes are nearly gone.

"Where to start?" Henrietta says. "That time when we spoke on the phone was my low point. I just couldn't see any way ahead. I'd been to my doctor twice in that week about my sore neck, and I got a note to be off work for two weeks, which I just can't afford because I've got no paid sick leave. I was

## HENRIETTA'S DIARY ON PROGESTERONE THERAPY

Name: Henrietta    Month: June    Year: 2004

| Cycle Day | 1 | 2 | 3 | 4 | 5 | 6 | 7 | 8 | 9 | 10 | 11 | 12 | 13 | 14 | 15 | 16 | 17 | 18 | 19 | 20 | 21 | 22 | 23 | 24 | 25 | 26 | 27 | 28 | 29 | 30 | 31 |
|---|---|---|---|---|---|---|---|---|---|---|---|---|---|---|---|---|---|---|---|---|---|---|---|---|---|---|---|---|---|---|---|
| Date | | | | | | | | | | | | | | | | | | Same as date | | | | | | | | | | | | | |
| Tampons/pads/day | 0 | 0 | 0 | 0 | 0 | 0 | 0 | 0 | 0 | 0 | 0 | 0 | 0 | 1 | 0 | 0 | 0 | 0 | 0 | 0 | 0 | 0 | 0 | 0 | 0 | 0 | 0 | 0 | 0 | 0 | |

Record 0 = none, 1 = minimal, 2 = moderate, 3 = moderately intense, 4 = very intense

| | 1 | 2 | 3 | 4 | 5 | 6 | 7 | 8 | 9 | 10 | 11 | 12 | 13 | 14 | 15 | 16 | 17 | 18 | 19 | 20 | 21 | 22 | 23 | 24 | 25 | 26 | 27 | 28 | 29 | 30 | 31 |
|---|---|---|---|---|---|---|---|---|---|---|---|---|---|---|---|---|---|---|---|---|---|---|---|---|---|---|---|---|---|---|---|
| Amount flow | 0 | 0 | 0 | 0 | 0 | 0 | 0 | 0 | 0 | 0 | 0 | 1 | 1 | 2 | 1 | 1 | 0 | 1 | 0 | 0 | 0 | 0 | 0 | 0 | 0 | 0 | 0 | 0 | 0 | 0 | |
| Cramps | 0 | 1 | 1 | 0 | 0 | 0 | 0 | 1 | 1 | 1 | 0 | 1 | 1 | 2 | 0 | 0 | 0 | 0 | 0 | 0 | 0 | 0 | 0 | 0 | 0 | 0 | 0 | 0 | 0 | 0 | |
| Breast Sore: Side | 0 | 0 | 0 | 0 | 0 | 0 | 0 | 1 | 2 | 2 | 2 | 1 | 2 | 1 | 1 | 1 | 1 | 0 | 1 | 1 | 0 | 0 | 0 | 0 | 0 | 0 | 0 | 0 | 0 | 0 | |
| Breast Sore: Front | 0 | 0 | 0 | 0 | 0 | 0 | 0 | 3 | 4 | 2 | 3 | 2 | 2 | 3 | 4 | 3 | 2 | 2 | 1 | 0 | 0 | 0 | 0 | 0 | 1 | 1 | 0 | 0 | | | |
| Fluid Retention | 1 | 0 | 0 | 1 | 0 | 0 | 0 | 1 | 1 | 2 | 1 | 2 | 2 | 2 | 2 | 1 | 1 | 0 | 0 | 0 | 0 | 0 | 0 | 1 | 0 | 0 | 1 | 0 | | | |
| Hot flushes - day | 0 | 0 | 0 | 0 | 0 | 0 | 0 | 0 | 0 | 0 | 0 | 0 | 0 | 0 | 0 | 0 | 0 | 0 | 1 | 0 | 0 | 0 | 0 | 0 | 0 | 0 | 0 | 0 | | | |
| # of flushes - day | 0 | 0 | 0 | 0 | 0 | 0 | 0 | 0 | 0 | 0 | 0 | 0 | 0 | 0 | 0 | 0 | 0 | 0 | 1 | 0 | 0 | 0 | 0 | 0 | 0 | 0 | 0 | 0 | | | |
| Hot flushes - night | 0 | 0 | 1 | 0 | 0 | 0 | 0 | 0 | 0 | 0 | 1 | 2 | 0 | 0 | 0 | 0 | 0 | 0 | 0 | 0 | 0 | 0 | 0 | 0 | 0 | 0 | 0 | 0 | | | |
| # of flushes - night | 0 | 0 | 0 | 1 | 0 | 0 | 0 | 0 | 0 | 0 | 1 | 1 | 0 | 0 | 0 | 0 | 0 | 0 | 0 | 0 | 0 | 0 | 0 | 0 | 0 | 0 | 0 | 0 | | | |
| Mucous Secretion | 0 | 0 | 0 | 0 | 0 | 0 | 0 | 0 | 0 | 2 | 1 | 2 | 3 | 3 | 4 | 2 | 1 | 1 | 1 | 1 | 0 | 0 | 0 | 0 | 0 | 0 | 0 | 0 | | | |
| Constipation | 1 | 0 | 0 | 2 | 0 | 1 | 1 | 0 | 0 | 0 | 1 | 0 | 0 | 1 | 1 | 2 | 0 | 0 | 2 | 2 | 0 | 0 | 0 | 0 | 0 | 0 | 0 | 0 | | | |
| Headache | 1 | 0 | 0 | 0 | 0 | 0 | 0 | 1 | 2 | 2 | 3 | 2 | 2 | 1 | 2 | 3 | 1 | 0 | 0 | 0 | 0 | 0 | 0 | 0 | 0 | 0 | 0 | 0 | | | |
| Sleep Problems | 0 | 1 | 0 | 0 | 0 | 1 | 0 | 0 | 0 | 0 | 1 | 1 | 0 | 0 | 0 | 0 | 0 | 0 | 0 | 0 | 0 | 0 | 0 | 0 | 0 | 0 | 0 | 0 | | | |
| Feeling Frustrated | 0 | 0 | 0 | 0 | 0 | 0 | 0 | 0 | 1 | 0 | 0 | 0 | 1 | 1 | 0 | 0 | 0 | 0 | 0 | 0 | 0 | 0 | 0 | 0 | 0 | 0 | 0 | 0 | | | |
| Feeling Depressed | 0 | 0 | 0 | 0 | 0 | 0 | 0 | 0 | 0 | 2 | 0 | 0 | 1 | 0 | 0 | 0 | 0 | 0 | 0 | 0 | 0 | 0 | 0 | 0 | 0 | 0 | 0 | 0 | | | |
| Feeling Anxious | 0 | 0 | 0 | 0 | 0 | 0 | 0 | 0 | 0 | 0 | 0 | 1 | 1 | 2 | 0 | 0 | 0 | 0 | 0 | 0 | 0 | 0 | 0 | 0 | 0 | 0 | 0 | 0 | | | |

Record M = much less, L = a little less, U = usual, Y = a little increased, Z = much increased

| | 1 | 2 | 3 | 4 | 5 | 6 | 7 | 8 | 9 | 10 | 11 | 12 | 13 | 14 | 15 | 16 | 17 | 18 | 19 | 20 | 21 | 22 | 23 | 24 | 25 | 26 | 27 | 28 | 29 | 30 | 31 |
|---|---|---|---|---|---|---|---|---|---|---|---|---|---|---|---|---|---|---|---|---|---|---|---|---|---|---|---|---|---|---|---|
| Appetite | L | U | L | L | U | U | U | U | U | L | U | U | U | L | L | U | U | U | L | U | U | U | L | L | U | U | U | U | U | U | |
| Breast Size | U | U | U | U | U | U | U | U | Y | Y | Y | Y | Y | Y | Y | U | U | U | U | U | U | U | U | U | U | U | U | U | | | |
| Interest In Sex | not much — no partner | | | | | | | | | | | | | | | | | | | | | | | | | | | | | | |
| Feeling Of Energy | U | U | U | U | Y | U | U | U | U | U | U | U | U | L | U | U | L | L | U | U | U | U | L | U | U | U | U | U | | | |
| Feeling Of Self-Worth | Y | U | U | Y | U | U | U | U | L | U | L | L | L | U | L | U | U | L | U | U | U | U | U | Y | Y | U | Y | Y | | | |
| Outside Stresses | Y | U | Y | Y | U | Z | U | U | U | Y | Y | Y | Y | Y | Y | Y | Y | U | U | Z | Z | U | Y | Z | U | U | Z | Y | Y | Y | |
| ~~Basal Temperature~~ Meditation | ✓ | ✓ | ✓ | ✓ | ✓ | ✓ | ✓ | ✓ | ✓ | ✓ | ✓ | ✓ | ✓ | ✓ | ✓ | ✓ | ✓ | ✓ | ✓ | ✓ | ✓ | ✓ | ✓ | ✓ | ✓ | ✓ | ✓ | ✓ | ✓ | ✓ | |
| Progesterone | 3 | 3 | 3 | 3 | 3 | 3 | 3 | 3 | 3 | 3 | 3 | 3 | 3 | 3 | 3 | 3 | 3 | 3 | 3 | 3 | 3 | 3 | 3 | 3 | 3 | 3 | 3 | 3 | 3 | 3 | |
| Comments (Temperature Taken Late, Feeling Sick, Poor Sleep, Etc.) | | | dinner with friends | | | | | | | | | | | | | | | | | | | | | | | | | | | | |

really mad when the hospital social worker kept calling about my mom. Finally I told my boss I'd work extra but I needed to get off at two to meet the social worker. To my surprise, the social worker turned out to be helpful and supportive. From all her phone messages I thought she'd be pushy. She said Mom had apparently forgotten to take her pills. That's why she got so manic. She wondered if I could stay with Mom for a while and see that she had her medicines and stuff. I told her about John and little Sonny staying with me. And that I had medical problems right now. She could see I was distressed. I don't know how she did it, but she made an appointment that very afternoon with a counselor at the hospital.

"Anyway, I now realize that part of the trouble is I am still, deep down, very angry at my mom. As I told the counselor, sometimes I just hate her. She had nothing to give me when I was little and now I have to mother her!"

"Those are very strong emotions," I say. "They bring out the scared little girl in you, don't they?"

"Yes, they do," she says. "And I'm feeling a bit guilty for my anger. But the social worker and the counselor both said it was natural to feel that way. The counselor has seen me several times since. Still, I'm stuck with the responsibility for Mom and getting her house fixed up and all that insurance stuff."

She pauses. "Then, a miracle happened. I guess it was when I was started doing my yoga-breathing again. I was meditating and I suddenly thought of my Aunt Tilly. I hardly know her. But Mom had mentioned a while ago, that Tilly is now retired and had been widowed. So I looked through Mom's address book and called. I asked Aunt Tilly whether she would come and be with Mom for a while."

Henrietta pauses and takes a long, deep breath before resuming. "Aunt Tilly seemed very happy at the chance. After she arrived, I went and stayed with her and Mom for a few days. It was amazing—like a little-girl party. I think my mom is like me—she didn't know how to ask for help. Aunt Tilly was the professional one. Mom felt like the black sheep—as though it were her fault that Dad left her. I'd forgotten how neat Aunt Tilly is. All the memories they share!

"Anyway, back to the medical stuff. I started the Prometrium right away and immediately began to sleep. I still occasionally wake somewhat sweaty, but I can go back to sleep more easily. You are right that my neck settled right down once I started getting good sleep. I was able to keep working. John, my son, pitched in at home and really made things easy for me there. And I've started jogging three times a week and walking the other days. I take my lunch to work and eat it as I walk." Henrietta pauses for breath.

"I'm anxious to know the results of my bone density and urine tests," she says.

"Well, let's see," I say. I open the envelope with the bone density results and turn the page so that Henrietta can also see. "In your lower back, you have a slightly low bone density with a T score of −1.4. In your hip, your bone density is lower with a T score of −2.0. Let me explain what those numbers mean by drawing a little picture. Average T scores are between +1 and −1."

### HENRIETTA'S BONE DENSITY RESULTS—T SCORES

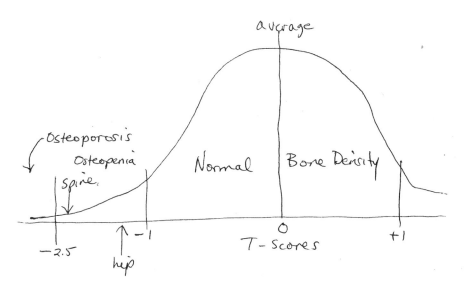

"Well that's good! At least I don't have osteoporosis according to the bone density. What about the urine?" Henrietta looks more relaxed now.

I take the pink lab slip out of her chart. "Not surprisingly, given all the stresses you've been under, this shows bone loss or high bone resorption. The normal deoxypyridinoline value is between 3 and 7.4—yours is 8.2. Remember that the goal level is 5 or below. If resorption is controlled, progesterone can cause you to gain bone density."

"I also ordered a test for cortisol in your urine. Although measuring cortisol in overnight urine isn't a standard test, we monitored it in about 20 normal women. Based on that, the upper limit of normal is about 25. That information is on the instruction sheet I gave you. As would be expected from your stresses, cortisol was high at 43 nmol/mmol of creatinine. That will also get better.

"How have you been doing with calcium and vitamin D?"

"I've been taking 1,000 mg of calcium from tablets with at least three or four high-calcium foods. And I did get just a cheap multivitamin and I am taking the 1,000 IU vitamin D that you recommended. Plus I eat eggs once or twice a week now."

"Unfortunately," I say, "eggs won't give you any calcium unless you eat the shell!" We both laugh and she looks a bit embarrassed. "But eggs are a very good source of protein," I finish.

"I don't think I've gained any weight yet," Henrietta says. "But why haven't the 2,000 mg of calcium and the 1,400 IU of vitamin D a day stopped my bone loss?"

"For a start," I answer, "you're still in perimenopause and in Phase D when probably *nothing* will prevent high bone resorption and loss of bone. We'll repeat that urine test in six months. If it is still elevated, we'll talk about a non-hormonal medication to stop you from losing bone."

"I don't like taking medicines that aren't natural, Dr. Madrona," Henrietta warns.

"I know," I say. "That's not a decision we need to make today. Just remember that I wouldn't suggest it to you if I didn't think it was better to try to prevent bone loss when you are young and can easily regain bone. It's hard work to fix up bone after you're menopausal or have another fracture."

"By the way," I add, "how are you feeling now about taking progesterone?"

"I still have a little caution. But it has been a lifesaver!" Henrietta exclaims. "And besides, it's a bio-identical hormone."

I nod as I finish completing the history on Henrietta's follow-up form, and look up to ask, "Tell me about your food in the last day."

"I thought you'd ask, so I ate especially well!" Henrietta laughs. "I had almond butter on a toasted whole-grain bagel with a glass of soymilk before I left for work. Then I had a decaf soy latte at the coffee shop near work when I was on my break. For lunch I had a big cheese-and-sprouts sandwich with butter on brown, and also an apple. This afternoon I had snack of granola as well as a honey-nut-seed-fruit bar. (John knows I need to gain weight, so he bought me a small case of them at one of those huge bulk food stores.) And yesterday's dinner was with Mom and Aunt Tilly. I had roasted chicken, baked potatoes, and a big salad. I even ate the chicken skin, put butter on my potato and poured lots of dressing on my salad. And I plan another soymilk warmed with cocoa in it before bed."

"Good for you!" I exclaim. "I'm getting hungry just listening. If you haven't gained any weight yet, I guess that's because you are doing a lot more exercise. Are you?"

"Yes, I'm walking every day for at least a half an hour except for the days that I do some 'wogging'!" She laughs. "I call it that because I walk fast and then jog a bit and then walk again. But I can already feel I'm getting stronger."

"Good for you," I say. "Now let's review everything you're taking."

"The progesterone, three at bedtime," says Henrietta. "Remifemin, the 250-mg calcium pill with each meal and at bedtime, a multivitamin and the 1,000 IU vitamin D are all the things I'm on now. By the way," she interrupts herself, "you were right about that magnesium. The diarrhea went away as soon as I stopped taking it with all of my calcium. I've also stopped the oil of evening primrose, black cohosh and dong quai, partly so I can afford the progesterone." She makes a wry face. "But I don't think they were helping. I'll soon stop the Remifemin also. Oh, I forgot, I still take 400 IU of vitamin E."

"You can stop that, too, now, Henrietta. Ok," I say, taking notes. "From your Diary it doesn't look as through you've had another period. If you do get one, you'll likely know it's coming because you'll get some breast tenderness and bloating. But progesterone results in a thinning of the endometrium. That means that you are less likely to get a period than if you weren't taking progesterone. And, I'm sorry, but it also means that you will need to go without a period for *two* years rather than one before you will know for sure that you are menopausal! Now, I'd like to examine you again, but more briefly this time. You can leave your slacks on."

~

After I finish the examination and Henrietta is dressed, she asks, "What did you say my weight was now?"

"You have increased a little to 54.8 kg—an increase of about 6 lb—even if we take a pound off for your slacks. Your blood pressure is great at 110 over 62 and your pulse is down to 74. I did find a few trigger points still."

I pause because Henrietta looks puzzled.

"Those are particular places where muscles join bone that get sore when deep sleep is interrupted," I explain. "When I first saw you, you had many positive trigger points. All of those are better now. And your hands are only cool and not icy cold."

Henrietta puts her fingers against her cheek and looks pleased. "So, am I seriously at risk of breaking bones like my mom? You better give me some information about that bone medicine you were talking about. I'll need to think about it before I see you next."

"Ok, good idea," I say. "Here's an information sheet on Cyclic Etidronate Therapy. This is the weakest and the first of the family of bone medications called bisphosphonates that prevent bone loss and decrease spine fractures. This one is the easiest of all to take and the safest. Even though estrogen is a natural therapy that slows bone loss, I won't prescribe it now because you are still making estrogen—and in big amounts, at least some of the time. Estrogen would be a possible option to take for about four years once you are truly menopausal.

"As for your Diary, things look so much better that I don't think you need to fax it anymore. Just bring it when you come next time."

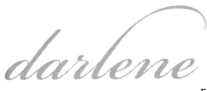

red river flooding

I call out Darlene's name as I walk into the waiting area in the Division of Endocrinology. She looks up at me. She already appears upset or angry to me.

She gets to her feet.

"Hi! Did you find something good to read?" I ask, trying to start on a light note as we walk together down the hall toward my small examination room-office.

Darlene scarcely nods. "I'm taking those pills of yours and still bleeding. It's like I'm spotting all the time now—without a break!"

"I'm glad I had a cancellation so soon after the seminar," I say, feeling myself getting defensive. "I remember that you had very heavy flow. You'd tried various kinds of Pills and the progestin-IUD. I did phone your doctor. I suggested he read the article, 'Managing Menorrhagia without Surgery,' that menorrhagia word means very heavy flow. That article is posted on the health care provider section of the CeMCOR website. I also recommended medroxy-progesterone—one 10-mg pill morning and evening continuously for three months. . . ."

"Well they're not working!" she interrupts.

"What's not working, Darlene? What are you *actually* taking?" I ask, trying not to sound exasperated.

"I'm on the Provera, the blue, 5-mg ones, for ten days a month, only I never know what's a period and what's just bleeding-all-the-time!"

"I wondered, when I talked with your doctor," I say, "about whether he would follow my suggestions. He didn't. He gave you the kind of progestin I suggested, but in *too low a dose and for too short a time* to be effective for heavy flow. It puzzles me why some doctors are worried about giving progestin yet prescribe estrogen without a second thought."

In the small exam-office, I motion Darlene to a seat beside the desk, then I sit in the desk chair and open her file.

"Birth control pills didn't help my flow," Darlene continues. "That experimental IUD caused wicked cramps. And now Provera has made it worse. I'm about ready to give up!"

"Are you taking ibuprofen during flow?" I ask.

"No, I don't like pills."

"In the seminar," I say, "I told you that ibuprofen decreases flow by about 25 percent (10). As a matter of fact, I'd suggest that you go to the Centre for Menstrual Cycle and Ovulation Research website (www.cemcor.ubc.ca) and look up 'Very Heavy Menstrual Bleeding.'" I watch Darlene shrug.

"Why do you think you're bleeding so hard, Darlene?"

"Just my luck, I guess."

"No ideas?" I ask. "Let's review the reasons for heavy flow in perimenopause—we talked about them in that group session. Too much estrogen and not enough progesterone cause heavy flow (22). Estrogen's normal job is to thicken the endometrium or uterine lining—progesterone's role is to make the endometrium both more mature and thinner. It is thick and juicy endometrium that bleeds too much and too long (22). Progesterone thins the endometrium and decreases flow. Too much estrogen with too little progesterone also causes an abnormal endometrial overgrowth that is a precursor to endometrial cancer."

"The Pill's got progestin in it—why didn't that thin my endometrium?" asks Darlene.

"The progestin in the Pill didn't help because it also has such a high dose of estrogen, Darlene," I reply. "The high estrogen level is likely why you had side-effects."

I pause a second to see if she is following my explanation. "I don't have enough experience with Mirena, the new progestin-containing IUD, to know why you got cramps from it. IUDs often increase cramps, but usually progestin treatment decreases cramps. I've read the published literature on this IUD and don't recall bad cramps as an important side-effect."

"But that progestin didn't slow my flow!" Darlene declares, again. "My doctor prescribed it on your recommendation."

"The low-dose cyclic Provera," I say slowly, consciously trying to be calm and positive, "was simply not strong enough to counterbalance effects of the high estrogen your body is making in perimenopause."

"What do you mean, 'counterbalance'?" This time Darlene seems to be asking a genuine question.

"I mean that the doses of the estrogen and progestin need to be similar for progestin to do its job and prevent estrogen from over-thickening the endometrium. That medroxyprogesterone blue pill is a low dose and not powerful enough to overcome the effects of your high estrogen levels. I recommended *daily* medroxyprogesterone in a dose four times higher than your doctor actually prescribed. Daily progesterone or progestin in a high enough dose can make the endometrium thin and inactive."

"I don't care why or what you do—just make this damned red river stop!" Darlene demands.

"Pretty soon we'll get to treatment for your heavy flow," I say. "But before that I need to review your medical history, do a general physical exam. . . . "

"You can't do a pelvic. I'm on my period!" Darlene interrupts.

"I wasn't planning on a pelvic exam," I answer, "because I assumed you'd had that and a Pap when you saw the gynecologist, or at your first visit with your GP, Darlene." I take a big breath and look seriously at Darlene. "When I've finished gathering data, we'll put everything together to understand any other reasons besides perimenopause that could be causing you such a tough time with bleeding. After that, we'll both be ready to discuss some choices about therapy."

"I've had a million physicals!" Darlene objects. "My GP did one before he sent me to the gynecologist. I had another for that IUD research study. . ."

"Darlene," I interrupt gently, "I wouldn't be a responsible physician if I didn't do a thorough history and physical examination before I prescribed for you. I know you are impatient and upset, but this is necessary if you want me to help you."

"Yeah, I know. Oh—here's my Diary." Darlene plunks two brown-stained sheets from her purse. "I only recorded flow. The rest of it was just too f-ing much. I'm so bagged when I get home from work."

"Great to have this, Darlene," I say. "It'll help us understand your bleeding and cramps." I study the second sheet. "Which days did you take the Provera?"

## DARLENE'S RECORD OF FLOW ON NO TREATMENT

Name: Darlene          Month: January – February   Year: 2004

| Cycle Day | 1 | 2 | 3 | 4 | 5 | 6 | 7 | 8 | 9 | 10 | 11 | 12 | 13 | 14 | 15 | 16 | 17 | 18 | 19 | 20 | 21 | 22 | 23 | 24 | 25 | 26 | 27 | 28 | 29 | 30 | 31 |
|---|---|---|---|---|---|---|---|---|---|---|---|---|---|---|---|---|---|---|---|---|---|---|---|---|---|---|---|---|---|---|---|
| Date | 9 | 10 | 11 | 12 | 13 | 14 | 15 | 16 | 17 | 18 | 19 | 20 | 21 | 22 | 23 | 24 | 25 | 26 | 27 | 28 | 29 | 30 | 31 | 1 | 2 | 3 | 4 | 5 | 6 | 7 | 8 |
| Tampons/pads/day | 8 | 7 | 6 | 9 | 7 | 5 | 8 | 9 | 5 | 7 | 4 | 3 | 3 | 4 | 3 | 2 | 2 | 1 | 0 | 0 | 2 | 4 | 1 | 1 | 0 | 0 | 0 | 0 | 0 | 0 | 0 |

Record 0 = none, 1 = minimal, 2 = moderate, 3 = moderately intense, 4 = very intense

| Amount flow | 4 | 4 | 3 | 4 | 2 | 3 | 3 | 2 | 2 | 2 | 2 | 2 | 2 | 2 | 1 | 1 | 1 | 6 | 0 | 1 | 2 | 1 | 1 | 0 | 0 | 0 | 0 | 0 | 0 | 0 | 0 |
|---|---|---|---|---|---|---|---|---|---|---|---|---|---|---|---|---|---|---|---|---|---|---|---|---|---|---|---|---|---|---|---|---|
| Cramps | 3 | 3 | 4 | 2 | 2 | 1 | 2 | 2 | 1 | 1 | 0 | 0 | 0 | 0 | 0 | 0 | 0 | 0 | 0 | 0 | 2 | 3 | 0 | 0 | 0 | 0 | 0 | 0 | 0 | 0 | 0 |

Darlene pulls the sheets around so they are facing her. "It looks like it was those ticks up at the top, there." She points. "I didn't get Provera until the second month."

## DARLENE'S FLOW ON LOW-DOSE CYCLIC MEDROXYPROGESTERONE

Name: Darlene          Month: February – March   Year: 2004

| Cycle Day | 1 | 2 | 3 | 4 | 5 | 6 | 7 | 8 | 9 | 10 | 11 | 12 | 13 | 14 | 15 | 16 | 17 | 18 | 19 | 20 | 21 | 22 | 23 | 24 | 25 | 26 | 27 | 28 | 29 | 30 | 31 |
|---|---|---|---|---|---|---|---|---|---|---|---|---|---|---|---|---|---|---|---|---|---|---|---|---|---|---|---|---|---|---|---|---|
| Date | 9 | 10 | 11 | 12 | 13 | 14 | 15 | 16 | 17 | 18 | 19 | 20 | 21 | 22 | 23 | 24 | 25 | 26 | 27 | 28 | 29 | 1 | 2 | 3 | 4 | 5 | 6 | 7 | 8 | 9 | 10 |
| Tampons/pads/day | 0 | 0 | 0 | 7 | 9 | 8 | 8 | 7 | 4 | 3 | 3 | 3 | 1 | 1 | 2 | 3 | 2 | 0 | 0 | 1 | 0 | 0 | 0 | 0 | 0 | 0 | 0 | 0 | 0 | 0 | |

Record 0 = none, 1 = minimal, 2 = moderate, 3 = moderately intense, 4 = very intense

| Amount flow | 0 | 1 | 1 | 3 | 4 | 3 | 4 | 3 | 2 | 2 | 2 | 2 | 1 | 1 | 2 | 2 | 1 | 1 | 1 | 2 | 1 | 1 | 0 | 1 | 1 | 1 | 1 | 1 | 1 | 1 | |
|---|---|---|---|---|---|---|---|---|---|---|---|---|---|---|---|---|---|---|---|---|---|---|---|---|---|---|---|---|---|---|---|---|
| Cramps | 2 | 2 | 2 | 3 | 3 | 2 | 2 | 1 | 0 | 0 | 0 | 1 | 0 | 0 | 3 | 2 | 2 | 1 | 0 | 0 | 0 | 0 | 0 | 0 | 0 | 0 | 0 | 0 | 0 | 0 | |

"You know, Darlene," I say. "It looks to me like your flow is improving. Yes, I see that you've still got a lot of spotting this second month. But comparing the first and the second cycles, it looks to me as though the number of soaked pads and tampons and the heaviness of flow are both better."

"Really?" Darlene asks. I point to the changes on her Diaries that she hadn't noticed.

"I have a letter from your family doctor," I continue, "who, I see, has recommended iron, and I also have a blood test result from January after you had been on the iron for a while."

"I'd taken them damned iron pills for a month before I had that blood test," Darlene says. "My doctor said my counts were fine, so I stopped."

"Yes, the tests are normal," I say. "But that only shows what is going on in your blood, not what is happening where iron is stored in the bone marrow. By the time your blood count gets low and you have anemia, the essential storage iron in your bone marrow is all used up. Because building back to a normal iron stores takes time, but the blood count becomes normal quickly, your bone marrow iron stores will still be low. It takes about a year of iron at a dose of one therapeutic-sized pill a day before the bone-marrow iron stores are back to normal."

"You mean I have to take iron *again*? It gave me black stools and constipation!" Darlene frowns.

"Sounds like you were on a full dose of three pills a day," I say. "One pill a day is all you need to take—that dose doesn't cause most women any problems.

"Now let's recap what I already know from your doctor's letter and the seminar. You are 43, had irregular periods most of your life, and have been on the Pill, right? How long now have you been having heavy bleeding?"

"I've soaked 25 or more tampons each period for more than a year. But I didn't think anything about it. Then it got really heavy with flooding, and I had a period that didn't stop for weeks—I remember, that was at Thanksgiving last fall. Since then, I've had everything you docs can offer and I'm still bleeding to death!"

"Your doctor initially treated the heavy flow with the birth control pill?" I ask. As Darlene nods, I go on. "What kind of Pill was it and how long did you take it?"

"I had the usual low-dose birth control pill," says Darlene. "I can't remember its name, then the doctor tried a stronger one in a maroon case, then he sent me to a gynecologist who put me in that research IUD study."

"Tell me what happened on birth control pills," I request.

"I continued to have heavy bleeding that would start before I had finished my pack of pills. And I started getting migraine headaches and really bad bloating. I took the Pill for three months, hoping everything would get better. I don't know which kind of pill it was, but my doctor said it was the lowest dose pill. I think it was called Ministron."

"Do you mean MinEstrin?" I ask.

"Yeah, that sounds right," Darlene says. "Reminded me of a kind of soup. Anyway, it isn't really the lowest dose Pill because I looked it up in the doctor's drug book that we have at work. Then my doctor thought that dose wasn't strong enough, so he gave me some samples. I can't remember what they were called."

"Did you ever have an endometrial biopsy?" I ask, concerned about her increased risks for endometrial cancer.

"God, yes. Hurt like heck! The gynecologist did that and also did a vaginal ultrasound that showed I have some fibroids. He said something about my heavy flow and the fibroids and suggested I have surgery to take them out."

"Did he mean a hysterectomy?" I ask. Darlene nods.

"How do you feel about having your uterus removed surgically?" I ask.

"I'd like to keep all my parts, thank you!" Darlene says emphatically. "But I've had it up to here"—she gestures to the top of her head—"with this flow."

"Do you know the results of that endometrial biopsy?" I ask.

"No. My family doctor just told me the biopsy was normal. That means the fibroids are causing my bleeding, right?"

"No, not right," I say. "That's a common misunderstanding. The high estrogen and low progesterone levels of perimenopause not only make the endometrium thick and cause heavy flow, they also make the fibroids grow. Fibroids are *associated* with heavy flow but rarely *cause* it. Fibroids are a benign growth of muscle cells inside the wall of the uterus. They are usually a long way away from the endometrium. Less than 10 percent of the time fibroids grow right under or into the uterine lining. These rare fibroids could cause abnormal bleeding."

"Would you please ask your family doctor, or the gynecologist you saw, to send me the consult letter and your biopsy results?" I ask. "I don't know why I don't have them."

"Isn't that what your secretary's for?" Darlene almost shouts. When I look up, startled, she slumps in her chair.

"If I ask for your report from your doctor," I say, feeling annoyed but trying to keep it from showing, "he will ask you for consent to release it. It's just easier if you ask, yourself."

"Oh, ok, I'll do it," she says, sounding resigned. "But I'm just fed up. I really don't think that you can help either. I'd just rather skip this menopause thing altogether!"

"I know *peri*menopause is frustrating, Darlene," I say. "But you and I need to work together or the bleeding will continue to be heavy, and whether you like it or not, you'll end up with a hysterectomy."

I review out loud. "You've already had the Mirena IUD with a high dose progestin imbedded in it. You said you used it for about a month before severe cramping made you to ask for its removal?"

"I was on it from October to November," Darlene replies. "That was just before the group meeting. Then I was on nothing for a month and things weren't any different—I just bled heavily for two weeks. Then I started the Provera for ten days every month."

"So during this first flow on your Diary, you hadn't been on anything during the month before?" I ask.

"Nothing. Then I started doing the Provera and spotting all the time. You can see from here that I'm still spotting," Darlene points to the Diary. "My vagina is getting too sore to wear tampons and the panty-liners give me candidiasis!"

"Yes," I say, "yeast grows well in a warm wet spot, especially when estrogen levels are high."

"I'm using some white cream the pharmacist said is for diaper rash!" Darlene blurts.

"Zinc oxide is an old-fashioned remedy that does keep yeast from growing," I say. I can't help grinning at the idea of a grown woman with a "diaper rash." To my surprise, Darlene smiles back.

"Ok, let's go back to the beginning," I say. "How old were you when your period first started?"

"I was just past my tenth birthday. I was the first of all the girls I knew to get it. After that my flow was pretty regular, especially after I started taking the Pill for bad acne and cramps. My periods started being irregular and farther apart after I got into nursing school. I didn't have regular periods again, unless I was on the Pill, until I hit 40. After my doctor made me stop the Pill, I was surprised that my periods were regular and heavier."

"How many years in total did you use the Pill?" I ask.

"I started in my teens, I guess around 15. I was off a couple of years during my marriage in my mid-twenties. My former wanted a kid," Darlene grimaces, then she continues.

"My flow was every six weeks or so in my twenties. I never got pregnant, and we divorced after three years. I started the Pill again and took it except for a month here or there when the doctor wouldn't renew it until I came in for my Pap. Then he wouldn't give me the Pill any more after I turned 40."

"So that makes about 25 years on the Pill," I say. "Have you ever been seriously ill, hospitalized, in an accident or broken any bones?"

"I fell out of a tree when I was a kid," she says, "but I don't think I broke anything and anyway there was no hospital where I lived in Ocean Falls. I just didn't wake up for a while. I was pretending to be a logger and top the tree like my dad, only I wasn't wearing spikes or a harness!" Darlene laughs.

"That must have been an interesting place to grow up!" I exclaim, recalling my own childhood in a remote place.

"Not really. It was raining and blew all winter, there was nothing to do, and I couldn't wait to leave."

I shrug and resume my history. "Are there any serious illnesses in your family—heart attacks, diabetes, tuberculosis, high blood pressure, osteoporosis?"

"My aunt, who is huge"—Darlene gestures widely with her hands—"has diabetes mellitus but is ok, I guess, when she takes pills. She's also getting a shiny scalp—soon she'll be as bald as my grandpa! My dad probably has emphysema and chronic bronchitis. He smokes a lot, wheezes, and coughs and spits all winter. My mom's fine, and not overweight."

"How much did you weigh when you were 18?" I ask.

"Let's see, that would have been around the age when I left home to go to nursing school. I guess I was about 170 pounds then."

"Who's at home with you?"

"I'm on my own, except for the odd fellow now and then who sleeps over. I've got no one regular."

"Are you taking any medicines, vitamins, herbs, supplements or other things besides the Provera?"

"Nope."

"What exercise do you regularly do?"

"I walk a lot at work. It is so busy, I run my full 12-hour shift. And I walk from my car to the ward. . . "

"I have no doubt you are busy at work. But for good health, everyone needs to walk at least half an hour a day. And it's better if once or twice a week you do something that makes you work up a sweat," I say. "That exercise will help with your weight."

"What do you do for fun?" I ask next. Darlene looks startled.

"Sometimes, if I'm bored I listen to the police/ambulance/fire radio. And I go dancing with the girls some weekends when I'm off."

"If you're dancing, you *do* get some exercise!" I exclaim.

"What do you do for fun, Doc?" Darlene asks me right back.

"I like to kayak, run, and play the recorder," I reply, deciding to be straightforward with her.

"Do you mean, a record player?" she asks with a quizzical grin.

"No, it's a wooden kind of flute they played in the Middle Ages, only you hold it up and down like a clarinet," I say. "Do you regularly check your breasts?"

"My doctor used to check them every year before he'd refill my Pill. And the research doctor did. That's plenty."

I take a deep breath and explain, "No one but *you* can tell if something has changed in your breasts, Darlene. They belong to you. That's why you need to check them yourself—so you'll know when something's different. I examine hundreds of breasts a year. I can't possibly remember what any given woman's breasts used to feel like!"

"I know I should," Darlene says. "But if I'm going to die of breast cancer, I'd just as soon not know."

"How many cigarettes do you smoke a day?" I ask.

"I'm only smoking about half a pack now." Darlene stares at me. "How did you know I smoke?"

"I can smell it," I reply, equally directly.

Darlene looks chagrined. I try not to smile, guessing that Darlene has been hanging her clothes outside, avoided her morning cigarette today, and also used a breath freshener.

"I smoked about 20 or 25 a day," Darlene continues, "from the time I was 18. All the girls in nursing school were smokers. I've never been able to quit. Once I tried, and I gained 20 pounds that I can't seem to lose."

"So you are 43 now," I say. "When did you decrease to ten cigarettes a day?"

"That must have been last winter when I had bronchitis. I tried to stop, but I couldn't. I ended up smoking fewer anyway."

"Good for you," I say, smiling. "One day, when the bleeding is over and you are regularly walking, you'll be successful at stopping. Let me know when you're ready to quit and I'll help."

I do some calculations on my form. "You have 43 minus 18 years of a pack a day which is 25 pack-years plus a couple of extras for those years when you smoked 25 cigarettes a day. That gives you a total of 27-plus pack-years of cigarettes. That clearly puts you at increased risk for lung cancer, Darlene."

She shrugs.

"Are you allergic to anything?" I ask.

"Nothing except bleeding! I'll be glad to be menopausal and done with all of this crap. Oh, I just remembered. My aunt had a hysterectomy when she was about my age. I'm fixing to be just like her!" Darlene shudders.

I raise my eyebrows, start to explain the interactions of lifestyle and heredity, but decide to skip it.

"How much caffeine do you drink a day?" I ask.

"About four cups of coffee at the start of a shift and then about two or three diet colas for the rest of the day."

"That's way too much caffeine to be healthy!" I say. "Believe it or not, caffeine could be part of the reason you have heavy flow. Caffeine amplifies high estrogen effects. I'd suggest gradually decreasing to one or two coffees and one diet cola a day. Do you think you could manage do that?" I ask. She shrugs. "It may well make a difference in your flow. How about alcohol?"

"I'll have a Scotch or two on the rocks when I get home from work," Darlene says, "and sometimes drink a bottle of wine with dinner. I drink more if I'm out with the girls or on a date, which doesn't happen often nowadays."

"On average how many drinks would you have in a week?" I ask.

"I'd guess three or four times seven or about 21–28," Darlene answers. "And I don't feel guilty, and I don't have a drink before breakfast. And I am not talking about quitting!" she states belligerently, reciting a common set of questions used by health care providers to identify those who have problems with alcohol.

I listen, and decide there's no use at this point mentioning that more than eight drinks a week is associated with an increased risk for breast cancer (61).

"Did you know that alcohol increases estrogen levels or estrogen's actions?" I ask. When she shakes her head I go on. "Has anyone in your family had a problem with alcohol?"

"My dad drinks a lot. But so do all loggers! Especially when they're out of work. Now he handles it fine. Better than when I was a kid."

"Did he ever hurt you?" I ask.

"No, he'd just come home drunk and would cuss and throw things," Darlene replies offhandedly.

"Ok, have I missed anything important from your history?" I ask. "If I have, just tell me as I'm doing the exam." I pull back the curtain and lay out a gown. "I'd like you to take off everything except your panties, put on that blue hospital gown, and lie down on this table. Relax so I can get a good blood pressure reading. While you're changing, with your permission, I'd like to make a copy of your diaries for your chart. Ok?" She nods. "I'll knock when I come back in," I add as I leave the room.

～

A while later, after I've examined Darlene, we are again sitting at the desk. "Ok, Darlene," I say, "let me recap what I've learned from your history and your exam. You started flow early and had bad enough acne that you needed treatment. You couldn't get pregnant and had cycles that were far apart. I think you have what many doctors call Polycystic Ovary Syndrome."

"PCOS! I know about that. No way! No one ever said that before," Darlene protests.

"I call PCOS, Anovulatory Androgen Excess or AAE for short. Not everyone with AAE gets troublesome facial hair, Darlene. You had enough trouble with acne to need the Pill as a young teen. When you were off the Pill, your periods were regular but far apart."

"I know, oligomenorrhea!" Darlene interjects.

"And you didn't get pregnant after trying for three years and using no protection," I say. "Your weight history also suggests you haven't ovulated regularly. That's the key problem in AAE. Your weight and height at age 18 together give a body mass index of 29 at that age. Any BMI over 24 at age 18 carries an increased risk for infertility related to ovulation disturbances (62)."

I lean back in my chair. "A further important family history is that your maternal aunt may also have AAE—it is definitely hereditary. AAE puts women at greater risk for hysterectomy, insulin resistance, obesity and type 2 diabetes mellitus. The higher insulin levels increase the hormones made in the ovary, make you more hungry, and eventually cause blood sugars to go high."

"Ok, but what does insulin resistance have to do with my heavy bleeding right now?" asks Darlene.

"Higher insulin levels seem to stimulate the ovarian follicle to make more estrogen. You see, despite oligomenorrhea, your estrogen levels have likely been too high all of your life. And with no ovulation, that means little or no progesterone. So your endometrium doesn't shed normally, has become too thick, and may have abnormal proliferation. In my experience, women with AAE who have not had regular ovulation or a pregnancy get into real difficulty with bleeding early in perimenopause." More to myself than to Darlene, I mutter, "Actually, I should look at all my charts of perimenopausal women with heavy flow and examine past and family histories."

I lean forward in my chair. "Darlene, I need to know that biopsy result because you are at increased risk for endometrial hyperplasia. That leads to endometrial cancer, but is reversible with high-dose progesterone or progestin therapy. Endometrial cancer is caused by too much estrogen and not enough progesterone."

"You gotta die of something, Doc!" declares Darlene.

"On your exam just now you weighed 97 kg, which means your current BMI is 36, given your height of 165 cm (five feet, four inches). That's officially Class II Obesity, Darlene. That, along with your smoking puts you at high risk for an early heart attack." I pause and notice Darlene's shrug.

"Your forehead is high at the temples on either side. Alopecia or head-hair loss is something else besides acne that male hormones cause. They have likely caused the problems your aunt has."

"Now you're telling me I'm going to go bald!" Darlene frowns.

"Don't panic," I say. "There are medicines that block the action of male hormones at the hair root. It turns out that one of the best is a medicine called spironolactone, a drug developed to treat high blood pressure, but that turned out to be an androgen receptor blocker (63;64). And it may well be needed for your blood pressure—it was initially 154 over 98 with a large cuff even though you had been lying down about five minutes. The second blood pressure reading was 142 over 92. That value, as you know, is still borderline high.

"Also on your examination, I noticed that your breasts are nodular and have a thickening, like a ridge, along the bottom part of both breasts. That's something else that I've come to associate with insulin resistance. You also have skin tags that are often the first skin sign of insulin resistance. You have them under your breasts and along your neck. Finally, your waist circumference of 109 cm is way more than the highest normal of 88 cm. That increased waist is diagnostic of insulin resistance."

"Oh, god! I am going to get diabetes like Aunt Betty," Darlene moans.

"Not if you make some changes in your life, Darlene. From two well-designed studies, we know that people at high risk for diabetes who began an exercise programme decreased their risks for developing diabetes by more than half (65;66).

"I think we need to order a fasting glucose or first morning blood sugar before breakfast—since you work nights and sleep in the daytime, you will need to have that test when you first wake up in the afternoon. I ordered fasting lipids because of your risks for heart disease. And a ferritin level that is a good measure of bone marrow iron stores. I've put your name as well as your doctor's on the lab slip so you will get copies of these results. I expect that the ferritin levels will be low. I hope seeing that result will convince you that you need to take one iron pill every day for a year." I finish writing out the laboratory order form and hand it to Darlene.

"Let's talk about how you are going to start your exercise," I say firmly.

"I'm not doing a darn thing until this bleeding is gone," Darlene says.

"Fair enough," I agree. "For the flow, although that 5-mg dose of Provera for ten days a month has helped, it's obviously not strong enough. You need an increased dose and a longer duration of progestin or the bio-identical oral micronized progesterone called Prometrium. I want you to take either medicine *daily* for three months. I'll prescribe either the full 10-mg medroxyprogesterone dose in the morning every day for the next three months or 300 mg of Prometrium at bedtime daily. I'm worried about endometrial cancer, that's why I've prescribed daily therapy with full-dose progesterone. You can start it today!"

Darlene nods.

"In order to interpret flow on your Diary, I need to know how much progestin or progesterone you are taking. So I've put 'Provera 10' on one line and 'Prometrium 300' on another line at the bottom of your Diary where basal temperature usually goes. Please put a check each day on the appropriate line to indicate whichever you take. You're a good nurse—this is just like charting! You can use up your 5-mg medroxyprogesterone pills by taking two-a-day—that's equivalent to the 10 mg I prescribed. On either progesterone or progestin medicine, because your own estrogen production is high, you will probably still get a regular period. But flow should not be either heavy or long."

"Well! I'll fax you my diaries if this spotting doesn't stop soon," Darlene declares.

"That's a good idea," I say. "My secretary will give you our fax number. Let me know if you have any more episodes of flooding. If you do, you will need to *double* the dose of medroxyprogesterone to one 10-mg pill in the morning and one in the evening. I'd like to see you again in three months."

"How come I get to see you in three months when your secretary says your waiting list is nine?" Darlene asks.

"Only new patients have to wait that long," I explain. Then add, "just so you know, after I first see all the women in your seminar, I'm not taking new patients anymore. I'm going to study the history of medicine. I'd like to see you sooner than usual because we'll need to make a decision then about whether you can start cyclic progesterone therapy on days 14–27 of your cycle.

Taking a big breath, I continue. "So, let's review the plan. You're going to take one ibuprofen pill every 4–6 hours while you have heavy flow. You will restart iron and take one pill a day for one year. You'll get that blood test about the risk for diabetes. And you will start taking full luteal-phase-equivalent medroxyprogesterone or Prometrium daily and take it for three months. Finally, before I see you again in three months, please look up 'Cyclic Progesterone Therapy' on the CeMCOR website."

I notice that Darlene has finally started jotting down a few things. "When I see you again, we'll also review things like your fasting blood sugar, waist circumference, exercise, weight and blood pressure," I say.

"Ok, so what will you do if the bleeding doesn't stop?" Darlene asks.

"We can certainly increase the progesterone dose. . . " I start to say, but Darlene interrupts.

"But Provera has side-effects of depression and hirsutism and bloating. . ." Darlene again looks angry. "I found that in the doctor's drug book!"

"Look, Darlene," I say. "Those side-effects appear in the Canadian and USA drug books only because they occur with extremely high doses of medroxyprogesterone, or with androgenic progestins or when a progestin is used with estrogen. They are listed there only for medical-legal reasons—they don't occur in normal dose, placebo-controlled trials of medroxyprogesterone alone" (67).

Darlene doesn't relax into her chair.

"Although I wrote both prescriptions," I add, "medroxyprogesterone is stronger against flow. But once flow is better, I'd prefer that you used Prometrium because it is natural and in fact decreases the effects of male hormones in the skin."

"How the heck can it do that?"

"Progesterone blocks a little chemical trigger called 5-alpha reductase enzyme (68) that testosterone needs to become dihydrotestosterone, the hormone that causes head hair loss and hair on the chin. Right now, while you are finishing up the Provera pills you have, I'd prefer that you take three of the Provera pills a day that your doctor prescribed. That will give you 15 mg a day until you finish the 5-mg pills. Then you can switch over to Prometrium. Oral micronized progesterone will also help you sleep during the daytime when you are working the night shift. The dose of progesterone I'm prescribing for you is about a tenth of the level it reaches during pregnancy."

"But you do think my bleeding will stop?" Darlene actually sounds, this time, as though she is asking for reassurance.

"Yes, I'm sure it will," I say with confidence. "Remember to use ibuprofen at least every six hours during heavy flow. I've also got more tricks up my sleeve if this treatment isn't strong enough. As long as you don't want a hysterectomy and we are working together, I know your flow will get better." I pause for a moment to let this register.

"But I can't make perimenopause go away, Darlene. Nor can I magically fix your risks for lung cancer, heart attacks and diabetes. You have to deal with those yourself."

"Well, Doc, I've had nothing but a run-around with this and no one seems to know anything."

"You're right, Darlene," I say. "We don't know a lot about medical therapy to control heavy flow in perimenopause. If you complete more of the lines on your Diary, it will help both of us to better understand how your estrogen levels are misbehaving. See you in three months."

In three and a half months I see Darlene again. "Hello, Darlene, how are you?"

Darlene grimaces. "I'd be better if I weren't having to work so many extra shifts and overtime. It's been a beautiful spring and I've not had a chance to enjoy it."

"How's your flow?" I ask.

"It's been perfectly regular for about five days every month, and only one day is sort of heavy."

"That's great! Here, let me see your Diary."

Darlene pulls four folded, dirty sheets from the back pocket of her green nurses' scrubs and hands them to me.

I scan the pages of her Diary. "It's amazing the power of high estrogen in perimenopause," I say. "If I gave that much progesterone to a premenopausal woman she wouldn't even have a spot of flow. Your flow is definitely better. But, Darlene, look. It's still too heavy—you used 5 plus 4, 9 plus 4. . . You're still soaking more than 16 tampons. Thanks for recording the 300 mg of Prometrium you are taking every day. It's been four months. I was hoping we could switch to *cyclic* progesterone now."

"I'm happy the way it is," Darlene says. "Don't bugger it up now, Doc. I get flow regularly and I can count on it not being a flood."

"It would be helpful for me if you put zeros in each box when you didn't experience something, Darlene," I say. "I can't tell whether you had sore front of your breasts except on June 23 through 25. What do those sore breasts before your flow mean?"

## DARLENE'S FLOW ON DAILY PROGESTERONE THERAPY

Name: Darlene    Month: June–July    Year: 2004    July

| Cycle Day | 1 | 2 | 3 | 4 | 5 | 6 | 7 | 8 | 9 | 10 | 11 | 12 | 13 | 14 | 15 | 16 | 17 | 18 | 19 | 20 | 21 | 22 | 23 | 24 | 25 | 26 | 27 | 28 | 29 | 30 | 31 |
|---|---|---|---|---|---|---|---|---|---|---|---|---|---|---|---|---|---|---|---|---|---|---|---|---|---|---|---|---|---|---|---|
| Date | 7 | 8 | 9 | 10 | 11 | 12 | 13 | 14 | 15 | 16 | 17 | 18 | 19 | 20 | 21 | 22 | 23 | 24 | 25 | 26 | 27 | 28 | 29 | 30 | 1 | 2 | 3 | 4 | 5 | 6 | 7 |
| Tampons/pads/day | 5 | 4 | 9 | 4 | 2 | 1 | 0 | 0 | 0 | 0 | 0 | 0 | 0 | 0 | 0 | 0 | 0 | 0 | 0 | 0 | 0 | 0 | 0 | 0 | 0 | 6 | 7 | 8 | 3 | 2 | 2 |

Record 0 = none, 1 = minimal, 2 = moderate, 3 = moderately intense, 4 = very intense

| | 1 | 2 | 3 | 4 | 5 | 6 | 7 | 8 | 9 | 10 | 11 | 12 | 13 | 14 | 15 | 16 | 17 | 18 | 19 | 20 | 21 | 22 | 23 | 24 | 25 | 26 | 27 | 28 | 29 | 30 | 31 |
|---|---|---|---|---|---|---|---|---|---|---|---|---|---|---|---|---|---|---|---|---|---|---|---|---|---|---|---|---|---|---|---|
| Amount flow | 2 | 2 | 3 | 2 | 2 | 1 | 0 | | | | | | | | | | | | | | | | | | | 2 | 2 | 3 | | | |
| Cramps | 0 | 0 | 2 | 1 | 1 | | | | | | | | | | | | | | | | | | | | | 2 | | | | | |
| Breast Sore: Side | | | | | | | | | | | | | | | | | | | | | | | | | | 1 | | | | | |
| Breast Sore: Front | | | | | | | | | | | | | | | | | | | | | | | 2 | 3 | 3 | | | | | | |
| Fluid Retention | | | | | | | | | | | | | | | | | | | | | | | | | | | | | | | |
| Hot flushes - day | | | | | | | | | | | | | | | | | | | | | | | | | | | | | | | |
| # of flushes - day | | | | | | | | | | | | | | | | | | | | | | | | | | | | | | | |
| Hot flushes - night | | | | | | | | | | | | | | | | | | | | | | | | | | | | | | | |
| # of flushes - night | | | | | | | | | | | | | | | | | | | | | | | | | | | | | | | |
| Mucous Secretion | | | | | | | | | | | | | | | | | | | | | | | | | | | | | | | |
| Constipation | | | | | | | | | | | | | | | | | | | | | | | | | | | | | | | |
| Headache | | | | | | | | | | | | | | | | | | | | | | | | | | | | | | | |
| Sleep Problems | | | | | | | | | | | | | | | | | | | | | | | | | | | | | | | |
| Feeling Frustrated | | | | | | | | | | | | | | | | | | | | | | | | | | | | | | | |
| Feeling Depressed | | | | | | | | | | | | | | | | | | | | | | | | | | | | | | | |
| Feeling Anxious | | | | | | | | | | | | | | | | | | | | | | | | | | | | | | | |

Record M = much less, L = a little less, U = usual, Y = a little increased, Z = much increased

| | 1 | 2 | 3 | 4 | 5 | 6 | 7 | 8 | 9 | 10 | 11 | 12 | 13 | 14 | 15 | 16 | 17 | 18 | 19 | 20 | 21 | 22 | 23 | 24 | 25 | 26 | 27 | 28 | 29 | 30 | 31 |
|---|---|---|---|---|---|---|---|---|---|---|---|---|---|---|---|---|---|---|---|---|---|---|---|---|---|---|---|---|---|---|---|
| Appetite | | | | | | | | | | | | | | | | | | | | | | | | | | | | | | | |
| Breast Size | | | | | | | | | | | | | | | | | | | | | | | | | | | | | | | |
| Interest In Sex | | | | | | | | | | | | | | | | | | | | | | | | | | | | | | | |
| Feeling Of Energy | | | | | | | | | | | | | | | | | | | | | | | | | | | | | | | |
| Feeling Of Self-Worth | | | | | | | | | | | | | | | | | | | | | | | | | | | | | | | |
| Outside Stresses | | | | | | | | | | | | | | | | | | | | | | | | | | | | | | | |
| Treatment or Supplement Prometrium 300 / Provera 10 | ✓ | | ✓ | ✓ | ✓ | | ✓ | ✓ | ✓ | ✓ | | ✓ | ✓ | ✓ | ✓ | ✓ | ✓ | | ✓ | ✓ | ✓ | ✓ | | ✓ | ✓ | ✓ | ✓ | | ✓ | ✓ | ✓ |
| Basal Temperature | | | | | | | | | | | | | | | | | | | | | | | | | | | | | | | |
| Comments (Temperature Taken Late, Feeling Sick, Poor Sleep, Etc.) | | | | | | | | | | | | | | | | | | | | | | | | | | | | | | | |

"I guess they mean they were sore!" snorts Darlene, shrugging.

"They tell me that your estrogen levels were very high. That usual luteal phase dose of progesterone is enough to prevent all but super high estrogen levels from causing breast soreness.

"Well," I say, when she doesn't respond, "I got your endometrial biopsy results. They showed endometrial hyperplasia with proliferation and no evidence of atypia. If you have to get an abnormal endometrial biopsy result, that's the best result you could have. You understand, don't you, that your uterine lining is at the step before endometrial cancer?"

"Yeah, but it's *not*, is it?" Darlene says. She folds her arms.

"Now that your flow is under better control," I continue, " I'm glad you're taking Prometrium rather than Provera, because I know for sure that higher doses of the natural, bio-identical progesterone don't act like male hormones. I doubt also that Provera does, but I'm less sure of that. Prometrium isn't as strong against flow as Provera. See, your cycles are still too heavy and are short—that one in June-July was only 25 days long. So we need to increase the dose of Prometrium to at least 400 mg a day. What medicines are you taking now, Darlene?"

"Just the 300 mg of Prometrium every day. That's all," she replies.

"So you haven't been using ibuprofen during days of heavier flow?" I ask. Darlene shakes her head.

I look right at Darlene as I speak. "Ibuprofen decreases flow by 25 percent (14). I'd suggest you take ibuprofen." I pause, checking the Diary for the cycle days of heaviest flow. "Take two or three ibuprofen pills on cycle days 2 and 3. Would you please do that?"

"Ok, if I remember," she says.

"Please also start a new sheet when you start bleeding again. Did you restart taking iron as we had discussed?" I ask.

"No, I guess I didn't," she replies. "And, damn! I forgot to get those blood tests, too. I just remembered."

"That was one of our reasons for meeting now, Darlene, to go over those results. Have you eaten or had a coffee or a cola today?" As she shakes her head 'no,' I continue, "Why don't you go right now and get that blood drawn, so you don't forget again? What exercise are you now doing?"

"Same as usual, except I haven't been dancing for about six months. When my cousin came from Duncan for a few days we did walk around Lost Lagoon."

"Good," I say. "How many cigarettes now?"

"The same—10 or 12 a day. And I haven't checked my breasts—I knew you would ask, so I almost did it before bed this morning!" Darlene laughs.

I smile ruefully. "How are you doing with coffee and colas?" I ask.

"I still have three or four coffees when I wake up, but I've decreased to one cola and it's usually diet."

"That's progress," I say. "How about alcohol?"

"I'm most of the time having Scotch with soda now and just one. Plus, if I open a bottle of wine I usually drink it over several nights." She pauses a second. "You know, before you asked about it, I never thought about my dad's alcohol problem possibly being related to me."

"I'm glad you've decreased your alcohol, Darlene. More than eight servings a week is associated with an increased risk for breast cancer (61). I'll do your examination now. Just a short one this time. Please just take off your scrubs on top and your shoes and lie down there." I pull the curtain aside and lay out a gown. "Try to relax so I can get a good blood pressure. I'll go out and copy your Diaries for your chart."

~

Later after we've both sat down again, I begin, "Ok, Darlene, let's review things. Your blood pressure is still high at 162 over 94. But you are just going to work, right? Nevertheless, that's not a good blood pressure.

"And, I'm more impressed than when I first saw you with your signs of androgen excess. You have some thickened red skin on your neck and chest, and a little palpable facial hair. There is definite and probably worsening hair loss at your temples. Your weight is up two kilograms at 99 kg and your waist is slightly bigger at 110 cm. The good news is your breasts are much softer although they are still full and continue to have inferior ridges.

"I think, given your history of anovulatory androgen excess and heavy weight, that you need higher than normal doses of progesterone. One study showed that high-dose progestin days 5–26 of the month was equivalent to the Mirena IUD in control of heavy flow (69). I think the best thing for you would be to take 300 mg of Prometrium every bedtime plus 10 mg of Provera days 12-27 of the month. Or I could prescribe 400 or 500 mg of Prometrium days 5–26 of the month. What's your preference, Darlene?"

"I guess I'd like to take only one kind of pill," she says. "I remember to take

Prometrium because it helps me sleep. Can't I take it every day? Why would you say to take Provera days 12–27 of the cycle rather than days 14–27 like your 'Cyclic Progesterone Therapy' handout suggests?"

"I'm glad you read that handout," I say. "But your situation is different—you have heavy flow. The days 5–26 of the month is a schedule that was effective for heavy flow (69;70). But I would be happy if you took 500 mg of Prometrium every day before bed."

"Good," she says. "As they say, 'Keep it simple, stupid!'"

"Ok, I'm happy to prescribe 500 mg daily at bedtime. Also, given your high blood pressure, I'd like you to start spironolactone at 100 mg a day. It will serve the dual purposes of helping to lower your blood pressure and also treating your androgen excess."

"How do you know that I have androgen excess?" demands Darlene, frowning. "You didn't even do a blood test!"

"As I mentioned earlier, you have several things in your skin that show me the actions of male hormones," I say. "I think that these signs are more accurate than any blood test, Darlene, because they show the effect of the hormones over a long period of time. A blood test only captures a single point in time."

"I think you're making a big deal of nothing," Darlene says. "I believe you, but I don't trust you."

"What do you mean by that?" I ask, feeling both puzzled and kind of hurt.

"That's just the way I feel, Doc!" Darlene says, offhandedly.

"Would you like me to explain or to just drop it?" I ask. Getting no indication from Darlene, I continue. "The signs of androgen excess are first, thinning of hair at your temples. And second—here, feel your neck. Do you feel that bumpy skin, a bit like a plucked chicken? That's another one of the actions of male hormones. You've heard of 'red necks,' haven't you?"

"Oh, god. Don't let me get like my dad!" Darlene looks horrified. "But I don't want to take any more pills, Dr. Madrona. You want me to take four or five of those round guys at bedtime and now to start another one!"

"I hear that you don't want to take pills," I say. "But I am worried about not treating things that will get you into trouble later. What you decide to take is, of course, your choice. I'll write you the prescriptions and explain the reasons to your family doctor. I think you need some treatment for high blood pressure, given your family history, heavy weight, and your other risks for heart attack. I've prescribed spironolactone rather than the usual diuretic or beta-blocker blood pressure pill because it's very effective for high blood pressure and will also help with androgen excess. You can talk it over with your doctor and decide whether you want to take it."

"Yeah, ok," says Darlene, shrugging.

"Any questions?" I ask. "No? We're about finished for today. I'd like you to keep recording your flow on the Diary. Fax it to me if you have problems. If you can make the time to record other things like breast tenderness and mucus, you'll start seeing when your own estrogen levels are high." As we enter the secretarial area, I ask Lana to book Darlene an appointment in three months.

"Bye, Darlene," I say.

"See ya, Doc," she says, abruptly turning away from me toward Lana.

Three months later, I'm waiting for Darlene whose appointment is next. "I confirmed Darlene's appointment with her about a week ago, but she hasn't shown up yet," Lana tells me as she comes back from looking in the waiting room. "I'll let you know when she comes."

A while later, Lana speaks to me from the doorway of my office. "Dr. Madrona, because it's getting so late, I called Darlene's physician. He said she is off on disability with a bad back." She pauses, and then she asks, "Shall I make her another appointment?"

"Let me look at her chart a second," I reply.

After leafing through her file, I say, "I'm concerned about her heavy bleeding, and her risks for diabetes. And she is very distrustful of doctors, so I suspect she's not taking the high-dose progesterone I prescribed. Let's make her an appointment for six months if she calls." I flip through more pages. "Oh—I see that she phoned to say she'd lost her prescription, and we called a new one in to her pharmacy. It's amazing that the most demanding people can't do the simplest things for themselves!"

I hand Lana the chart. "I feel helpless with people like Darlene," I mutter to myself. "I'm afraid that she'll end up having a hysterectomy," I say more clearly. "Then she'll go on estrogen treatment and have an even worse time. Eventually, given her obesity, androgen excess, heavy smoking and risks for diabetes, she's likely to get an early heart attack. And all of those problems are preventable. But she has to take some responsibility for her own health."

"We've got all different kinds of patients, Dr. Madrona," says Lana. "Don't let her get you down. She's a grown-up."

# 7

*jennifer*  seasick on dry land

"Jennifer?" I call as I enter the endocrinology waiting area.

Jennifer looks up from the book she is reading and smiles at me as she gets up.

"I'm sorry you've had to wait," I say. "An earlier patient today was upset and I hadn't seen her for ten years—both caused her to take more than her allotted time. I've been behind all morning," I add ruefully.

"No problem, I know what it's like to work with troubled people," Jennifer replies. "I came prepared—I brought a good book."

We settle into my small examination room-office. Smiling in welcome, I ask, "I know we talked about it in the group session, but tell me again what I can help you with."

"My big problem is nausea," she says. "And sometimes I actually vomit. It's worse in the morning and some times are worse than others, but basically it's there all the time. Did my doctor send you results for all those tests? They've all turned out to be normal," she grimaces.

I nod, looking through her lab results. "Your gallbladder ultrasound was normal," I say, "and liver tests are also ok, but he didn't order alkaline phosphatase. Hepatitis tests are all negative, and the only abnormality is a slightly elevated creatinine level." I push back the papers and look at Jennifer.

"How long has this nausea been going on?" I ask.

"I can't exactly remember, but I know that at Christmas a year ago I was brushing my tongue when I gagged and vomited. So that's more than 15 months ago. It's gradually gotten worse since then."

"Does the nausea change with anything besides time of day?" I ask.

"Sometimes it's triggered by smells, and it's usually worse either a week before my flow or sometimes also during my period."

"At those times in your cycle do you notice anything else?" I ask.

Jennifer pulls out a sheaf of dog-eared pages on a magenta-coloured clipboard. "Since I've been charting, I've noticed I get sore breasts, swollen breasts, often bloating, and sometimes a bad headache." She turns the Diary so that I can see. "I made a new line under the basal temperature. I call this Nausea and I've scored it 0-4, with a '4' meaning so bad I am vomiting."

"That's excellent!" I exclaim.

### JENNIFER'S APRIL DIARY SHOWING NAUSEA

Record M = much less, L = a little less, U = usual, Y = a little increased, Z = much increased

| | | | | | | | | | | | | | | | | | | | | | | | |
|---|---|---|---|---|---|---|---|---|---|---|---|---|---|---|---|---|---|---|---|---|---|---|---|
| Appetite | U | Y | U | U | U | Y | Y | U | U | Y | U | Y | Z | Y | U | U | U | Y | U | U | U | |
| Breast Size | U | Y | Y | Y | U | Y | U | U | U | Y | U | U | Y | U | U | U | U | Y | Y | Z | Z | Y |
| Interest In Sex | L | H | L | L | L | M | L | L | L | L | M | L | L | L | U | L | L | L | C | L | U | L |
| Feeling Of Energy | L | L | U | M | L | L | L | U | L | M | L | M | M | L | U | L | L | M | L | L | U | |
| Feeling Of Self-Worth | Y | U | U | U | Y | U | U | Y | U | Y | U | U | U | U | U | U | Y | U | U | U | U | |
| Outside Stresses | Y | Y | Z | U | U | U | L | L | Y | Y | Y | Z | Y | U | L | Y | Y | Z | Z | U | U | |
| Basal Temperature | | | | | | | | | | | | | | | | | | | | | | | |
| Nausea 0-4 | 4 | 3 | 3 | 2 | 2 | 2 | 2 | 1 | 3 | 4 | 3 | 4 | 4 | 2 | 2 | 3 | 3 | 4 | 3 | 2 | 2 | |
| Comments (Temperature Taken Late, Feeling Sick, Poor Sleep, Etc.) | | | | | | | | | | | | | | | | | | | | | | | |

I look closely at the page, "I notice that this cycle is 21 days long. Thankfully flow isn't heavy. Is this cycle different in length than your usual?"

She fans out the four pages in front of us. "I used to be a regular 30-day person. I think they've been shortening over the last four or five years."

"Have you ever skipped a period?" I ask.

"No, but a couple of times,"—Jennifer takes her clipboard and looks back in her calendar at the winter months—"I've had cycles that were only two weeks apart. As I recall, those were the very worst months for nausea."

"That is more confirmation of my hunch that it is the high estrogen levels that are causing you to feel sick to your stomach," I say. "Short cycles mean that estrogen levels are so high that the thickened endometrium just has to start shedding early. I've seen this before in a couple of women. All of them, like you, were young at the start of perimenopause.

"A few more questions about the nausea before I go on to gather the rest of your history. Does the nausea change when you change position?" At Jennifer's "No," I continue. "Have you noticed any change in your vision during the worst nausea attacks?" Jennifer shakes her head.

"Those answers," I say, "indicate that the nausea isn't from your inner ear or a kind of migraine."

"You're a detective, Dr. Madrona! A medical detective—am I ever glad I got to see you!"

"And I'm glad that we can work together to find a solution," I say. "Let's see, you're 38, aren't you? And you do something—is it social work—with handicapped children?"

"No, I'm a teacher and counselor for differently abled kids in the schools," she corrects.

I nod. "Have you ever been ill, or hospitalized, or injured?"

"No, I've never darkened the doors of a hospital, except briefly when my two kids were born and"—she pauses a second—"when I was born!"

I grin at her humour. "How old were you when you had your first period?"

"I was just 12," she says, her voice trailing off.

"Do you remember what your cycles were like back then?" I ask.

"I don't rightly know, but I think they were regular. I know that I skipped a few after high school. That was when I went away to university. It was a shock going from a little mill-town like Quesnel to the big city, Vancouver! I got a scholarship. Then, after my first year of university I got married, much to my parents' chagrin, and had two babies in a row. I did what they wanted anyway—I kept up my schooling. My former wasn't good for much, but he did take shifts with the two babies so that we both could continue our studies. I got my first degree in psychology, my second in teaching, and my third in counseling—all while my boys were toddlers, grade-schoolers, and then high-school students!"

She laughs at the look of astonishment and respect on my face. "When you have a strong and positive goal, almost anything is possible."

She pauses, suddenly sober. "However, my goal to help needy kids was not something my husband shared. We grew apart and eventually divorced. He got a good job as an engineer back at one of the mills in Quesnel and wanted me to return with him and quit my schooling. Instead, the boys and I managed to stick it out here in the city, and the oldest is in university now. The second has just gone up to live which his dad to finish high school.

"Thankfully, their dad is helping our eldest with university. Plus he got scholarships. He comes over now and then to do a load of wash, or bring a new girl friend for supper, but I feel like both my sons are pretty grown and gone. That's a relief. With the neediness of the kids at work, I couldn't manage to give my heart out at home too."

"What do you do for fun?" I pause. "Or, to ask what I really want to know—who takes care of Jennifer?"

"Nobody special," she replies. "But I've got an old fixer-upper house in East Vancouver and quite a community of people around me. I've known most of them since we traded childcare and demonstrated together about local parks. Now we often help each other with home renovations and make a party out of it. At least every weekend I'm doing something with one or several of them. I'm really lucky to be so well loved and supported."

"How are things financially? Are you at risk of losing your job?" I ask.

"I'm ok for now. My house, such as it is, is paid for. But, like most people in the school system, I'm always at risk of lay-off. If I didn't have the extra skills for disabilities and special learning needs, I'd have been let go long ago like most other school counselors. Instead, my client-load just gets bigger and bigger.

"I've been training a few Grade 12 students with exceptional maturity to run support groups for the children I'm supposed to counsel. That does two things at once. It helps me with my load, and it gives these able youngsters a chance to give. But it takes just about every ounce of my energy. Some days when the nausea is wretched, I wonder how long I can keep up this heavy schedule."

"How's your sleep?" I ask.

"Oh, it's bad! I get to sleep before I've even opened my book. I wake a few hours later to pee and then count sheep and still have trouble getting to sleep again. Just when I am into a deep sleep, the alarm goes! I'm ready to vomit, and wonder what hit me!"

"I see constipation is also a problem," I say, "and it seems to worsen at the same time as the nausea."

"I hadn't thought of that, but I see that you're right," she says.

"Are you taking anything?" I ask. "Any herbs, pain medicines, vitamins? No? And do you have any allergies?"

"I'm allergic to penicillin and to peanuts. I nearly died with both of those as a kid. For me they introduced a 'peanut-free zone' in my hometown Quesnel school district. But I try to avoid medicines except for the occasional aspirin."

"Do you have any illnesses that run in your family?" I ask.

"My dad drove logging trucks—he was killed in a truck crash when I was in high school. I think he had high blood pressure, but he never went to the doctor. My mum is well, still teaching, but will soon retire and plans to start her own educational daycare. She's very healthy. My older brother had TB as a kid, but as far as I know he's fine now. My paternal grandparents both died in their sixties—one with heart failure and the other with a stroke after some little procedure. My mother's parents are running a bed and breakfast in the Okanagan—they have loyal guests from around the world. They used to travel lots and took me with them when I was a teenager. I'll spend a relaxing week with them shortly over spring break."

"That's great, Jennifer," I say. "Are you sure that you don't go there to help them renovate, or scrub floors, but to really relax yourself?" Jennifer looks a trifle sheepish and opens her mouth to protest.

"Don't bother to explain," I say gently. "I know that you feel more comfortable when you're helping others. You must learn to feel good about taking care of *yourself*. That's the lesson from perimenopause for you!

"This is a good place to stop. I need to examine you now. As I do, feel free to tell me anything else that's important. Here's a gown—you can change behind that curtain. Take off everything but your panties, lie down and relax. I'll make a copy of your Diaries for your chart if that's ok. I'll knock when I return."

～

As I'm examining Jennifer, I ask, "Has your doctor ever told you your blood pressure is high? You've seen him a lot in the last while about the nausea, haven't you?"

"Yes, I've been back and back," says Jennifer. "But I don't remember him taking my blood pressure."

"The reason I ask is that your pressure is quite high right now." I grab her hand, feeling that her fingers are warm. "Was your blood pressure ok during your pregnancies?"

Jennifer looks dismayed. "I forgot. When I was pregnant with my first son, I was a bit puffy, and the doctor wasn't too happy with my blood pressure. During my second pregnancy, I had to take a blood pressure medicine that made my heart race. I had to lie down a lot and they put me on an impossible low-salt diet. But I was fine, and my babies were ok. I'm still sticking to my low-salt diet. I guess my blood pressure hasn't really been checked since."

"Lie quietly and try to relax. Now shut your eyes, take a slow deep breath and let it seep out," I say soothingly as I set up a special blood pressure instrument. "I'm going to ask this machine to measure your blood pressure six times, each a minute apart," I explain. "I'll go out of the room and leave you in peace and quiet. That's the best way to accurately document your blood pressure." I start the instrument and quietly walk out.

When I return, I note the average blood pressure in my record and tell Jennifer, "It was 156 over 97 just now—you can write that down in a minute. Your hands are warm and you seem to be relaxed. You say the nausea is about a 2 today—I wonder what your blood pressure is like when you're really feeling sick? Your breasts are very full and engorged. Do they feel different than usual to you right now? Wow, if ever there were a sign of high estrogen, that's got to be one! From the feel of your breasts I'd think you were about ready to nurse or were taking a high-dose birth control pill.

"Ok, go ahead and get dressed." I draw the curtain closed and sit at the desk, writing in Jennifer's chart. "I notice that you covered your bra with your top, Jennifer," I muse. "I think there are two kinds of women in this world, those like you and me, who are quite proper. And then those who just fling off their underwear and leave it where it lands!" I laugh.

Jennifer, emerging from behind the curtain, is giggling. "I didn't even think about it," she exclaims. "There's not much you don't notice, is there?"

As Jennifer buckles her sandals, I begin to review. "Let's summarize what we know so far. You're 38 and early in perimenopause, probably in Phase B, with short cycles, nausea and sore, firm breasts. Plus today at least you have edema or leg swelling. You have a personal history of pre-eclampsia—high blood pressure and edema during pregnancy. It sounds as though you have strong risks for high blood pressure from your father's side of the family. You thought your father had it—the stroke and heart failure his parents died from are common consequences of untreated high blood pressure. High blood pressure—given the risk factors you have—often first becomes visible in perimenopause. And some, but not the majority of women, tend to have high blood pressure when estrogen levels are high.

"You're allergic," I continue, "to peanuts and to penicillin. All that said, you're basically a healthy young woman."

"That leg swelling I have right now," Jennifer bends and examines her ankles. "I wouldn't even give that a '1'! You should see it when I have a long day of standing and it's hot, especially when the nausea is bad. Then I can't even get my shoes back on!"

"That's interesting," I say, "because you have definite edema today. Your heart is fine and the retina in the back of your eyes, as best as I can see, doesn't show high intracranial pressure or evidence of damage from longstanding high blood pressure. Your weight is perfect for your height, and your liver and spleen are normal. I could feel what I think is a fibroid in your left pelvis, but it's not causing problems. I think high estrogen plus your strong family and personal history are the reasons for your high blood pressure. Good for you for sticking to a low-salt diet! The other non-drug things besides low salt that help blood pressure are being of normal weight, which you are, exercising regularly and practicing some form of relaxation."

"Oh," says Jennifer. "I get that you think I'm having high estrogen levels. That is causing periods that are close together, nausea and high blood pressure as well as swelling. But what can we do? This nausea is wearing me down!"

"We'll talk about that in a second," I say. "First I want you to collect a 24-hour urine sample so we can be sure that your kidneys are working fine. I'm going to order another serum creatinine, a potassium level and an estradiol or estrogen level the morning you start your urine collection. I'll repeat the estradiol level the day you bring your urine collection to the lab. Plus I'll give you a slip so that you can get a liver and kidney test as well as an estradiol level when you are having a '4' nausea day. I'm suggesting that your family doctor refer you to an eye doctor. An ophthalmologist can look into your retina and test to be sure that glaucoma is not a reason for your nausea and to confirm my normal findings. Finally, I'd like you to start a blood pressure record at the bottom of your Diary in the Comments section. Put down the average reading we got today and then take your blood pressure at a drugstore once or twice a week. We want the average for the systolic blood pressure, the top number, to be less than 140. It is healthy for the diastolic blood pressure average to be less than 90 mmHg. When you have a dozen or so readings from different times of day, workdays, and weekends, see your family doctor and bring him your pressure record."

"I think I'll do that average of my blood pressures before I see him," she says. "He's too busy to take the time. To get an average I just add all the top numbers together and divide by the number of readings, right? Then I do the same for the bottom number?"

"That's right," I confirm. "I'll suggest that he start you on spironolactone, a kind of medicine that interferes with estrogen's stimulation of the salt-retaining hormone, aldosterone. This medicine tastes like peppermint and isn't too expensive. It isn't a very commonly used BP pill, but is very good for high estrogen-caused blood pressure. Dr. Prior told me that in the early 1970s she helped out with a study that first used spironolactone for high blood pressure. So it is a medicine we've known about and used for a long time." Jennifer is busily writing in her flower-print covered clothbound journal.

"You said 140 over 90 is the upper limit of normal blood pressure?" she asks. I nod and she writes those numbers down.

"Now," I say, "Let's talk about what to do about the nausea. I think you should take one or two dimenhydrinate 25-mg tablets at night." I spell it out for her. "These will help your nausea and are long acting. You can take them at bedtime, and because they cause drowsiness, they will also help you sleep. Dimenhydrinate is an old-fashioned antihistamine that is used for seasickness or stomach flu. You can buy it over the counter, and it's inexpensive. The other thing I'd like you to do is to get vitamin $B_6$ and take 25 or 100 mg a day. When estrogen's high, our bodies need more $B_6$. It also helps with nausea. Actually, $B_6$ was part of an old-fashioned medication I took for morning sickness when I was first pregnant back in 1982."

"Great!" Jennifer exclaims, smiling, "I'm so glad there's something we can do. But can anything make the high estrogen levels better?"

"I don't have much hope of that for now," I say. "Remember we talked in the group session about lower Inhibin B levels, higher pituitary hormones and more stimulation of ovarian follicles to make the chaotic and increased estrogen levels? FSH is without its inhibin brake-hormone, so it increases. There isn't much to stop its over-stimulation of the ovaries. I would be so delighted to be able to *treat* you with Inhibin B! But so far, we don't have Inhibin B available as a therapy."

I pause a moment, thinking. "For the sake of completeness, not because either choice is appropriate or practical, if pushed by your symptoms, we could temporarily use a medicine called 'GnRH' that blocks the signals to FSH and causes a medical menopause—but it causes rapid bone loss and bad hot flushes. Or if we really *had* to, your ovaries could be surgically removed."

"Forget that!" declares Jennifer. "I can live with this nausea if I know that it will eventually stop."

"Yes, perimenopause—with its high estrogen levels—will eventually be over," I say reassuringly. "But I can't tell you exactly when. It will likely last at least five more years. Given that we can't take away the high estrogen, we can block its effects in tissues by using estrogen's partner hormone, progesterone. For this to be successful, you will need to take progesterone in high doses."

"But I'm still making my own progesterone!" Jennifer asserts.

"You may be," I reply, "but regular periods don't tell us that."

"Oh, no, I'm not going by periods," she insists. "I didn't get one of the sheets your secretary gave Beverley on how to figure out about ovulation. But when she had trouble understanding it, she called asking for help. I analyzed mine, too. I almost forgot to give you that record." Jennifer looks rueful as she pulls out a sheet of paper folded into her notebook. "Here are my last two. This April one is that short cycle when I didn't ovulate. But, see! Here in May

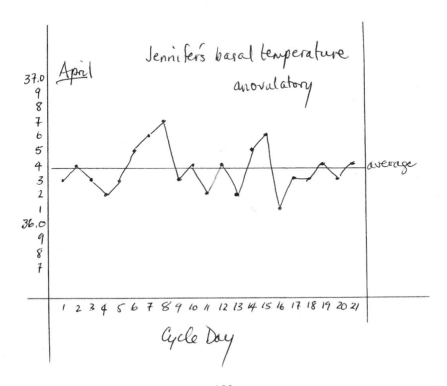

I definitely had a temperature increase on Cycle Day 17. I've ovulated every cycle except that one in April," she says, showing me four other records.

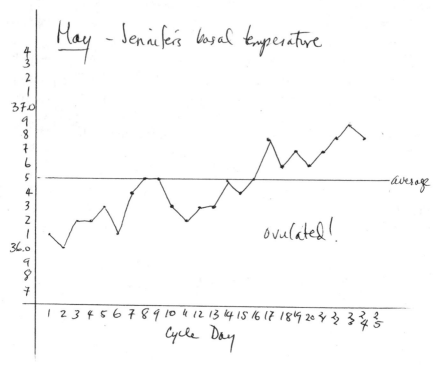

"I'm happily surprised that you're ovulating, Jennifer," I say. "*And* that you have kept this excellent record. I didn't even think to ask you about your temperature results because I expected we'd need to analyze the temperature data for you. You are right that you have ovulated, but the time from ovulation until flow is too short. Look, here in May your temperature went up on Cycle Day 17 and your period began after Day 25. That makes only eight days. That is called a short luteal phase cycle—they are typical in early perimenopause. The minimum normal luteal phase length, the time from the temperature rise until the next period (71), is ten days and the ideal is more like 14 days. So you *are* ovulating, but with only eight instead of 14 days of high progesterone levels."

I ponder a minute. "My suggestion is still to give you a full luteal phase dose of progesterone. Because your nausea looks like it bothers you throughout your cycle, I'll prescribe progesterone every day. The reason for *daily* rather than *cyclic* progesterone is that we are trying to decrease estrogen's effects throughout the whole cycle. Progesterone, through a complex set of actions, causes less estrogen action in all of the tissues in which estrogen works."

"But won't that mess up my periods and ovulation?" She asks.

"I think that your own estrogen levels are high enough that you will continue to have regular periods despite daily progesterone treatment," I say. "And your own ovulation is not reliable or normal. If you wanted to get pregnant . . ." At Jennifer's emphatic headshake, I stop that line of thought. "I'll write the prescription so that you could double the dose for the few days a cycle when you are really feeling nauseated or are vomiting. Prometrium treatment isn't acceptable because it is dissolved in peanut oil to which you're allergic. So I'll prescribe compounded bio-identical oral progesterone—if you go to a local compounding pharmacy they will measure and mix micronized progesterone with olive oil and put it into capsules. Take one capsule of 300 mg at bedtime—you can take two on the super-bad nights. Only take progesterone when you are actually on your way to bed. Slim women like you are at increased risk for its drowsiness side-effect."

I write out the prescription. "Progesterone in this dose has also been shown to lower high blood pressure (72). "Be sure to get your first couple of estrogen blood tests before you start taking progesterone. Let's see. Your last period started two and a half weeks ago. Give me back that lab slip." Jennifer searches in her bag and brings out the folded paper. "Your cycle day is right to get a progesterone level now, too. I've asked the lab to send these results to your family doctor as well as directly to you. And please remind the eye doctor you see to send me a copy of her/his consult letter."

Jennifer writes down these instructions, then pauses, looking thoughtful. "Dr. Madrona, I don't want to be stubborn, but I'd like to honour my own cycle. Although you make a good point that the nausea is all the time, I'd like to take progesterone only when I should be in the progesterone time of my cycle."

"Ok, Jennifer," I say reluctantly. "Have you had a chance to read the 'Cyclic Progesterone Therapy' handout I gave you?"

Jennifer nods. "I will follow your wishes," I begin again. "I will write your progesterone for 300 mg taken cyclically during the last 14 days of your cycle. Because your cycles are so short, I've moved the days you take progesterone to Cycle Days 12–25 instead of cycle days 14–27.

I pause, watching her writing, and knowing that I need to review this complex information with her. "What will you do if you start having your period

## CYCLIC PROGESTERONE THERAPY DIAGRAM (45)

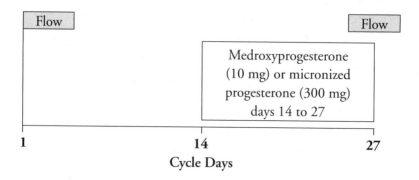

before Day 25 of your cycle? In other words, you get flow while you are still taking your 14 days of cyclic progesterone?"

"I don't know. Stop it, I guess," she answers.

"No," I reply firmly. "We want progesterone levels to be able to 'catch up' with your high estrogen levels. Flow before you finish 14 days of progesterone means that estrogen levels are very high. Therefore, I want you to take progesterone for a full 14 days, in every cycle." I say slowly, and with emphasis. "So let's imagine that the flow came early, say on Cycle Day 22. You'd start a new Diary sheet, and take progesterone days 1 through 3 of your next cycle. Look at this diagram so that we are both clear about this."

## CYCLIC PROGESTERONE THERAPY AND EARLY FLOW (45)

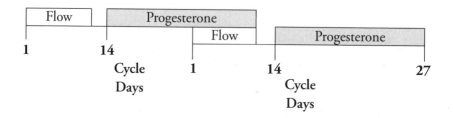

We both bend over the diagram. "Taking progesterone for a full 14 days, and having fewer days off progesterone allows the progesterone level to increase to match up with your own high estrogen production."

"Ok," she nods, writing. "I see. Because of high estrogen levels, even if I want to take progesterone cyclically, I may end up taking it nearly all the time!"

"You got it!" I laugh. "Any questions? No? It will be interesting to see what happens with your nausea. Be sure to record the $B_6$ and the dimenhydrinate dose as well as spironolactone and progesterone on your Diary sheet. Ok?"

"You bet!" Jennifer exclaims, looking excited. "Dr. Madrona, you need to know that I came here feeling there was nothing much you could do to help. But I'm leaving assured that we have a plan." Her eyes fill with tears, then she blinks, pulls herself to her full height and holds out her hand. "Thank you so much."

"You are very welcome, Jennifer." I give her a handshake and a little hug. "Remember that your biggest job is to feel good about taking care of yourself. I should know, because that's my hardest job, too." We walk down the hall together.

"Lana, please make Jennifer an appointment for three months. Jennifer, if there's anything from your lab results that changes what we're thinking, I'll call you. Be sure to bring your blood pressure record when you next come, too."

"Will do!" she exclaims. "'Bye!"

Three months later, I go to the waiting room to call Jennifer. "Jennifer? Hi! It's good to see you again," I say. "How are you doing?"

Jennifer smiles and settles back in her chair. "I guess the good thing is that my blood pressure's better. But the nausea is getting me down. It's relentless and wearying. I can't stand the heat, my legs are swelling, and I didn't think I'd make it to summer break. My principal strongly requested that I teach summer school, but I almost lied by saying I had other commitments."

"You need a break, Jennifer." I say, feeling empathetic. "You teach differently abled kids, don't you, and do counseling for your full school. What a load!"

"It's too much. . ." Jennifer pauses, looking weary. "Here's my record,

Dr. Madrona." Jennifer pulls out her magenta clipboard and tells me she's put the last Diary before therapy on the top.

"This is an incredibly meticulous record, Jennifer. I'm sure it will help us figure things out. Let's look at the nausea first. It seems like it continued to be '3s' and '4s' for the first two weeks after you started taking cyclic progesterone. But since then it seems a little better with only a rare '3' and mostly '1s' and '2s.' What do you think?"

"Yes," she sighs, "I do think that progesterone is helping—just not enough for me to have a *life*. I have to go to bed at eight at night, and I still feel exhausted in the morning."

"You've had almost a month now of summer holidays in which to recover. Are you starting to have more energy?"

"Yeah," Jennifer says. "I guess I didn't realize how much stress I was under. I just vegetated for the first two weeks. My blood pressure averaged 143 over 96 during the school year. Now it's down to about 135 over 92."

"Oh, I was wondering about your blood pressure," I say. "Looks like you started on only 25 mg per day of spironolactone. I thought,"—I check my notes—"yes, I did write 100 mg per day."

"My doctor said he wasn't familiar with spironolactone," she replies. "So we decided to try a smaller amount. I'm ready now to increase it to 50 mg and see how that goes."

"Did you see your estrogen levels?" I ask. "They're sky-high! One is 1860 and the other of 1235 picomoles per litre—the usual midcycle estrogen level is between 500 and 800, for comparison. And, as I suspected, your progesterone level is a low-normal ovulatory level at 22 nanomoles per litre. I see your flow started five days after that blood test. That progesterone level is by no means high enough to counterbalance your triple-high levels of estrogen. The ideal progesterone level is over 45 nmol per litre five days before flow."

"So you're saying that even if progesterone didn't help my nausea, I need it to be in balance with the excess estrogen that my ovaries are making?" Jennifer asks.

I nod.

"Does taking progesterone suppress my own progesterone?" she asks.

"Probably, but perimenopausal changes and all your life stresses already are suppressing your own progesterone production," I say, trying to explain complex things simply. "Progesterone therapy just adds to your own levels to make them better able to offset the tissue effects of your high estrogen levels.

I see that you're taking the $B_6$ 100 mg a day and that you gradually increased that from 25 mg. Also you're taking one dimenhydrinate at night. Do you think that either of these is helping with your nausea?"

"Yes, probably," she says. "I'm sleeping better. But whenever I think about it, I feel sick to my stomach. Most of the time I can ignore it, but surprisingly, on holiday it's even harder because I'm not so busy. When it intrudes, despite a busy life, it is really awful."

"I'm sure it is, Jennifer," I say reassuringly. "I still think that high-dose progesterone every day will help. And I'd also suggest that you increase the dimenhydrinate to two tablets at bedtime. The dose you are taking now is one we would give a child for stomach flu.

"It looks like your period is now coming the day you stop the progesterone," I observe. "That's better. But flow came on Day 5 of that second cycle. It looks like you handled that just right by continuing to take the progesterone for the full 14 days. You were off progesterone only five days that cycle. Good for you for sticking with the plan! Now it looks like the progesterone has 'caught up' with the high estrogen at least in terms of flow."

"If I've got such high estrogen levels, why didn't I ever have heavy periods?" she queries.

"I don't know, Jennifer, except that I think you've been ovulating normally most of your life. There are also hereditary differences in tissue sensitivity to estrogen (20). That's the best explanation I have for why high estrogen levels give some women migraines or heavy flow, others nausea, some women sore breasts, and yet others bad hot flushes."

"You know," she says quickly, "I think I've been having some hot flashes. I get suddenly warm after my shower and before bed, but I don't sweat much. First I thought it was just the warm summer evenings. But it can come even if the air is cool. And I'm damp when I wake at night to urinate."

"That's interesting," I say. I am scrutinizing Jennifer's Diary records, glancing at the bottom to see which days she had taken progesterone. "You've started getting daytime and night-time sweats, but not bad ones. Looks like they are on about days 8–10 of your cycle. Whoa! What's this very bad three-day headache, Jennifer?"

"I don't know, but it was wicked! I've actually had two. One as I was just finishing grading and reports, and the other for no reason, started on a weekend. They're not like anything else I've ever had. The nausea was super bad those days. My eyes were sore, I was irritable, and my head just pounded."

"They sound like migraines to me," I assert. "Look, one started the day after you stopped your progesterone, and the other one is about a day after you restarted progesterone that next cycle. Jennifer, tell me again how they started and what they were like."

"These were the worst headaches I've ever had. The first came on in the middle of the night. I felt so rough in the morning that—for almost the first time ever—I stayed in bed. I was ok as long as I just lay in bed in a dark room. But aspirin, ibuprofen and acetaminophen—everything in my cupboard—was useless to treat the throbbing pain that was right here." She points to her right temple. "That lasted for about two days. The next one started on the weekend, and I felt weird, as though I were looking through wavy glass. Then the throbbing and bad nausea started. I vomited and had to lie down in the women's washroom in a store before I could drive myself home."

"Those sound like classical migraine headaches to me, Jennifer. They will get better when you are through perimenopause. But in the meantime I think the onset of new migraine headaches is a very strong reason for you to take your progesterone *every day*," I say with emphasis. "You see, Jennifer, progesterone doesn't *cause* migraine headaches, but the brain of someone with migraine headaches responds to sudden changes in any hormones. Stopping or starting progesterone is enough to trigger a migraine when your estrogen levels are very high. It probably didn't help that you had changes in stress levels with a maximum level during final marking and reports, and the sudden relaxation with a restful weekend."

"You think that if I took it every day I would be less likely to get another migraine?" At my definite nod, she continues, "But I wanted to take progesterone in a natural way, like the normal cycle." This time her objection sounds less intense to me. "Ok, I guess you're right. I'll agree to your original suggestion that I take progesterone every day. But do I still have to take such a high dose?"

"Three hundred milligrams of progesterone is a normal luteal-phase-equivalent dose, Jennifer. Although it's still considered high by some pharmacists—ones who are accustomed to treatment of menopausal women with a third of that dose—you need that dose to keep your progesterone blood level in the normal luteal phase range for 24 hours (73). And given how high your estrogen levels are, you are going to need at least that much. It also looks as though you'll start needing it for hot flushes (74). Unfortunately, based on the usual history of hot flushes and night sweats, they are likely to get worse over the next few years."

"Why do you say they'll get worse?" she asks.

"First, because that's what has been reported in a study of perimenopausal women observed over perimenopause (39). The reason is that you've had high estrogen levels for the last four or more years and your brain has gotten used to them. The pattern in perimenopause is that now and then estrogen levels drop from high back down to normal. As they do that, your brain will react to that drop with a hot flush or night sweat."

"So *that's* what causes them!" she says. "I wondered. Some of the teachers in my school are having a hard time. Especially the women who stopped their Premarin after the Women's Health Initiative results came out." I nod with understanding. "I've told a few of them about your CeMCOR website," she finishes.

"Thanks, Jennifer," I reply. "For hot flushes in women who've been on estrogen, I think it really helps to start full-dose progesterone and then taper estrogen very slowly over months to years. Tell them there are detailed instructions in the 'Stopping Estrogen Therapy' article on the CeMCOR website."

I pause. "I guess I should explain that Dr. Prior's research shows medroxy-progesterone, a cousin of progesterone, is as good for hot flushes as estrogen (75). And progesterone doesn't carry the risk of rebound increase in flushes when you stop it, like estrogen does. By the way, if you know of any women with bad flushes who are not on hormones, we're doing a study of oral micronized progesterone or placebo for hot flushes and night sweats."

"You mean progesterone by itself might help with hot flushes?" Jennifer questions. "Everyone always talks about estrogen!"

"Because estrogen's what most people think about," I answer. "But lots of studies from the 1970s and the 1980s have shown that progestins effectively treat hot flushes (74;76;77). We did a blinded and randomized comparison study between conjugated equine estrogen, Premarin, and the synthetic progesterone-derivative, Provera. We tested full doses of each daily for one year—38 women completed diaries much like yours. These women were most likely to have a difficult time with hot flushes because they were menstruating before a hysterectomy and removal of their ovaries, just prior to starting the study. It's quite clear that Premarin and Provera are equivalent and both effective in control of night sweats and hot flushes (75)." I pause, look rueful and continue, "Dr. Prior and I've gotten five rejections on that paper so far."

"Why?" Jennifer asks. "Why would they reject it? Because they don't believe you? Or maybe because the Premarin lobby is so strong? Why do you think?"

"Editors and reviewers are just like most of us," I say. "Once we believe something, we don't want anyone changing our minds."

"I thought medicine was supposed to be about *science*, not about prejudice," Jennifer declares.

"It is," I say. "That's why I'll keep revising and resubmitting that paper until we do get it published. And that's why we're now doing a study of progesterone and hot flushes even though we don't have funding for it. I keep hoping that, one day, these fixed and unhelpful concepts will change. That will be much better for women."

"It sure will," declares Jennifer.

"Before we solve all the problems of the world, you'd better get yourself changed so I can examine you, " I say. We both laugh. "Just a short check this time. You don't need to take off your shorts, just your bra and top and your shoes. I'll go copy these Diary pages."

～

After I've examined Jennifer and she is dressed, I hand back her pages and start to review.

"Well, your blood pressure is better but still not good enough, especially since you are well into your summer holiday. I got 144 over 92 just now. I think your breasts are a bit softer. What do you think?"

"They haven't had any sore-as-a-boil times for several months," she replies. "And I can check them more easily."

"The rest of your exam is just fine," I say. The little puffiness in your ankles probably relates to the heat. You're doing a bit better, Jennifer."

She looks a bit doubtful. "I don't know. I'm only 38, I've got a load of pills, high blood pressure, nausea that no one can fix, and now migraine headaches. Enough diseases to last a lifetime!"

"Remember that these are temporary!" I declare. "And your high estrogen levels in perimenopause are causing most of these symptoms. They'll soon start getting better." I pause to reflect. "From your new daytime flushes I think you may be getting toward Phase C of perimenopause. That would mean that you are within about four years of becoming menopausal."

"Great! So you think I'll be at a normal age at menopause?" she asks.

"I expect that you'll be about 42 or so, which is on the young side of normal but still normal," I reply.

"I tend to blame myself for the high blood pressure, although I know that's crazy. . . ," her voice tails off.

"Yes it is!" I exclaim. "You've got a high blood pressure history in your family, and you are one of those women whose blood pressure is sensitive to high estrogen levels—you had high blood pressure during pregnancy. Given your sky-high estrogens, it's no wonder that your blood pressure is high right now. Your high blood pressure may well get better during menopause and even get completely better. However, all your life you'll need to stick to a low salt-diet, keep up good exercise, and keep your weight normal."

"I'm doing all of that and my blood pressure is still high. I guess you're right that I need more spironolactone, especially since you found I've still got some swelling in my legs."

"I'd be happier, for now, if you took 100 mg of spironolactone a day. Our goal for your blood pressure is to be lower than 135 over 85 to be optimal. There are proven, non-medical ways to treat high blood pressure. Any guesses, Jennifer?"

"Let's see," she says, counting on each finger of one hand, "low-salt diet, regular walking, normal weight, and avoiding alcohol?"

"Almost right," I reply, smiling. "I do think it is good to avoid excess alcohol. But the fourth one, besides diet, exercise, and normal weight is meditation or relaxation. A professor of Dr. Prior's, Dr. Herbert Benson, did a controlled trial showing that relaxation practice significantly decreased blood pressure. I suggest you learn to do relaxation or meditation and then practise it for about 10–15 minutes twice a day. I've found it very helpful, even though I don't do it as regularly as I should."

"That's a good idea," Jennifer says. "I'll look for a book on meditation. So being menopausal at age 42 or 43 is normal?"

"Yes, the normal range is from 40 through to about 58. If your bone density were low, however, with menopause at that age, many doctors would recommend hormone therapy until you are 50."

"Ok," she says. "You've convinced me. I'll take progesterone every day. I feel fine on it. Now I have hot flushes and migraines, besides my nausea, as strong reasons to take it daily."

"In addition to what you're already doing, Jennifer, the higher dose of spironolactone and the progesterone daily, I have another job for you."

Jennifer looks somewhat startled.

"I'd like you to think about ways that you could decrease your load at work in September," I say. "I think things will start to get better soon, but you will need to guard your energy. Some women have to take a medical leave of absence for a few months."

Jennifer looks dismayed. "I couldn't do that. I might not get back on again. And the kids would suffer."

"I know that you are conscientious, Jennifer," I respond. "But your union should protect you during short-term sick leave. Or you could go on a part-time schedule for a while. I'm not saying this will be necessary, but it may be. So I want you to think about it. I don't want you to get into total burnout. I'm just warning that your impossible work load and the physical and emotional stresses of perimenopause increase your risks for that."

Jennifer looks sober. "I don't think I'm that bad. But I hear you."

"Let's meet again in six months, Jennifer. And you know that you can fax me your Diary if things are not good."

"Thanks, Dr. Madrona," she says. "I'm not likely to fax or phone, but I really appreciate your willingness to respond if I need you. A couple of times I've called Lana who has hauled out my chart and read things to me or reassured me. Somehow you folks are the only ones who 'get' what an awful time I've been having." She shrugs and looks at Lana's empty chair. "I guess Lana's at lunch. You took a long time with me. Better go get some lunch, yourself! I'll call in for an appointment. See you in six months."

# 8

## *beverley*  turning the tide of infertility

I round the corner of my office and look into the crowded waiting area. All of the chairs are occupied. At first glance I can't see Beverley. Then I find her hidden behind a large plant. I say her name. She stands up, smiling in recognition, and introduces me to her husband, Victor.

"Ok he come too?" she asks. "My English not good—Victor help."

"That's fine with me, Beverley," I answer, "but I'll talk to *you*. I think you understand perfectly well, but may have trouble saying what you mean. If you can't figure out what I mean, or I can't understand you, we'll ask for his help." Beverly and Victor smile and nod politely.

After we are all seated in my small examination room-office, I tell Beverley that I will take her history, examine her, and then review things with both her and Victor.

I begin. "I remember from the group meeting that you are having trouble getting pregnant, Beverley. Tell me again how old you are, how long you have been trying to become pregnant, and what tests you've had."

"I'm 39. We use nothing"—she stops, says a Chinese word that Victor translates as "condom"—"for two years. Don't get pregnant."

I wait while Beverley consults with Victor, then she says, "Dr. Lam send me to special doctor. He do sound test." She moves her hand across her abdomen.

"A pelvic ultrasound?" I interrupt, and they both nod.

"That ultrasound ok," she continues hesitantly. "He do internal. . ."

"A pelvic examination," I say, interrupting to show her I understand.

"Ok too."

I glance down at her file in front of me. "Dr. Lam, your family doctor, sent me some information. He says that you had a consultation with a gynecologist who did the ultrasound and an endometrial biopsy, and he also did something called a hysterosalpingogram."

I look up and see that Beverley's face transiently furrows in pain; she holds her lower abdomen.

"Tung! Right?" I use the Chinese word I think means pain. She nods.

"Unfortunately, I don't have the results of these tests and I really need them. The endometrial biopsy will tell us about how much progesterone effect there is on your endometrium—if it were full of glands, it would show us that you ovulated and made an egg that cycle. And the hysterosalpingogram will tell us if your tubes are open for carrying an egg to the uterus. You would probably know if your tests were not normal. But I'd like to see them myself. Would you please call Dr. Lam and ask him to fax me those results?"

Beverley takes a pad of paper and an expensive-looking large green pen from a well-organized black leather binder and makes a note.

"Many things besides a woman's illnesses or diseases can cause infertility or trouble getting pregnant," I say, turning to Victor. "Did the gynecologist ask you to do a sperm count?"

"No." He seems surprised.

"That's not right!" I exclaim. "Beverley shouldn't have had those painful and expensive tests before your sperm was shown to be normal, Victor. Problems with getting pregnant and having a normal baby can come from either the man or the woman."

They look startled at my vehemence.

Victor quickly says, "Ok, I'll do the sperm count."

I nod to Victor and continue with Beverley. "Tell me where you were born," I ask, looking at her as I change the subject. "Where have you lived, and when did you come to Canada?"

"I born in China, in Hunan Province," Beverley says. "My whole family, all brothers and sisters, they stay in China. I go to Hong Kong, then come to Canada with Commonwealth Scholarship, study at UBC. Now married." She looks at Victor. "Have good Canadian business."

"Tell me about your work," I ask.

"She has two stores," Victor interjects, "one in Metrotown and a new one at City Square. She sells silk sweaters knitted in China. We also have a warehouse in Burnaby. Twenty-one people work for her."

"You sound very busy!" I exclaim, turning to Beverley. "Now, new questions. Have you ever been very sick, in the hospital, in an accident, or had surgery?"

Beverley looks uncertain. She talks briefly in Cantonese with Victor. She gestures at her chest.

"Mother says bad cold when baby," she says. "Otherwise ok."

"Were the chest X-rays normal that they did when you came to Canada?" I ask, wanting to be sure she didn't have tuberculosis or TB, and knowing that the X-rays would show it.

"Yes, ok," she replies.

"That's good. Are there any medical problems or illnesses in your family?"

"My father died." She points to her throat. "Cancer—smoke too much. Sisters have babies; brothers have babies. Mother, eye surgery, ok." Beverley hesitates a minute and finishes with, "Mother want Canada grandson."

"That's a normal thing for a Chinese grandmother to want, Beverley." I say, having heard from other patients about the family pressure on a Chinese woman to bear a son. "What do you do for fun?"

She looks startled and almost asks Victor for help. Then she starts, hesitantly. "I work," she says, pausing. "Like work. Sing at North Burnaby Choir. Sometimes translate at MOSAIC, Eagle Ridge Hospital—Chinese people."

Victor murmurs to Beverley. "Oh!" she says. "Play tennis on weekend, visit family, sometimes mahjong."

"Good," I say, nodding. "How are your menstrual cycles, Beverley?"

Beverley pulls Diary sheets from her black leather organizer and gives them to me. I see that she also has graph paper on which she has plotted her cycle and luteal phase lengths from the past six months. Beverly points to the graph. "Ask Jennifer—help me with the temperature. Not enough progesterone. Why?"

I look appreciatively at the graph. "This is great! Tell me how you did it!"

Beverley looks pleased.

Victor answers. "We read the paper you gave Beverley. She needed help, so she called Jennifer, a woman from that group session. All the thermometers from flow to next flow make average."

I interrupt briefly. "That's right, all of the temperatures divided by the days of the cycle give the average that's usually above 36.6 if you have ovulated (2)."

"See, this one 36.8." Here Beverley points to where the temperatures are all above 36.6, starting five days before flow. "Ovulate, but no baby." She shakes her head.

## BEVERLEY'S CYCLES OF TEMPERATURE DATA
### SHOWING LUTEAL PHASE LENGTHS

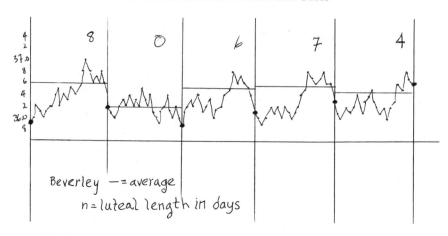

Beverley —= average
n= luteal length in days

"You are clearly ovulating," I agree, "but you have too short a time of progesterone—that's a short luteal phase cycle. It doesn't prepare the endometrium enough to allow the egg to implant. You've done a very good job of figuring out your quantitative basal temperature (2). Although some people argue about this, I think the reason you haven't gotten pregnant is that the luteal phase is too short. That means you are making too little progesterone. If progesterone isn't making the uterine lining rich and juicy for at least ten days, a fertilized egg can't grow inside you."

"Why luteal phase short?" she asks.

"The reasons aren't always clear," I say. "One big reason is that a woman has too much stress. Or maybe she works too hard, or is sick, or is losing weight, and with those things may be exercising too much (78)."

"Maybe menopause?" she asks.

"Perhaps *peri*menopause," I say feeling again that I'm up against common misconceptions. "But you have eggs, you have regular periods, and you ovulate. We don't know why short luteal phases occur in perimenopause but it is probably because the high estrogens don't produce the LH peak that normally triggers ovulation (33;34). Do you remember talking about that in the group session?"

"Right," she says. "I remember. Perimenopause."

"Now," I say, "do you notice any changes in how you feel?"

"I wake up and worry," she says. "Right, Victor?"

Victor looks from Beverley to me and back before speaking hesitantly. "She always wanted to do things perfectly. Now she worries a lot and feels her heart jumping. Could that be perimenopause?"

"Well," I say, "someone who already works very hard, who starts to have sleep problems and heart palpitations—can become very fatigued and stressed. Yes, that definitely sounds like perimenopause. Those feelings also have something to do with who you are, as a person. And they may be part of why you are having short luteal phase cycles. I need to find out more about you. Have you lost any weight?"

Beverley shrugs. "Don't know. Don't make attention. Usually 52 kg."

I nod, "What did you eat for breakfast?"

"Sometimes have toast. . ." Again she shrugs.

"What about today?" I persist.

"Leftover rice, vegetables. I go to City Square quick."

"So you were rushed. But that still sounds like a good breakfast. Are you allergic to anything?" I ask.

"Not eat milk—gives pain." She holds her stomach and consults with Victor.

He adds "And diarrhea."

Beverley continues, "Nothing else. "

"Are you taking any medicines or herbs or vitamins?"

"I start calcium for sleeping. Victor and I read paper." She holds up the "ABC's of Osteoporosis Prevention for Midlife Women" handout. "Also help bones. No pills."

"You need to take a special vitamin pill with lots of folate or folic acid in it to prepare for pregnancy and a healthy baby. I'm surprised that Dr. Lam or your gynecologist didn't suggest that."

"What kind vitamin? What name?" She asks, sitting at the edge of her chair.

"There are several," I say. "Just ask the pharmacist at the drugstore for a maternity vitamin." Beverley writes another note in her black folder.

"How old were you when your period started?" I ask.

"Fourteen or 15—age same as girls. No periods, wait until university done."

"We got married five years ago, Dr. Madrona," Victor interjects. "We haven't used condoms for at least two years."

"Have you ever taken the Pill?" I ask Beverley.

"No Pill," she shakes her head.

"Have you ever been pregnant?" I ask.

"No. You see?" She holds up her Diary records and says with frustration, "Monthlies regular, no misses. Always same. Never pregnant. "

"I know it's hard to have patience when you care so much, Beverley. I'm sure that if the three of us work together, we can achieve a pregnancy." I look at her and reach out to cover her small hand with mine. I feel that my belief, all by itself, is healing. "Is there anything else that I should know before I examine you?" I ask.

Beverley shakes her head. I turn to the Victor. "If it's ok with Beverley, you may stay while I examine her. Or you may sit out there in the waiting area. If you want to wait out there, I'll come and get you when we're finished. Then the three of us will talk things over and make a plan."

Beverly looks at Victor and says, "He go."

I hand Beverley a blue gown, ask her to take off everything except her panties, and show her where she can lie down on the examination table behind the yellow curtain. "You have already had a pelvic exam," I say, "so I will be checking everything else today."

"Ok," says Beverley, walking behind the curtain.

"I'll copy your Diaries and graph for your chart," I say. "When I come back, I'll knock first."

As Victor and I walk down the hall together, he says, "You talked about stress and how that affects ovulation. She feels guilty. . ."

"Why does she feel that way?" I ask.

"She decided to stay here instead of returning to China after university. We met at UBC. I persuaded her to stay, we got married, and I helped her start her import business. But I've been very busy with my own telecommunications company, I have to travel lots, and she is quiet." He pauses. "When we married, she was 34. And she said she needed to make a strong business before she would think about having children. Now she feels like maybe it is too late. She feels like she has to give her mother a grandson or she will not be a good daughter."

"Those are very deep feelings," I say, "and can keep a woman from getting pregnant. Body and feelings have to work together to create a pregnancy." I watch as Victor takes a seat in the waiting room. Then I copy Beverley's Diary records and head back to the examining room-office.

"I've had a good look at your Diary as I photocopied the records," I say after I return. "You have kept very good track!"

Beverley smiles, and I begin the examination.

"Do you check your own breasts once a month?" I ask as I begin examining her breasts.

"I never learn."

"They feel pretty firm and lumpy to me, although they are quite small. Has that firm area been there before?" I take Beverley's hand to feel a firm lump on the outer edge of her left breast.

"Don't think there—hurts!" she says.

"That's good," I say, breathing out slowly with relief. "A lump that's sore is not likely to be cancer. But you need to regularly check your own breasts, Beverley. No one can know how they feel better than you do. Want me to show you how?"

Beverley nods.

"Once a month at the end of your period, check each of your breasts. You need to do it regularly so you will remember what each felt like the month before. You want to use the opposite hand—the left hand on your right breast and your right hand for your left breast. Place your arm up over your head on the side you are checking, like this." I demonstrate by raising Beverley's arm. "You can check your breasts in the shower. My breasts, since perimenopause, are too big to do a good job in the shower so I have to check mine lying down. Use the soft part of your fingers to move over every part of your breast. I like to make a big circle starting up here under the armpit and then 'walking' my fingers around the outer edge of the breast. Walk your fingers in smaller and smaller circles until you finish under the nipple and have covered all of your breast tissue. Then do the other side. Will you do that?"

"Yes I do," she says. "I not know before."

"You can start having screening mammograms every two years once you are 45 or 50. That's another way to assess your breasts. But you still always need to check them yourself."

"Get Pap tests," she declares.

"That's good, Beverley. What exercise do you regularly do besides playing tennis now and then?"

"Do not much. Did Tai Chi—no teacher now."

"I'd like you to walk for a half an hour every day. Be sure to take Victor too. If you play some tennis, or hike, or swim, you can skip your walk that day. Exercise is good for your health and good for your heart."

"Ok we do," she says.

"Have you ever smoked?" I ask. "No, I didn't think so. And Victor doesn't either, does he? Any alcohol?"

"Don't like this. Drink tea—that good."

"Ok," I say, as I finish her examination. "Come over to the scale here. Let's check your weight and height. Take a deep breath and stand as tall as you can." I note that her height stays the same after my instruction—that shows her basic excellent posture. "You said your usual weight is 52 kg? Hmm. Now you weigh 46 kg! That's not enough for your height of 156 cm. Although it is normal, especially given your Chinese ancestry, for you to be light and small, your body mass index—that's a way of putting height and weight together—is too low for you to get pregnant easily. I'll show you what I mean after you are dressed."

"While you're dressing," I continue as I pull the curtain across again, "I'll go get Victor. He needs to be part of our discussion about how you can become pregnant."

~

All three of us are again sitting around one corner of my desk. I have spread out the copies of Beverley's Diary records, basal temperature analysis and all of her lab tests.

Victor says, "If you ask your secretary, she'll probably have a fax of the tests from Dr. Lam. I called while I was waiting."

"Great! Thanks for doing that, Victor" I say. Several pages mysteriously slide under the door. "Oh here they are now!" We all chuckle.

I add the new lab results to the display on the table. "Let's look at the results together. First, we'll go over the tests that your doctors ordered. Your endometrial thickness on the ultrasound test was 3.2 mm. That is a normal result—Asians normally have thinner endometrial lining results than Caucasians. I recently learned that 4 mm is the upper limit of thickness for a person of Asian heritage. That's different because the endometrium can be 5 cm and be normal for a Caucasian woman. Although endometrial thickness is not very reliable in a perimenopausal woman."

"What does having a thicker than normal endometrium mean?" asks Victor.

"If the endometrium is too thick after menopause, the woman might have endometrial hyperplasia, which means that the lining of her uterus is over-stimulated by estrogen and doesn't see enough progesterone action. If that goes on for a long time, it could cause endometrial cancer. That is why I am glad we have results of your endometrial biopsy. It shows 'patchy proliferation with some hyperplasia but no atypia,'" I read. "Translated, that means the estrogen effect is strong and isn't being affected by enough progesterone. 'No atypia' is the good news—it means that there is no hint of cancer."

Beverley looks at Victor who says, "I wish Dr. Lam or the gynecologist had explained that to us!"

"Yes, it would have been easier for you because they could have told you in Cantonese. That would be better than my trying to explain things in English."

"I don't think they like questions," comments Victor quietly. Beverley nods.

"Dr. Lam also ordered tests including estrogen, FSH and TSH levels and a prolactin on Day 3 of your cycle. The FSH is nice and low at 5.0 IU, your TSH is 2.1, and prolactin is also perfect. See, they are all in the middle of the normal range. But the estrogen level at 348 pmol/L is higher than normal for a premenopausal woman in that part of the cycle."

"Why doctor say no more eggs?" asked Beverley.

"Perhaps because of the higher estrogen level. But all it says to me is that you are in perimenopause. There are plenty of eggs in your ovaries. Now that you've kept such a fine record, and we can see that you've ovulated for four of the last five cycles, I am sure that you will be able to become pregnant!" I say confidently. Then I pause a second. "But I can't promise you a son!" We all laugh.

"All right," I say. "Let's review what else we've learned. Your breasts are a bit too firm, meaning again not enough progesterone for your high estrogen levels. And you have excellent posture—it must be your Tai Chi."

Beverley looks quizzically at Victor. "That means that you stand up straight, Beverley," I answer quickly. "Also, you seem to have lost weight. That makes you too slim to easily become pregnant. Everything else is fine," I look from Beverley to Victor reassuringly.

"Ok, let's make a plan. First of all you weigh too little for a woman who wants to become pregnant. Body mass index or BMI is the weight in kg divided by the height in metres squared. An ideal BMI for pregnancy is 22 or 23 and you're at 19." I reach for my BMI wheel and start looking it up.

Beverley pulls a calculator from her binder and starts entering numbers—46 divided by 156 times 156. "Ok," she mumbles, "for BMI 22, need weigh. . ." She very quickly solves the equation. We both come up with 54 kg at the same time.

"Ok, I eat," says Beverley. "Walking thirty minutes day." She looks at Victor. "You walk too." They exchange a small smile.

"Next, Victor, you need to get a sperm count," I say. I write out a lab slip and hand it to him. "I put your name on it as well as Dr. Lam's so you'll get the result. Let's hope that your sperm count is normal. Victor, only get that test when you are rested, relaxed, and haven't been travelling."

I turn back to Beverley. "I'd like you to start taking that special maternity vitamin tomorrow. It should have 1 mg of folate in it. A mother's folate levels must be normal in the first weeks of pregnancy or the baby might have a neural tube defect. That means a problem with the nerves in the base of the spine and sometimes not enough strength in the legs."

"In addition to the one 500-mg calcium tablet you are now taking at breakfast, I'd like you to take a second one at dinner and a third one at bedtime. Also, drink a couple of glasses of fortified soymilk a day. The soymilk will give you a few more grams of protein every day as well as providing about 200 mg of calcium in each glass."

I sit back in my chair and look at Beverley writing and Victor quietly observing. "You won't be able to become pregnant until you both feel 'at home' with yourselves, in Canada. As well you must feel at home with your choices, your friends and family, and your future. Victor mentioned to me, Beverley, that you sometimes feel bad about not returning to China after university. Instead of feeling sorry or sad, now you need to focus on feeling calm and confident. Maybe you can write down your feelings in a journal, or talk with Victor while you walk."

"When I sad make egg trouble?" asks Beverley.

"For every pregnancy to happen, your whole body, mind and spirit need to be in balance. A traditional Chinese doctor would explain it as balancing yin and yang. The brain senses your feelings. If they are sorry or sad, your brain decides it's not a good time for you to have a baby. So it doesn't send the full signals to your pituitary and ovary (79). The result, if intense, is low estrogen and no period. If less intense, then the result is a short luteal phase or no ovulation. That's why you didn't have periods when you were in university. At that time in your life you probably lost weight, so you didn't make enough estrogen either."

Beverley nods. I turn to Victor.

"Do you have to be away again soon, Victor?"

"I am scheduled to go to Singapore in July," he says, consulting his hand held computer. "Then I've no trips scheduled until October."

"That's good," I say. "You need to be here to do your part as well as to provide Beverley with support."

I look from one to the other. "Do you know when in your cycle to have intercourse so you'll be most likely to get pregnant?" I ask.

Both are quiet, then Beverley says tentatively, "Temperature up day?" she gestures.

"That would usually be too late," I reply. "Look here at your Diary. See that stretchy mucus that comes about Day 17 or so of your cycles? When the mucus gets to be quite stretchy, at a score of '2' or a '3,' that is the ideal time to have sex. You should wait until it is at least a '2,'" I add, pointing out the days of stretchy mucus in the several cycles.

"Because we know you are making an egg most cycles, if your endometrium were better prepared by progesterone, you would likely become pregnant. For that reason I will prescribe oral micronized progesterone 100-mg capsules, three a day. Always take them at bedtime. To mimic the luteal phase, I want you to take the progesterone on Days 14–27 of your cycle. Progesterone will make your endometrium secretory, which means that it will be juicy and supportive for the fertilized egg to implant in it and start to grow."

I pause. "Do you understand?" Both nod, and I continue. "You don't need to take your temperature any more, because the progesterone pills you start will make your temperature go up (80)." I realize I need to explain about absence of withdrawal flow. "However, if you don't get a period after you stop taking your progesterone, you could take your morning temperature. See, it's 36.7 Celsius or higher when you have ovulated." I point at the temperature graphs. "If it's 36.7 or more, and you're at least on Day 30 of your cycle, you'll have the first indication that you are pregnant.

"It looks like today is Day 21 of your cycle. Usually you get your flow on Day 26 to 28. So you could get a blood test today for estrogen and progesterone levels. Start taking the progesterone pills on the fourteenth day after your flow next starts."

Beverley looks puzzled. "This progesterone on website?" she asks.

"That's right!" I exclaim. "Look on the Internet at the Centre for Menstrual Cycle and Ovulation Research website—www.cemcor.ubc.ca—and find 'Cyclic Progesterone Therapy.' You will take it exactly like the website instructions. However, if you take the progesterone for 14 days and don't get a flow for two weeks afterwards, take your temperature and get a pregnancy test. If your temperature is low, and that test is negative, it means you are not pregnant that cycle. Take progesterone again for 14 days. Do you have any questions?"

Beverley shakes her head, scanning her notes.

"Are there any side-effects of the progesterone, Doctor?" asks Victor.

"That's an important question," I say. "No, progesterone has no serious side-effects. Progesterone doesn't cause blood clots, heart attacks, strokes, dementia, migraines or breast cancer, and it protects against endometrial cancer. Its good side-effect is that it increases deep sleep (81). One thing you may notice, Beverley, is that you feel tired in the morning after you first start taking it. That's because your body is trying to catch up on deep sleep. Progesterone may also help with bad dreams and worry. And, as I explained, I think because of your short luteal phase cycles in perimenopause, progesterone will help you get pregnant. The very first cycle, it may stimulate higher estrogen levels causing you to feel more soreness in your breasts and some bloating. That will go away in the second cycle."

"What if I tired?" asks Beverley.

"Just keep taking it for the full 14 days. If you feel tired in the daytime, it's because you need more rest, not because of the medicine." I pause.

"Are you really sure that progesterone is safe in pregnancy, Dr. Madrona?" Victor asks earnestly.

"I am very sure, Victor," I answer firmly. "Progesterone levels are *normally* very high during pregnancy—Prometrium is the same hormone. There are potentially serious effects, however, if Beverley *doesn't* take progesterone." I turn toward her. "Your endometrial biopsy shows warning signs that your estrogen is too high for the amount of progesterone your body is making, Beverley. That is a risk for endometrial cancer."

Beverley and Victor glance at each other. I smile and try to reassure them. "I've prescribed the progesterone that is one of the safest medicines there is. I think about it this way—progesterone levels are extremely high during pregnancy and the fetus is exposed to those high levels. If progesterone were harmful, the Great Creator wouldn't have allowed it to bathe the most precious of all treasures." Beverley and Victor now look more relaxed.

"Keep up the good record-keeping, Beverley. Down here where you wrote your temperature before, please put the number of 100-mg progesterone capsules you took that day."

"Thank you, Dr. Madrona," Beverley and Victor say in concert.

"You two have a great summer together!" I say. "I'll see you in six months!" I hand the lab slip and the progesterone prescription to Beverley. "Come with me to meet Lana, who will give you your appointment date. If you have more questions, you can call Lana. She'll answer them or ask me."

"Ok, Dr. Madrona," says Beverly. "'Bye!"

About six months later, I call Beverley's name as I enter the waiting area.

"Hi. It's me!" Beverley says brightly as she comes toward me.

"It's good to see you," I say as we walk together down the hall. "You're looking great. How are things going?"

"Victor in Texas now," Beverley says. "We're fine—not pregnant yet. One month no flow. Temperature high. Period late. Not pregnant."

"You could have been pregnant and had a very early miscarriage, Beverley. The good news is that means you can get pregnant. Although it is sad that pregnancy didn't stay. When that happens the fetus usually has something the matter with it," I say, pausing to gauge her feelings as we both sit down in the examination room-office.

She nods matter-of-factly and I continue. "What else is new in your life?"

"I do Tai Chi, mornings, Central Park. Walk there. Feel strong, ready make baby."

"That's great, Beverley. Tai Chi is a wonderful kind of meditation or relaxation. I used to run up to Queen Elizabeth Park in the early morning hours. I remember my awe seeing dozens of quiet people doing Tai Chi there. It looked powerful."

"Feel strong to me," Beverley says.

"How are you doing with the progesterone, Beverley?" I ask.

She gets out her Diary sheets and shows them to me. "I took two Prometrium the first time. Then three—feel fine."

"Your sleep looks a lot better and your flow is less." I compare the new Diaries with the old.

"Yes," says Beverley. "My heart not too fast at night."

"I'm glad you're not waking with palpitations any more. It looks like you were pregnant here, Beverley." I point to the cycle where flow didn't start until Day 31. "First morning temperatures on Days 28 and 29 were 37.2 and 37.6 and then dropped to 36.4 and 36.1 the day before flow and the day flow started. See? You had more breast tenderness and fluid retention in the last week of progesterone therapy and until the day before flow. That suggests the high estrogen levels of pregnancy."

"I pregnant. . ." Beverley says thoughtfully with a mixture of pride and grief in her voice. I wait, then reach out my hand. Feeling my support, she begins again. "Then Victor gone. He not here at right time."

"When does Victor get home?" I ask.

"He back tomorrow, then not away—maybe March."

"That's good," I say. "You need him here. Now—you look as though you've gained a little weight. Your cheeks are more full."

"Yes, fat! Eating sunflower seeds every afternoon. Eat soymilk every meal."

"Great," I say. "How's your work coming?"

"I not work much," she says. "Sold City Square. I make baby important job."

"That is a very wise decision, Beverley. How is your family?"

"Victor's family," Beverly replies, "very big." She gestures with her arms. "Many Canadian, all kinds!" She laughs. "Big picnic, big dinner, and big wedding. I play with babies!"

"You play with your little nieces and nephews?" She nods. "That sounds really good, Beverley. You seemed too busy before to enjoy family gatherings. And being around babies and children is a good way to get ready for your own. How is your mother?"

"She getting old. Work hard—cook, carry, sew, help. She lives with brother, oldest brother."

Beverley pauses. Then she leans forward in her chair. "Dr. Madrona, I check myself." I look puzzled. Beverley continues. "Not take Prometrium one month, October. See!" She points to the Diary showing the temperature increasing on Day 16 with a period starting on the Day 27. "Normal—12 days—by me! Progesterone blood 52—very good."

"That's great, Beverley. I believe that you can ovulate normally and get pregnant on your own. Learning about your own cycles, increasing your weight, decreasing stress, understanding perimenopause and ovulation, are all part of the healing."

Beverley looks both surprised and gratified. "You not mad."

"Good grief, no!" I laugh. "That means you are learning about your own body, Beverley. That's even more important than getting pregnant!"

"Need Prometrium, Doctor?"

"What do you think?" I ask.

"Probably yes. Next year,"—she points to herself—"40 year old. Not many chances. Prometrium—I like."

ir cycles, what other medicines or

bottles. I see that her multivitamin
is a 1-mg folate pill. "Take calcium

do?"
iis on weekend."
s?" I ask.

mention that Victor's sperm count
. And that estradiol level we did the
: that time your progesterone level
...too low at 17. That's what I suspected—too much estrogen and not
enough progesterone."

~

When we finish the exam and are settling into our seats again, I remark,
"You've done a very good job, Beverley. You have started regular walking and
doing Tai Chi, you've decreased your work stress, and you've gained weight.
With your weight now at 55 kg, your BMI is 23. I suspect you'll be pregnant
before we know it."

"Good!" exclaims Beverly. "Thank you, Dr. Madrona. Feel stronger. Much
hope baby. New friend—Jennifer."

As we walk down the hall toward Lana's desk, I say, "Let's meet in six
months. Call and give us the good news when you're pregnant!"

Estrogen's storm season :
stories of perimenopause

31227079162496

7340

Spri

Pickup By: 11/3/2020

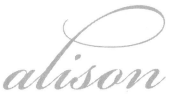 murderous migraines

"**G**ood morning, Alison."
"Whata ya' at!" She calls out cheerfully.

I smile in greeting, but must look puzzled.

"That's a Newfoundland greeting, Dr. Madrona."

"So that's what it is! I almost said 'Getsunt heit'!" I say, matching her jocular tone. "Come on in. How are you today?"

"Well," Alison begins, "this is not the best of days. But at least I'm here. I feel drugged, and my migraine is still a '2.' I woke at three or so with a screeching migraine, and it isn't tame yet. I went straight from a sound sleep to up-chucking!"

"'How many times in a month would you have a bad migraine like that?" I ask.

"More like two or three times a *week* rather than a month. I used to have a bad headache day during bleeding and another about a week after my period. But now it can last for a week at a time, and I'm never free of them for as long as a week."

"That's rough! As I mentioned in the group session, I know all about migraines," I grimace in sympathy. "Tell me when they started, and what you've tried to help."

"I was 43 when I had my first one. I thought I was getting the flu. I had night sweats, was vomiting, and my period started. That time I had no warning and no idea what was going on. I don't think I had another until the day before my next period. When I got the flashing lights and numb hand, I got scared. My family doctor gave me Immitrex, I took it and got chest pain. That scared the pants off me—but the headache went away. Since then I've tried seasick pills. . . "

"You mean dimenhydrinate?" I interrupt.

"Yeah, that's it. And I've tried all kinds of drugs for prophylaxis like propranolol, metoprolol, several kinds of old-fashioned antidepressant medicines called tricyclics and even some anti-anxiety pills. I've kept diary cards of migraine triggers. I avoid even a drop of wine, stinky cheeses, and all of the things that are supposed to make migraines worse. But I can't avoid one of my major triggers—the weather!"

"Nor can you, or any of us, avoid perimenopause!" I say.

"Since the first migraines, I've seen two specialists. One told me I should take estrogen during my flow." She stops in frustration. Then she decides to ask me about it. "Why would he say that? I thought estrogen made migraines worse."

"You're right that estrogen makes migraines worse. But so does going on and off of hormones," I say. "I guess his idea was that your estrogen levels drop during flow and that the change in estrogen levels was triggering a migraine. That would be an accurate idea if you weren't in perimenopause when estrogens can be stubbornly high any old time and don't suppress when you take estrogen treatment."

"Bet your bottom dollar I refused estrogen!" Alison says. "But the short answer is: Nothing has really helped these migraines." She shakes her head. "I'm lucky that I don't have to punch a time clock. And glad my job is taking care of my guys. So I can be quite flexible. Mostly *they* have to be flexible!" She laughs.

"You mentioned night sweats with your first migraine. Are you still getting them?" I ask.

"I do, but they are nothing compared with the time bomb in my head."

"Let's look at your Diary. Do you notice anything here that relates to your migraines?"

"I haven't thought about it for a while. But here,"—she looks at the December cycle—"the cramps were starting, then the night sweats and a migraine and then my period. But I got another migraine without cramps or flow and without night sweats three days later."

"What are you using now for the migraines?"

## ALISON'S DECEMBER DIARY AND DAILY MIGRAINES

Name: *Alison*        Month: *December*  Year: *January*

| Cycle Day | 1 | 2 | 3 | 4 | 5 | 6 | 7 | 8 | 9 | 10 | 11 | 12 | 13 | 14 | 15 | 16 | 17 | 18 | 19 | 20 | 21 | 22 | 23 | 24 | 25 | 26 | 27 | 28 | 29 | 30 | 31 |
|---|---|---|---|---|---|---|---|---|---|---|---|---|---|---|---|---|---|---|---|---|---|---|---|---|---|---|---|---|---|---|---|
| Date | 12 | 13 | 14 | 15 | 16 | 17 | 18 | 19 | 20 | 21 | | | | | | | | | | | 1 | 2 | 3 | 4 | 5 | 6 | 7 | 8 | 9 | 10 | 11 |
| Tampons/pads/day | 3 | 3 | 5 | 4 | 0 | 0 | 0 | 0 | 0 | 0 | 0 | | | | | | | | | | | | | | | | | | | | |

Record 0 = none, 1 = minimal, 2 = moderate, 3 = moderately intense, 4 = very intense

| | 1 | 2 | 3 | 4 | 5 | 6 | 7 | 8 | 9 | 10 | 11 | 12–20 | 21 | 22 | 23 | 24 | 25 | 26 | 27 | 28 |
|---|---|---|---|---|---|---|---|---|---|---|---|---|---|---|---|---|---|---|---|---|
| Amount flow | 2 | 3 | 3 | 1 | 1 | 1 | 0 | 0 | 0 | 0 | 0 | | 0 | 0 | 0 | 0 | 0 | 0 | 0 | 0 |
| Cramps | 3 | 2 | 2 | 0 | 0 | 0 | 0 | 0 | 0 | 0 | 0 | | 0 | 0 | 1 | 0 | 0 | 0 | 0 | 0 |
| Breast Sore: Side | 1 | 0 | 0 | 0 | 0 | 0 | 0 | 0 | 0 | 0 | | | 0 | 0 | 0 | 0 | 0 | 6 | 0 | 0 |
| Breast Sore: Front | 3 | 3 | 2 | 0 | 0 | 0 | 0 | 0 | 1 | 2 | 2 | | 6 | 0 | 1 | 1 | 0 | 1 | 2 | 0 |
| Fluid Retention | 2 | 1 | 1 | 0 | 0 | 1 | 0 | 1 | 2 | 1 | | | 1 | 0 | 1 | 2 | 0 | 0 | 1 | 0 |
| Hot flushes - day | 3 | 1 | 0 | 0 | 6 | 0 | 0 | 6 | 0 | 0 | | | 0 | 0 | 0 | 6 | 0 | 0 | 0 | 0 |
| # of flushes - day | 2 | 1 | 0 | 0 | 0 | 0 | 0 | 0 | 0 | 0 | | | 6 | 0 | 0 | 0 | 0 | 0 | 0 | 0 |
| Hot flushes - night | 2 | 0 | 0 | 0 | 0 | 0 | 0 | 0 | 2 | 0 | | | 0 | 0 | 0 | 0 | 0 | 0 | 0 | 0 |
| # of flushes - night | 1 | 0 | 0 | 0 | 0 | 0 | 0 | 0 | 2 | 0 | | | 0 | 0 | 0 | 0 | 0 | 0 | 0 | 0 |
| Mucous Secretion | 2 | 2 | 0 | 0 | 0 | 0 | 2 | 3 | 2 | 2 | | | 0 | 0 | 0 | 0 | 1 | 0 | 0 | 1 |
| Constipation | 0 | 0 | 0 | 1 | 0 | 0 | 0 | 0 | 0 | 0 | | | 0 | 0 | 0 | 0 | 0 | 0 | 0 | 0 |
| Headache migraine | 3 | 4 | 3 | 2 | 0 | 1 | 4 | 4 | 3 | 3 | | *most days + nights* | 2 | 3 | 2 | 0 | 1 | 4 | 3 | 3 |
| Sleep Problems | 3 | 2 | 3 | 1 | 0 | 0 | 3 | 2 | 0 | 0 | | | 0 | 1 | 1 | 0 | 0 | 3 | 1 | 1 |
| Feeling Frustrated | 1 | 0 | 0 | 1 | 0 | 0 | 2 | 0 | 0 | 0 | | | 0 | 0 | 2 | 2 | 0 | 2 | 1 | 1 |
| Feeling Depressed | 0 | 1 | 0 | 0 | 0 | 1 | 0 | 0 | 0 | 0 | | | 0 | 0 | 0 | 0 | 0 | 1 | 0 | 0 |
| Feeling Anxious | 1 | 1 | 2 | 0 | 0 | 0 | 0 | 0 | 1 | 0 | 0 | | | | | | | | | |

(handwritten notes across the middle of the chart: *forgot sheet*, *most days*, *no*)

"I still carry something, some pill like *Immitrex,* only it's a new and experimental drug. I forgot the name. I avoid it if I can help it. I start with a 50-mg dimenhydrinate and a couple of ibuprofen. If that doesn't work, I call my friend and ask her to pick up the younger two boys after school and I go to bed with a bucket."

"Except that the migraines have become more frequent, has anything else changed in the last couple of years since they started?"

"I'm getting more stretchy mucus and at any old time in my cycle, and I'm gaining weight. Amazing that I can gain when I'm vomiting and have eaten next to nothing. Whatever is making me gain, it's the fuel of the future!"

"It looks like some of your cycles are very short—the shortest I see is 20 days—no 18 days," I correct myself. "It also looks as though your migraines are more frequent in the shortest cycles compared with the longest cycles—although 25 days is not very long."

I look through more Diary sheets. "You've recorded some morning temperatures," I say, "but I see that you are not taking your temperatures some days. Oh, I get it! Those must be mornings when a migraine starts in the middle of the night. That's the right thing to do. Waking early and taking pills and vomiting are all likely to make your morning temperature reading inaccurate. If we need to, we can use a least squares analysis method for basal temperatures which will work in a cycle with a third of the data points missing, as long as they are not missing from the temperature shift time of the cycle (2)."

"Do you think ovulation might have something to do with the migraines?" Alison asks.

"I'm not sure," I reply. "People with migraines have brains that react to changes in hormones, in weather, in just about anything. I equate high estrogen levels and emotional tension with migraines, and I think your currently high estrogen levels are why you are getting them so badly. Often women will have migraines during adolescence that will go away until they start the Pill or until perimenopause. But you never had them before?"

"No, I was a happy, scrawny outport teen with not a care in the world!"

"When did you move to British Columbia?" I ask.

"Oh, I taught high-school math in Corner Brook for a couple of years. But I was restless and moved to St. John's. When I saw a job listed for a high-school math teacher here in Vancouver, I took it. I liked that job fine and became the head of the math department. Then I met Walter." She laughs. "We were married in Corner Brook, then came here to live. He's got a construction contracting business in Kitsilano. We both decided we wanted kids, so I took a leave of absence from teaching. Now I've raised three boys ages six to 13. I thought by the time my youngest was ready for school I'd begin working again, at least as a TOC." She sees my puzzled look and translates. "Teacher On Call. But with these migraines, I can't even count on taking care of my boys and my house. I can't even tutor."

"Tell me again about the lights you see, the aura," I ask. "Is it always the same or does it change?"

"Mostly now they come in the night," she replies, "so I don't know about anything before I wake puking. But I used to see flashing lights off to the left of my eyeballs and have a weird feeling in my right hand. They looked for a brain injury cause and even for seizures, but my EEG and head CT scan were perfect!"

"I need to find out about the rest of your history. Then we'll come back to the migraines and figure out what to try," I say. "Have you ever been really sick, hospitalized, injured or broken a bone?"

"I cracked my head good and proper when I was kid. My sled smashed into a rock. But I was only out cold for a minute or two. Just scrambled my brains a bit." Alison chuckles.

I'm about to ask my next question when Alison leans towards me. "You're pretty smart, Dr. Madrona," she says. "It's good to have someone like you helping me through perimenopause. If I thought this would never end and there was nothing I could do but live through it, I'd get awfully discouraged right about now." She pauses for a moment, "It's a bit like a Newfoundland winter! It never seems to end!"

"I wouldn't blame you a bit for feeling blue, Alison!" I say. "But if we put our two heads together we should be able to come up with something that will at least help. Now, are there any illnesses that run in your family?"

"Yeah, being overweight and having diabetes and heart attacks," she says. "My sisters, my mom and all of my aunts and uncles are, let's say, 'heavy set,' and two of my mom's sisters have diabetes—the kind that needs pills, not shots. The only skinny one is my brother Bill, who smokes like a chimney and is always of a twitch."

"Who had the heart attacks?" I ask.

"My dad, when he was in his mid-sixties. He lived until the year after my wedding and his sixty-sixth year—saw my firstborn I named after him. And my Grandma May, but when she was old. They think that my oldest sister is having angina and diabetes. But I've been fine. I have a normal before-breakfast blood sugar—I got tested for that a while ago—but at the time I weighed a bunch less. My blood pressure is fine, and I've never smoked."

"That's good. Do you do some regular exercise?"

"I used to be a real sport, but I haven't done a thing since having my second son. Having two babies in nappies wore me out. I walk the two youngest boys to school and back. Johnny, my oldest, takes the bus to high school or gets a ride with Walter. I know I need to start exercising again."

"What was your weight at age 18?" I ask.

"I think I was 145 pounds then. All solid, you know. I'm pushing 170 now and most of it I've gained since these migraines started. It defies the law of thermodynamics that I can gain weight when I eat so little."

"Do you feel hungry?" I ask.

"Not most of the day, or until the migraine has settled, and that might not be until late evening. But then I'm ravenous," she says.

"For any particular kind of foods?" I ask.

"I'll eat a whole pie or a jar of jam on a pancake. And then, I'm up all night peeing. It seems it's the nights I've gone overboard on sweets I'm for sure likely to wake with a migraine." She grins ruefully.

"Like you, I developed migraines in perimenopause," I say. "Before that, I was a real sweet tooth. I don't know how I figured it out, but I put myself on a low-carb diet and swear that staying away from sweets has made my migraines better. So you may be right about a connection between a load of sugar and your migraines. At any rate, an exercise program and a sugar-free diet would definitely decrease your risk for diabetes (65;66)."

Alison sighs. "Would you refer me to a dietician who can teach me about nutrition and what foods to eat and not?" she asks. "I'm totally ignorant. Mom cooked whatever she had, like her mother before her. We just ate bread and cakes and scones and biscuits and potatoes at home."

"Sure," I say. "I'll refer you to one here at the General who is also into exercise. I know that you are nauseated sometimes and can't eat. But not eating for a long while and then eating is one of the reasons you're gaining weight."

Alison looks skeptical.

"Let me put it another way," I said. "When we go without food for more than overnight, it's as though our brain decides we're in a famine. Our metabolism shifts so that when we next eat, we pack it straight into fat. It's the body's smart way of saving up for hard times."

"Go on!" exclaims Alison. "How did they ever show that?"

"Well," I say, "it has actually been experimentally proven with littermate rats. Half of them were fed a pellet an hour. The other half had the same number of pellets in the day, but all at once, once a day. The ones that 'grazed' kept their weights steady, but their identical siblings that ate the same amount of calories once a day gained significantly."

"I guess I could try eating some yogurt or crackers or something every few hours", she says. "I don't feel hungry, but maybe it would help with 'Endless Appetite,' '*she who must be obeyed.*' who comes to visit about nine at night."

I laugh. "You've got a droll way of saying things, Alison! New topic—are you allergic to anything?"

"Vegetables! No, not really. I serve them because Walter thinks a meal isn't complete without some veggies or a salad, but I just didn't grow up with them. Unless potatoes count!" We both laugh.

"On a night without a migraine, how is your sleep?" I ask.

"I have the usual tossing and turning from about 3 a.m. onward. I sometimes get frustrated because I know I'm exhausted, yet I'm thrashing about and awake."

"How about falling asleep?" I ask.

"Usually that's fine. I'm asleep in a nanosecond. It's staying asleep that is the problem."

"How about coffee or tea or caffeinated pop?" I ask.

"I have a couple of good strong coffees when I finally feel like I won't vomit. And then I keep the pot on all day. It's about my only pleasure."

"Any alcohol?"

"I was a fair drinker," she says, "screech and all that, when I was in university, but Walter doesn't touch the stuff. If we were out, I used to like a glass of white wine. One sip and I was flushing. Two sips and I've got a migraine aura! Like I said, no pleasures except coffee."

"How old were you when your period started?"

"I was younger than 11—well, almost 11," she says. "I think my periods were pretty much a month apart, but no problem. I got acne and cramps when I was about 14 and was put on the Pill. I took it until I got married. After my third child, I had a tubal ligation."

"What ages were you when you had your three boys?" I ask.

"I was 33 with Johnny, 35 with James, and 40 with Richard. I nursed each of them as long as they wanted. Johnny demanded hardtack at six months! James nursed until he was four and Richard quit at about nine months."

"All so different," I say, smiling. "How much did they each weigh at birth?"

"Johnny was 8 lb 5 oz, James was 8 lb 11 oz, and Richard was early at 9 lb. Thank goodness he was impatient, or they'd have had to dynamite him out! I know, they're all pretty big. I had that gluggy glucose tolerance test in all three pregnancies and never had to be on insulin. Thank god!"

"Sounds as though you already know that, unless Walter is a giant, those high birth-weights suggest diabetes risk. In my experience those at risk often become insulin-resistant in perimenopause because of the high estrogen levels (82). Because insulin isn't working effectively, insulin levels go higher to compensate. In turn, higher insulin levels can make you crazy with hunger.

"I'll order another fasting blood sugar now and a test called 'Hemoglobin A1C' that can tell us about your blood sugar night and day over the past three months."

"Really? How does that work?" she asks.

"Every red blood cell contains hemoglobin, the oxygen-carrying part of blood," I answer. "The cells are made regularly, and each lives about three months before being recycled. If they are being made at a time when your blood sugar is high, like it would be after a big meal, a funny glucose molecule is stuck to the hemoglobin and stays with that red blood cell its whole life. The normal range for hemoglobin A1C, HbA1C for short, is 4–6 percent. I'll make a standing order for HbA1c so you can go to the lab every three months over the next two years. You'll get a copy of the test as will your family doctor."

"That's a good plan," says Alison. "So, as I start exercising and reducing my sugar, we can see some progress."

"If we have to, meaning if the HbA1c goes to about 6 percent in spite of your best efforts," I say, "there is a medication we can use that helps insulin work better."

"I'd rather do it without pills if I can, you know," says Alison firmly.

"Of course," I say. "And you probably can. There's now experimental evidence from two randomized controlled trials, one in Finland (65) and one in the USA (66) that exercise decreases the risk for developing frank diabetes in people like yourself who are at high risk."

"Have we missed anything important in your history, Alison?" I ask. She shakes her head.

"Ok, why don't you take everything off except your underpants, put on this gown and lie down." I pull the examining room curtain shut. "I'll look at your Diaries and copy these pages while you're changing. Lie quietly and relax so I can get a good blood pressure! I'll knock when I return."

~

A few minutes later, I enter the examining room. "Hi again. It's just me. You've kept an excellent Daily Perimenopause Diary and temperature record! I've got a math-whiz colleague. With your permission, I'd like to enter the data and then do time series analysis or whatever she thinks is appropriate, looking for relationships between the other variables and your migraines."

"Great," says Alison.

"You are relaxed, almost asleep!" I exclaim. "Your blood pressure is 124 over 86—that's excellent, especially given your difficult and early morning. I forgot to ask if you are regularly taking anything apart from your migraine medicines. Any supplements? Vitamins?"

"Yes," says Alison. "I take a multivitamin tablet that I began so I wouldn't have to take cod liver oil. And I've taken to having a dimenhydrinate at bedtime. It helps me sleep and I think it helps prevent migraines."

"That's not a bad idea," I say. "I've recommended that to several women. I take a long-acting old-fashioned antihistamine like that myself for allergies and sleep. Do you regularly check your breasts?"

"Yep, the months I don't forget or they're not too sore."

"Good, then you can tell me if this feels the same as always to you," I say as I grab Alison's left hand and guide it to an area below the nipple on her right breast.

"That's always a lumpy spot," she says.

"And it's the same as the other side," I say, "which makes it unlikely to be worrisome. Do you remember how long ago you first felt that kind of ridge along the undersides of your breasts?"

"I noticed that. I thought it was just because I was getting to be a busty-crusty! I think it began in the last few years . . ."

"I've associated that bottom breast ridge with insulin resistance, Alison, although I don't know why that occurs or whether or not it's a reliable sign. Just interesting. . ."

"I wonder if you can see that as a more dense area on a mammogram?" Alison asks. "I'll ask a neighbour of ours—a radiologist—to take a look at my last mammogram. Actually, I've had a mammogram every April since I turned 40. I know they've been developing the scanning techniques to digitize mammograms and accurately assess breast density. If mine turned out to show that the 'foothills' were more dense, we could randomly pick mammograms from women aged 45 to 50 in this province's Mammographic Screening Programme, digitize them all, and send everyone a questionnaire about family history of diabetes."

"That's a great idea, Alison," I say. "A study like that would be a start toward determining whether or not I'm right that the bottom breast ridge is associated with insulin resistance. Let me know what you find. Of course, even if we do plan a pilot study, we still have to find funding for it." I shake my head.

"Well, I've worked hard on the Breast Cancer Foundation Board for years," says Alison. "Let's just see what comes of this first look. Makes me wonder if breast cancer is related to insulin resistance. I know that increased breast density is a risk factor for breast cancer (83). So it always bugs me that they don't let us know that density result."

"Let's continue," I say. "Are you warmer or colder than other people?"

"I tend to be warm, but it's because I have so much blubber. Why do you ask?"

"Your thyroid gland is easy to feel and rather firm. Your skin and reflexes suggest it's still working fine, but I'll order a TSH level anyway."

"I forgot to tell you that another of my mom's sisters has to take a thyroid pill because her thyroid was under-active. She used to have a big goiter. It's better now."

"Ok," I say. "The rest of your examination is fine, except that you didn't tell me about your gall bladder surgery!"

"Sorry! I had that when I was 34. I got heartburn, bellyache and nausea during my first pregnancy, toughed it out, and had the surgery about three months after delivery. I've been fine since."

"One more thing to check," I say. "Before you get your slacks done up come here and let me measure your waist size. No, I'm not a dressmaker! This is another indicator of insulin resistance. For women, the upper limit of normal is 88 cm. Over that size is highly associated with increased abdominal visceral fat and with insulin resistance. Yours is 94 cm. The good news is that waist size decreases more quickly with exercise than does weight. Your waist will decrease with either exercise or a lower carbohydrate diet, even if your weight is unchanged."

"Cool! I'll measure my waist with my sewing tape when I get home. And then maybe once a week."

"Ok, get yourself dressed while I write down these numbers. Let's see, weight 79 kg, height 168.5 cm, gives a BMI of 28. You are a pretty big-boned woman and have broad shoulders, so a maximum BMI for you would probably be 26. That would be a weight of 73 kg or 161 pounds for your height."

When Alison has dressed and sits down, I begin reviewing with her. "So let's summarize. You have horrid migraines mostly at night—on average twice or three times a week. You are probably in Phase A or Phase B of perimenopause now, with short cycles, some cyclic night sweats, sleep trouble, and weight gain. Your family history and your examination suggest insulin resistance and risks for diabetes. And you have early heart disease in your family.

"We've already got a plan that you will increase your exercise to 30 minutes of walking a day, for a dietician to help you achieve a diabetic-type diet with more protein, and that you continue your nightly dimenhydrinate pills. For the migraines, I think it would be worth trying another prophylactic medicine, if you've not used it before, and that is gabapentin. It is a medicine that acts on the brain. It was originally used for a peculiar kind of seizures or for nerve pain from neuropathy. Its primary side effect is drowsiness, it may help hot flushes (84), and it's listed as a migraine prophylaxis. Let's start with a dose of 300 mg, a single capsule, at bedtime. After two weeks, take two, and after four weeks, increase the dose to three capsules or 900 mg at bedtime. Gabapentin can be given in much higher doses than that, but with your excellent record we should know in six weeks if it's helping. Meanwhile, I'll order a progesterone level during the week before you expect your period and analyze your basal temperature data with our least squares program (2)."

Alison is nodding and writing things down in her small, dog-eared spiral notebook. "And I'll let you know whether my mammogram showed high 'foothill' density or not," she says.

"Ok," I say. "Finally, if the gabapentin helps, but you are still getting more than one migraine a week—or if it doesn't help—I'd like you to start a full luteal phase dose of progesterone and take it daily. I usually prescribe progesterone only for 14 days a cycle while a woman in perimenopause is still having regular periods. But remember that your brain is likely to react to the hormone changes, even to the changes of a hormone like progesterone that doesn't cause migraines. I would be using progesterone to prevent migraines because it has calming effects on brain action (81;85). It is such a good and safe sedative that you can anesthetize a rat with it. In fact, progesterone increases breathing in contrast with most anesthetics and sleep medicines that suppress respiration. I'll prescribe Prometrium 100 mg three at bedtime daily. You can start it as soon as you've finished the six weeks of gabapentin. Progesterone will also take away your night sweats and make menstrual cramps better. Both night sweats and the high prostaglandin levels causing menstrual cramps can either cause migraines or make them worse."

I pause as Alison writes in her notebook. "Does that sound like a good plan?" I ask.

"What will happen with my periods?" she says.

"As long as your estrogen levels remain high," I say, writing out her prescriptions, "you'll continue to have a regular period about every month. Progesterone is counteracting the effects of estrogen on the endometrium, so flow will become lighter. I've known quite a few women, early in perimenopause like you, who continue to have regular cycles for several years on this dose. What counts is if it makes your migraines better."

"You're darn tootin'!" Alison exclaims.

"Like perimenopause itself," I say, "the migraines will improve as you get closer to menopause. And I hope, for you, like for me, they'll go away totally after you reach menopause."

"That'd suit me just fine!" she says.

"Here, I'll give you a Diary sheet so you can record these medications." I write 'gabapentin 300' on one line, and 'Prometrium 100' on the other. "Write down the number of pills that you take at the bottom of the column for each day," I ask. "Then we will have a clear record of whether or not they help."

I stand up and smile. "I'll see you again in six months. If something important changes, and it's not for the better, let me know, and I'll fit you in sooner. I'd also suggest going to see your family doctor in the next couple of weeks. By then he'll have your laboratory tests and my consult letter."

Alison stands up and shakes my hand. "Thanks for your help, Dr. Madrona," she says. "I thought I was fresh out of options. Now I am hanging on to new hope."

"Keep up the good work," I say as I return her handshake. "This too will pass."

About six months later, I look around the waiting area, spot Alison and call, "Whata ya at!"

Laughing, Alison joins me. "I'm glad to see you again—I feel like I'm visiting an old friend, not having a doctor visit. But," she pauses a moment, "you put the emPHAsis on the wrong syLABle! It's 'whata ya AT!'" she says.

"At least I tried! Whata ya AT, whata ya AT," I chant softly as I lead Alison to the exam room. Alison continues to chuckle.

"How are things with you?" I ask. "I must say, you look better, less 'puffy and peaked' as my grandma would say."

"I am better—see for yourself!" she exclaims. "I'm not sure if the gabapentin helped or not. But I *know* that the progesterone did. I sleep like a baby now and don't even wake to pee. And if I get a migraine once a month, that's lots."

"I'm so glad," I say. "It's hard because we're working in an area of medicine that has few randomized trials. And the physiology of the perimenopause is

## ALISON'S JUNE DIARY ON PROGESTERONE AND GABAPENTIN

Name: **Alison**     Month: **June**     Year: **2004**

| Cycle Day | 1 | 2 | 3 | 4 | 5 | 6 | 7 | 8 | 9 | 10 | 11 | 12 | 13 | 14 | 15 | 16 | 17 | 18 | 19 | 20 | 21 | 22 | 23 | 24 | 25 | 26 | 27 | 28 | 29 | 30 | 31 |
|---|---|---|---|---|---|---|---|---|---|---|---|---|---|---|---|---|---|---|---|---|---|---|---|---|---|---|---|---|---|---|---|
| Date | 5 | 6 | 7 | 8 | 9 | 10 | 11 | 12 | 13 | 14 | 15 | 16 | 17 | 18 | 19 | 20 | 21 | 22 | 23 | 24 | 25 | 26 | 27 | 28 | 29 | 30 | 1 | 2 | 3 | 4 | 5 |
| Tampons/pads/day | 2 | 1 | 0 | 0 | 0 | 0 | 0 | 0 | 0 | 0 | 0 | 0 | 0 | 0 | 0 | 0 | 0 | 0 | 0 | 0 | 0 | 0 | 0 | 0 | 0 | 0 | 0 | 0 | 0 | 0 | 0 |

Record 0 = none, 1 = minimal, 2 = moderate, 3 = moderately intense, 4 = very intense

| | | | | | | | | | | | | | | | | | | | | | | | | | | | | | | | |
|---|---|---|---|---|---|---|---|---|---|---|---|---|---|---|---|---|---|---|---|---|---|---|---|---|---|---|---|---|---|---|---|
| Amount flow | 1 | 1 | 1 | 0 | 0 | 0 | 0 | 0 | 0 | 0 | 0 | 0 | 0 | 0 | 0 | 0 | 0 | 0 | 0 | 0 | 0 | 0 | 0 | 0 | 0 | 0 | 0 | 0 | 0 | 0 | 0 |
| Cramps | 1 | 0 | 0 | 0 | 0 | 0 | 0 | 1 | 1 | 0 | 0 | 0 | 0 | 0 | 0 | 0 | 0 | 0 | 0 | 0 | 2 | 0 | 0 | 0 | 0 | 0 | 0 | 0 | 0 | 0 | 0 |
| Breast Sore: Side | 0 | 0 | 0 | 0 | 0 | 0 | 0 | 0 | 0 | 0 | 0 | 0 | 0 | 0 | 0 | 0 | 0 | 0 | 0 | 0 | 0 | 0 | 0 | 0 | 0 | 0 | 0 | 0 | 0 | 0 | 0 |
| Breast Sore: Front | 0 | 0 | 0 | 0 | 0 | 0 | 0 | 0 | 1 | 1 | 0 | 0 | 0 | 0 | 0 | 0 | 0 | 0 | 0 | 0 | 0 | 0 | 0 | 0 | 0 | 0 | 0 | 0 | 0 | 0 | 0 |
| Fluid Retention | 1 | 0 | 0 | 0 | 0 | 0 | 0 | 0 | 0 | 0 | 0 | 1 | 0 | 0 | 0 | 1 | 0 | 0 | 0 | 0 | 0 | 0 | 0 | 0 | 0 | 0 | 0 | 0 | 0 | 0 | 0 |
| Hot flushes - day | 0 | 1 | 0 | 0 | 0 | 0 | 0 | 0 | 0 | 0 | 0 | 1 | 0 | 0 | 0 | 0 | 0 | 0 | 0 | 0 | 0 | 0 | 0 | 0 | 0 | 0 | 0 | 0 | 0 | 0 | 0 |
| # of flushes - day | 0 | 2 | 0 | 0 | 0 | 0 | 0 | 0 | 0 | 0 | 2 | 0 | 0 | 0 | 0 | 0 | 0 | 0 | 0 | 0 | 0 | 0 | 0 | 0 | 0 | 0 | 0 | 0 | 0 | 0 | 0 |
| Hot flushes - night | 1 | 0 | 0 | 0 | 0 | 0 | 0 | 0 | 0 | 0 | 0 | 0 | 1 | 0 | 0 | 0 | 0 | 0 | 0 | 0 | 0 | 0 | 0 | 0 | 0 | 0 | 0 | 0 | 0 | 0 | 0 |
| # of flushes - night | 1 | 0 | 0 | 0 | 0 | 0 | 0 | 0 | 0 | 0 | 0 | 0 | 1 | 0 | 0 | 0 | 0 | 0 | 0 | 0 | 0 | 0 | 0 | 0 | 0 | 0 | 0 | 0 | 0 | 0 | 0 |
| Mucous Secretion | 0 | 0 | 0 | 0 | 0 | 0 | 1 | 1 | 0 | 0 | 0 | 0 | 0 | 0 | 0 | 0 | 0 | 0 | 0 | 0 | 0 | 0 | 0 | 0 | 0 | 0 | 0 | 0 | 0 | 2 | 2 |
| Constipation | 0 | 0 | 0 | 0 | 0 | 0 | 0 | 0 | 0 | 0 | 1 | 0 | 0 | 0 | 0 | 0 | 0 | 0 | 0 | 0 | 0 | 0 | 0 | 0 | 0 | 0 | 0 | 0 | 0 | 0 | 1 |
| Headache | 0 | 0 | 1 | 0 | 0 | 2 | 1 | 0 | 0 | 0 | 1 | 0 | 0 | 3 | 0 | 0 | 0 | 0 | 0 | 1 | 0 | 0 | 0 | 0 | 0 | 0 | 0 | 0 | 0 | 1 | 2 |
| Sleep Problems | 0 | 0 | 0 | 0 | 0 | 0 | 0 | 0 | 0 | 0 | 1 | 2 | 0 | 0 | 0 | 0 | 0 | 0 | 0 | 0 | 0 | 0 | 0 | 0 | 0 | 0 | 0 | 0 | 0 | 1 | 0 |
| Feeling Frustrated | 0 | 0 | 0 | 1 | 0 | 0 | 0 | 0 | 0 | 0 | 1 | 0 | 0 | 0 | 0 | 0 | 0 | 0 | 0 | 0 | 0 | 0 | 0 | 0 | 0 | 0 | 0 | 0 | 0 | 0 | 0 |
| Feeling Depressed | 0 | 0 | 0 | 0 | 0 | 0 | 0 | 0 | 0 | 0 | 0 | 0 | 0 | 0 | 0 | 1 | 0 | 0 | 0 | 0 | 0 | 0 | 0 | 0 | 0 | 0 | 0 | 0 | 0 | 0 | 0 |
| Feeling Anxious | 0 | 0 | 0 | 0 | 0 | 1 | 0 | 0 | 0 | 0 | 0 | 0 | 0 | 0 | 1 | 0 | 0 | 0 | 0 | 0 | 0 | 0 | 0 | 0 | 0 | 0 | 0 | 0 | 0 | 0 | 0 |

Record M = much less, L = a little less, U = usual, Y = a little increased, Z = much increased

| | | | | | | | | | | | | | | | | | | | | | | | | | | | | | | | |
|---|---|---|---|---|---|---|---|---|---|---|---|---|---|---|---|---|---|---|---|---|---|---|---|---|---|---|---|---|---|---|---|
| Appetite | Y | U | Y | U | U | Y | U | Y | U | U | U | Y | Y | U | U | U | Z | U | U | U | U | U | L | U | U | U | U | U | U | U | U |
| Breast Size | Y | U | U | U | U | U | U | U | U | | | | | | | | | | | | | | | | | | | | Y | | |
| Interest In Sex | L | L | L | U | U | L | L | L | U | U | L | L | U | L | L | L | U | L | L | L | L | L | U | U | U | Y | L | L | L | U | U |
| Feeling Of Energy | U | U | U | U | U | U | U | L | U | U | L | U | U | U | U | U | U | U | U | U | U | L | U | U | U | U | U | U | U |
| Feeling Of Self-Worth | L | L | Y | U | U | U | U | U | U | U | U | L | L | U | U | Y | U | U | U | U | U | U | U | U | U | Y | U | U | U |
| Outside Stresses | U | U | U | Y | Y | U | U | U | U | Y | U | Y | Y | U | U | U | U | U | U | U | U | U | U | U | Y | U | U | U | U | U |

| Treatment or Supplement | | | | | | | | | | | | | | | | | | | | | | | | | | | | | | | |
|---|---|---|---|---|---|---|---|---|---|---|---|---|---|---|---|---|---|---|---|---|---|---|---|---|---|---|---|---|---|---|---|
| Prometrium 100 | 3 | 3 | 3 | 3 | 3 | 3 | 3 | 3 | 3 | 3 | 3 | 3 | 3 | 3 | 3 | 3 | 3 | 3 | 3 | 3 | 3 | 3 | 3 | 3 | 3 | 3 | 3 | 3 | 3 | 3 | 3 |
| Gabapentin 300 | 2 | 2 | 2 | 2 | 2 | 2 | 2 | 2 | 2 | 2 | 2 | 2 | 2 | 1 | 1 | 1 | 1 | 1 | 1 | 1 | 0 | 0 | 0 | 0 | 0 | 0 | 0 | 0 | 0 | 0 | 0 |
| Basal Temperature Waist (inches) | 36 | | | | | | | | | | | | | | 35 | | | | | | | 35 | | | | | | | | 34 | |

| Comments (Temperature Taken Late, Feeling Sick, Poor Sleep, Etc.) | | | | | | | | | | | | | | | | | | | | | | | | | | | | | | | |
|---|---|---|---|---|---|---|---|---|---|---|---|---|---|---|---|---|---|---|---|---|---|---|---|---|---|---|---|---|---|---|---|
| | | | | | | | | | | | | | | | | | | | | | | | | | | | | | | | |

not well described. I'm working from Dr. Prior's big review (8) and stuff I've learned for myself and from my patients."

"I'm glad I found an 'old salt' like you!" Alison says.

"Old salt, am I? What do you mean by that?" I ask.

"I mean someone who's wise by living and learning. At home in New-foundland it means someone who has studied the waves, wind and weather and makes good sense of them. Yep, you're an old salt! And that's highest praise from a Newfoundlander!"

"Thanks, Alison," I say.

"You were dead right about my flow," Alison says. "I get it once a month, nice and light and regular. My breasts are rarely sore and they're less lumpy. That progesterone is the best thing since sliced bread!"

"Good," I say. "I was going to ask you about flow. I see from your Diary record your cramps are less and you aren't having night sweats—except here. Any idea why this bad patch, in late June?"

"Oh, that. I was going through interviewing and stuff to get back into teaching. I applied for a part-time job. It's hard because I've been out of it for about 13 years. I don't quite feel like I belong in the working world. Like I'm not good enough. It's silly, I know. It's like my head knows. But it's real, and stress enough to sweat me at night!"

"I know exactly what you mean," I agree. "I didn't feel like I was a real doctor any more when I got back into medicine again after only six months away caring for my firstborn baby."

"I doubt that men would have that feeling," she says thoughtfully. Then we both laugh.

"It looks like you've successfully lost some inches and some weight," I say. "Did low-carb work for you?"

"Yeah, I feel much better with a little more protein and less starch. And I do think that's also helping my migraines. We went out for dinner for my birthday and I had crème brulee for dessert. It was my very first dessert in months. Wouldn't you know it! I woke in the morning and had to cram down a handful of ibuprofen and dimenhydrinate."

"How are you doing with exercise?" I ask.

"Great! I've started having a good walk early in the morning. I usually go with a friend, someone I used to work with at school. I just got re-acquainted with her after my job interview. I'm using a pedometer that I got from one of my sons' cereal boxes. I'm now doing about 8,000–10,000 clicks, I guess it's steps, a day. I'm really doing about double that because of bicycling with my boys or taking them swimming in the summer."

Alison puts her hands on her waist. "By the way," she says. "I found it really helpful to measure my waist. I can see progress, without holding my breath!"

She twinkles a smile at me. "I don't know what it will show in centimetres, but I think I've lost about 2 inches."

"Good for you, Alison. I admire you for taking the suggestions I made and running with them. If there's one thing I've learned it's that a lot of health is how we think about it."

"What do you mean?" she asks.

"There are three different approaches we can take to our own health called Health Locus of Control. Each approach has a fancy name but a simple meaning. One of them is *Chance* Health Locus of Control. That means you believe it's just your bad luck if you get sick. Another is called *External* Health Locus of Control, meaning that what the doctor/teacher/preacher says is law. You have what's called *Internal* Health Locus of Control. That means you decide your health is up to you, and you do something about it (86). In fact, just *believing* that you can cope with hot flushes makes them significantly better (87). Any guesses about which attitude turns out to be the most healthy, with the longest life expectancy and the least illness?" I ask.

"I guess if you do what the doctor says," she says.

"Nope!" I exclaim. "The most healthy attitude is the kind you have, where you take what you read and what the doctor says and integrate it with what you know about yourself."

"Aren't I the clever one!" Alison laughs. "By the way, I looked at my mammograms with my doctor-neighbour. We found out that my breast density, all over, has been increasing over the last six years. Because of the way they squish the breast, they thought, but couldn't say for sure, that my breasts also got more dense in my 'foothills,' as I call them!"

"You mean that ridge at the bottom? You have the funniest way of saying things!" I laugh. "I'll have to remember that one!"

"I guess we now need to find some women without that inferior ridge, but who are also in perimenopause, and see whether their breasts on mammogram look similar to yours or different. If you give me your neighbour's name and phone number I'll give her a call." I stop and make a note on the back of my prescription pad. "I'll also review your mammograms with her. Perhaps we have another important research idea here, Alison!" I stop a moment. "I'm starting to feel like there are too many good ideas for me to explore in my whole life. That's why we started the Centre for Menstrual Cycle and Ovulation Research—so that we can work together to learn more and to help women."

"I've been to your website a couple of times," says Alison. "I'd even like to do some volunteering now that I'm feeling better."

"That would be good," I say. "We can always use extra hands. Now, let's finish your history. How are you now doing with coffee?"

"I've cut down to two or three cups a day," she replies. "I sure miss it, but I'm doing it!"

"Any alcohol at all?" I ask.

"Not a drop," she says. "It isn't worth the pain and suffering!"

"Ok, let's check you. Here's a gown. Except for loosening the waist, you can leave your shorts on. Lie down and relax. I'll be right back after copying your Diary pages."

~

I've finished examining Alison and we're both seated again. "Well," I say, "I'm happy with how you're doing. Your blood pressure is great at 126 over 84, and your weight is down to 77 kg, which makes your BMI 27. Your waist is now down to 88 cm or the upper limit of normal. I'm impressed!"

"I didn't work to lose weight," Alison says. "I just focused on exercise and making sure I had something small with protein in it to eat regularly. I always carry almonds with me—in a vitamin bottle!" She produces the brown scruffy looking bottle from her bag with a flourish. "And I never miss a day of exercise. It's become my favourite thing to do—a day isn't complete without it."

"Most people," I say, "especially those with insulin resistance, find it almost impossible to lose weight in perimenopause. So I'm really impressed that you've managed. Keep up your exercising and eating well! Although your fasting blood sugar was 5.8 and your HbA1C was 6.2 in February, your HbA1C came down to 5.4 in these last three months. We'll get a set of fasting lipids and a blood sugar before I next see you in another six months. Here's your prescription. I've refilled your progesterone at 300 mg every bedtime for a year. Do you think I should also refill the gabapentin?"

"I don't really know if it's helping. I've decreased it to two at bedtime, then to one and finally stopped it without noticing any difference. I don't want to be on anything I don't have to take."

"Ok," I say. "I'll just prescribe the Prometrium. Ok, let's make another appointment for six months from now."

"I forgot. We, the gang of us that met for that seminar back almost a year ago, would like to have a get-together to see how we all are doing and stuff. We'll do a potluck supper on a Saturday night in February. We'd really like you to come. Would you?"

"I'll have to see, Alison. Sometimes I feel pulled so many ways that when I have a weekend free, all I want to do is curl up with a book and listen to a Bach fugue. But it would be fun to see all of you and the others in a social rather than a medical setting. Let Lana know the date, time and place."

"You don't have to do anything or bring anything," Alison says. "Just come. We want to have you, Dr. Madrona. We all owe you so much."

# 10

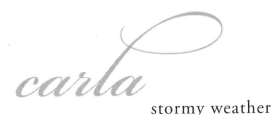

*carla*

stormy weather

"Hi, Carla. I didn't realize it'd be almost a year before we met again. How are you doing?"

"I'm just barely hanging in, Doc. If it's not the sweats, it's the moods. I can't notice any improvement either since my doctor gave me that progesterone like you suggested."

"So what are you taking now, Carla?"

"I've got that candy-coated reddish purple estrogen pill again," she says.

"That's Premarin—the 0.625-mg one, right?" I ask.

"Yeah, I stopped it after the group, cold turkey," she says. "What you said about my own estrogen being too high made sense. Bad idea! If I thought night sweats were awful, they doubled and started coming all day too. I had a really rough time, Doc. So I went back on that estrogen. Then I saw my doctor and he reluctantly gave me that little peach progesterone pill."

"The 2.5-mg medroxyprogesterone pill."

Carla nods. "Since that, even though I went to your website and know how to stop estrogen, I'm chicken to try going off it again."

"Did you do any diary-keeping?" I ask.

"I forgot. I can't remember shit," she says.

"That's ok. Let's start with your history. If I remember right, you had a hysterectomy because of heavy bleeding, but you kept your ovaries. Then you got night sweats and your doctor started you on Premarin 0.625. When we met in that group session, you were feeling very angry plus you had night sweats in spite of being on full-dose estrogen. Did I get that right?"

"Yep," says Carla. "You left out the bit where my partner, Jane, threatens to leave me every other day, and I can't remember my name. I stand in the middle of the room, wondering what I'm doing there. They chopped my uterus out when I was 43. My periods had gotten closer and closer together until I had fulltime flow. My crotch got chapped from soaked pads. They tried me on the Pill, but that made my moods worse and didn't touch the flow. I thought, like a fool, that if I had my uterus out I could skip perimenopause!"

"Not a chance!" I say. "How old are you now, Carla?"

"I'm 45 going on 70. I remind myself of my great Aunt Edna—off my rocker and crotchety."

"Skipping perimenopause is not something any of us can do," I say, "although a few women hardly notice anything. You and I are in the 10–20 percent who have a really rough time of it. But we'll figure this out and get you feeling better soon. I'd hoped your doctor would follow my suggestion and give you a large enough dose of progesterone or progestin to take care of the hot flushes so you could go onto a half-strength green estrogen pill." I take a deep breath. "What you're on is too little progestin and more than plenty of estrogen."

"Why do doctors dish out estrogen like the elixir of life and seem scared of progesterone?" Carla demanded.

"I don't really know, Carla. But I know, since the Women's Health Initiative randomized, controlled trial results, that Premarin with low-dose progestin, in exactly the same doses and kinds of pills you are taking, causes serious problems like breast cancer, blood clots, strokes, dementia and heart attacks (23;27;88)."

"Oh, god. What was my doctor thinking?" She pauses momentarily. "Maybe he wasn't!"

"Doctors, like most of us, get into habits, I'm afraid," I say. "So, back to you. I use progesterone to help women stop estrogen because it is as good for hot-flush control as estrogen. I believe that because of a randomized double-blind study Dr. Prior did (75) comparing Premarin with full-dose medroxy-progesterone at 10 mg per day. That study was in menstruating women and began just after they became surgically menopausal with removal of their uterus and ovaries. However, most doctors never learned or don't know about the effectiveness of progestins for hot flushes (74;89).

"The other reason I want you to have natural progesterone is that oral micronized progesterone doesn't have any bad effects and it has a really great side-effect—it helps sleep (81). When you are sleeping better and are less stressed by the flushes, your memory will return to normal, and your aches and pains will go away."

"Bring it on, Doc!" says Carla. "I could use a little sleep. All I know is that nothing changed with that peach pill I'm taking."

"No wonder!" I say. "It's a baby dose. You need a *full* dose of progesterone."

"I think not sleeping is the worst. I'm so tired. I fall asleep pronto. Then I wake. If I'm not worrying about whether I can make ends meet, and whether Jane really means it about leaving me, I'm soaking the bed and wiggling."

I nod. "I know what you mean. Progesterone's been a lifesaver for me. Now, tell me where you grew up and what you do."

"I grew up in Campbell River. My dad was a fisherman until they made him sell his license to save the salmon. I'm now in Victoria. I've batted from deck hand to shelf-stocker to corner-store clerk. But what I really like is computers and the computer courses at Camosun College. Right now I'm still learning and fiddling. I've been helping in a sort of a fly-by-night computer-repair place. What I'd like to do, if I can get my act together, is start my own computer shop. I'd mostly repair, sell parts and fix up and sell older computers, maybe even teach grannies to use 'em for email. I like teaching. I even got my 73-year-old landlady to be a fair hand at her little PC."

"How are you and Jane managing financially?" I ask.

"She's got a regular job at a daycare, and her benefits include some prescription medicines. Plus she earns extra by gardening for other people. She loves mucking in the dirt. I'm not earning much now, but we've got what we've saved and her pay stub. We do ok."

"How old were you when you had your first period?" I ask.

"I was finishing Grade 7, so I was 12, I think. It was just a bother. I never really had much trouble, but I knew from day one that my periods were simply a nuisance. I never did have any plans to have a passel of kids and settle down with Mr. Right. I went on the birth control pill when the doc and my mom thought I'd get pregnant. I felt ok and just took it. One time I went moose hunting in the fall with a bunch of my buddies. I knew that the bears were busy, and I didn't want them sniffing me out. So I just kept taking the Pill to avoid my period." She laughs. "Now that's all the rage. The CNN website reported a few years ago that you could take the Pill every day for three months at a time. I was fine with four instead of 14 periods a year. My doctor wasn't too happy, but refilled the Pill and I just took it. When we moved to Victoria, I didn't tell my new doctor what I'd been doing. I think I went because my breast was really sore. My new doc got upset. She said we didn't really know the results of daily Pill schedules (90) and that I was over 40 so I should stop the Pill. It wasn't too long after that when the really heavy flow started. You know the rest of the story."

"So you were never pregnant," I say. She nods. "And did you ever have a serious illness, hospitalization, broken bone, or injury?"

"When I worked for Dad on his seiner, I barked my ankle on a gaff and ended up with blood poisoning. We had a load of fish to take in, so it was a day or two before the health nurse in Alert Bay gave me a big shot in the bum. I still ended up with a red streak up my leg and a wicked fever. It took a week in the hospital with intravenous to get rid of that infection. I also fell off a shed when I was 11 and broke my leg." She points just above her ankle. "Crazy kid," she mutters, shaking her head. "I never could turn down a dare!"

"Ok," I say. "Are there any health problems that run in your family, Carla? Like TB, diabetes, heart attacks, cancers?"

"Mom's older brother died of lung cancer," she replies. "Consequently she was dead set against smoking and finally got Dad to quit when I was a kid. Mom died, I think, from bleeding too much after she had my brother, but don't think that's something I could inherit. I was in Grade 8." She pauses a minute, then starts again. "Dad's still got bad lungs—he says it's from quitting smoking! He's hacking up stuff all winter, but he never sees a doctor. Grandpa Earl died in a logging accident. And Dad's dad was drowned somewhere off the Charlottes."

"That's where I grew up—I know about rough seas up there."

"I don't think my grannies," Carla continues after nodding, "who died in their eighties, had anything except old age and too many babies.

Carla pauses again. "However, homophobia runs in my family, and it's a contagious disease up-island!" She looks away, and then looks back at me again.

"Does your family know about you and Jane?" I ask gently.

"Naw!" she says. "They live their lives and I live mine. I was close to Mom, but not to Dad or my brothers. They sort of know—I guess they just want to think we're roommates."

"Fair enough," I say. "But it's hard if family doesn't know who's really important in your life. How are your brothers and sisters?"

"I have a kid brother 13 years younger than me who's running a bunch of city folks out fishing and growing pot on the side, and two older brothers I hardly know. One moved to Port Hardy when I was in grade school and the other to Kelowna. They wanted to get as far away from Dad as possible."

"I'm sorry that you lost your mom, Carla. You must have had a lot of work taking care of your baby brother."

"I don't often think about Mom," Carla says, "but if I smell bread fresh out of the oven, I want to cry."

"That is hard. It's rough to lose someone like your mom when you're in your teens. That and other old sadness tend to surface during perimenopause (41). As far as you know, are your brothers and dad well?"

"The boys, they are the wild type, always boozing and bragging. I'm not sure they've settled down yet. If the smokes don't do them in, the liquor will."

"What about *you* and cigarettes and alcohol?" I ask.

"I used to booze," she says, "and I was bumming smokes from the time I was ten, but I wheezed and coughed. I think I'm allergic. And I know Mom would be happy I don't smoke. I quit drinking for the first few years after I met Jane. She rarely has any. Sometimes now I'll have a beer on the weekends."

"Besides cigarettes, are you allergic to anything else?" I ask.

"I got the yellow jaundice when I was about six. My neck was all swollen, it hurt to swallow, and I was given some kind of antibiotic. I think they figured it wasn't allergy when several other kids got hepatitis."

"As far as you know your liver's fine now?"

"Yes," she says. "I don't think anyone but you has asked! Doctors today give you five minutes, including walking from the door to a chair and out the door again. I hardly know Dr. Hall, so I rarely ever go. He was Jane's doctor and had room, so I see him if I have to."

"It sounds like you were pretty active as a kid," I say. "What about now? What exercise do you regularly do?"

"I ride my bike, rain or shine, because we can't afford a car. Jane and I play softball in the spring with a zany team. I'm a pretty damn good shortstop and can hit it out of the park if I have an aluminum bat. Plus I like curling. I learned in Kamloops in college. Then it was mostly an excuse to get together and party. But I always watch it on TV. I like it, and am trying to get Jane to have a go."

"What did you weigh when you were 18?" I ask.

Carla shifts in her chair. "I was a pretty hefty one already, but it was mostly muscle from the work I did. I must have been 150 pounds, easy. Now I've been gaining, starting maybe five years ago when I went on that everyday Pill. I'm probably over 180 now. Everyone in my family is—let's be 'politically correct'—stocky!

"Speaking of weight—I can't face food in the mornings. It takes three or four coffees to get me going. But by about two in the afternoon I'm so crazy hungry I could eat a hard drive. Plus after dinner I need more coffee and something to eat to keep me awake because I'm not sleeping worth shit. Ok, well, all the more of me for Jane to love!"

I shake my head. "It sounds like you're drinking six or more cups of coffee a day. That's a lot, Carla. And it can make you more irritable and also more hungry. But, like estrogen, don't decrease your coffee intake suddenly or you'll get withdrawal—stopping caffeine quickly causes wicked headaches!"

"You think I should cut down, eh? That and milk is all I drink. I have at least a litre of milk a day."

"That's good," I say. "You're probably getting enough calcium. If you can get down to two or three coffees in the morning, that'd be fine. Anyway, you won't need it soon when you're sleeping better."

"I hope you're right," says Carla.

"Do you regularly check your breasts?" I ask.

"Nope. Never pay them any mind. Never had a mammogram either. And Dr. Hall doesn't ask, so I don't think I've ever had a Pap test. Not that I'd like his paw up there anyway."

"Have you ever been sexually active with men, Carla?" She shakes her head. "Then you need a Pap far less than the rest of us. The virus that causes cervical cancer is primarily passed by heterosexual sex. Although your risks for breast cancer are decreased because of your hysterectomy (18), you should learn to check your own breasts. No doctor can remember what a woman's breasts feel like from one year to the next. And it's *change* that's the clue to breast cancer. So you are the only one who can spot a change, and that's only if you are checking them yourself, every month."

"I'll get Jane to do it!" Carla laughs. I feel like she's trying to make me uncomfortable.

"Well you can get Jane's help," I parry, "but she'll be doing well to remember to check her own breasts!" I smile and go on. "I'll remind you how to check your breasts when I'm examining you. Now," I say, glancing at her record, "are you taking anything else besides the 0.625 Premarin and the 2.5 mg very low-dose medroxyprogesterone?"

"I take a handful of aspirins a couple of times a day," she replies. "I'm stiff and sore a lot—I walk on pilings, like poles on docks, when I first get up. We buy the cheap aspirin in big bottles. I probably eat four to eight a day."

"That's a lot. Ever get heartburn?" I ask.

"Yeah," she says. "Most mornings my little guts are arguing with my big guts. Not good, eh? Black-coffee-and-aspirin for breakie. I guess I'll have to add a little food to that."

"Good idea," I say, smiling. "At least drink a glass of milk. Ok, Carla, I've run out of questions. I'll examine you now. Please change into this gown. Take everything off but your underpants, lie down there, and try to relax." I pull the curtain shut behind me.

~

A short while later, I return to find Carla sitting and staring at the curtain. "Oh, you're not relaxing!" I say.

"Did you tell me to lie down? Sorry," she says, and lies back.

I check Carla's reflexes and listen to her heart before putting on the blood pressure cuff.

"Your blood pressure's on the high side, Carla, at 152 over 96. I'll check it again before I finish.

You've got a normal-sized liver," I say after percussing the upper border. I feel under Carla's rib cage on the right side. "Is that tender? No? That's good. And your spleen's ok. When you haven't had too much coffee and aspirin do you ever feel nauseated?"

"Sometimes, in the mornings," she replies.

"I'll check your liver tests, because either leftover effects from hepatitis or high estrogen levels can cause nausea."

I begin to check Carla's breasts; I try to keep my face neutral even though I feel alarmed. "I'm worried, Carla. Your breasts are so firm they're almost woody. And there's a lump here." I'm feeling high on the left breast under her arm. "I wish you had checked them before so you could tell me if it was always like that. Is it sore?"

"Nope."

"Here, feel this," I say taking her right hand. "Do you feel something like a marble under there? It moves around, so it's probably a cyst. To check your own breasts, you need to lie down, like you are now, with your arms up over your head. Use your opposite hand to check each breast. Then just walk your fingers around the outermost part and make smaller and smaller circles until you are under the nipple and have felt your whole breast. Because you've had a hysterectomy, you can remember to do it by using,"—I glance at her chart—"the thirteenth, your birthdate, every month."

"That's not too hard," Carla says. "Could you do my Pap for me?"

As I check Carla's blood pressure again, I say, "Ok, I will, but I don't usually do pelvic exams because I don't want to seem to be taking work away from family doctors. Paps are something that family doctors are supposed to do."

"Thanks so much for doing it. I don't know," she pauses, "I'm just funny about a male doctor and a pelvic. And I've never told a doctor—except you, now—about Jane and me. I don't trust them, I guess."

I put the stirrups into the exam table and warm a speculum as I ask Carla to take off her underpants and move her bottom to the end of the table. "Everything looks and feels fine here, Carla. If this Pap test turns out perfect, you won't need another one, ever. Unless you suddenly switch kinds of partner."

"No chance of that!" she says.

"We're about done," I say. "Let's get your weight and height. Your guess on your weight was close: 81.4 kg, which is 179 lb, and your height is 167.6, or 5 feet, 6 inches. Does that sound right to you? You are muscular with a normal waist circumference so I think that your BMI of 29 is only a bit high. If you keep up your activity and start eating regularly and sleep better, you'll lose a little weight. Go ahead and get dressed while I write stuff down."

As she sits down, Carla shrugs. "I don't care about weight anyway," she says as she finishes throwing on her shirt and buttoning her jeans. "I just want to get out of this damned stormy weather."

As we're both sitting in our chairs again, I look at this sturdy energetic woman in front of me and reach out to take her hand, noticing that it feels cold. "You've not had it easy, Carla. But in spite of everything, you're making something for yourself," I say as I let go of her hand.

Carla looks as if she could cry. Instead she says, "Most of the kids in my computer classes are sappy guys. But computers can really help women. I'd like to start some kind of computer network for women. Get information to them. Help them not feel scared of bytes and software and modems."

I lean back in my chair. "That's a great idea," I say. "For a start, you can let women know about the Centre for Menstrual Cycle and Ovulation Research website—www.cemcor.ubc.ca—we've been putting things there that we've learned over the years. I think the Internet is a great way to share information. And with your business, let me know when you start it. I'll certainly send any Victoria folks I know your way for computer repairs.

"Now, let's get a plan going to help you feel better. Remember that you are in perimenopause even though your periods have gone away with the hysterectomy. It was probably higher estrogen levels that were not suppressed by the Pill that originally took you to the doctor with a sore breast. That was also why you bled heavily, and you probably rarely ovulated normally given all the rough things in your life (79). Maybe that continuous birth-control pill contributed. We really don't know it's long-term effects."

"I just thought—well—guess I didn't think," Carla says. "I only wanted to get rid of periods."

"Because your ovaries are still making high estrogen levels, that extra estrogen in the Premarin pill you're taking is too much. That's why you're feeling so stressed (91). Did you know that high estrogen amplifies your stress hormone responses to stressful things? Believe it or not, that was shown in a wacky randomized controlled experiment in young men. Half of them wore an estrogen patch and half wore a placebo patch. Each came back a couple of days later for a stress test in which they spoke in front of a group and had to do math out loud with an audience! Before, during, and after that stress test, hormones were measured—stress hormones like cortisol and norepinephrine went up in all the men, but went up significantly more in the men wearing the estrogen patch (91)."

"Way out!" laughs Carla. "Serves them right—now they know how we feel on estrogen!"

"It's the estrogen magnification of your stress hormones that is making your hands cold and your blood pressure a bit high, "I say. "By the way, your blood pressure came down to 142 over 96 when I took it a second time. That is still on the high side.

"Anyway, back to estrogen. Although estrogen treatment is good for hot flushes after menopause, there aren't any randomized trials showing it helps during *perimenopause*. And since the big USA studies showed a doubling of clots in women on estrogen pills, I will never again prescribe estrogen in the form of a pill. If, and when, someone needs estrogen, I only give it as a gel, a patch, or a cream that's less likely to cause blood clots (92). But you don't need any extra estrogen—your perimenopausal ovaries are cranking out plenty. Instead, I think progesterone, the hormone that's in short supply in perimenopause, is the right treatment for you."

"How will I know when I become menopausal?" Carla asks. "I can't wait!"

"That's a good question," I say. "The best way I know is for you to keep that Daily Perimenopause Diary. When you've been a year without any bloating, breast tenderness, or mood swings, you will be menopausal."

"Sure, I'll try to keep that Diary. I could put it on my computer notebook. I'll computerize it and send you a copy you can give to other women who want to complete it on a computer. If you wanted to make a discussion section on your website, you could ask women for their code, and you wouldn't have to enter Diary data before you could analyze it." Carla takes a hand-held computer out of her bag and makes a couple of entries.

"That would be great," I say. "Good idea! Now—I'd like to review a few things. You need to check your breasts every month, decrease your coffee to two or three cups a day, and continue your good bicycling exercise—make sure you get 30 minutes a day of something active. I'll give you the phone information to set up an appointment at the Breast Screening Centre nearest and most convenient for you. Just ask for routine screening. Otherwise you'll get the diagnostic mammogram that has triple the amount of radiation. Ask the centre to send a copy of the results to me as well as to Dr. Hall."

I watch as Carla clicks away, taking notes, then I continue. "You're going to have a mug of milk after your first cup of coffee in the mornings. I think that the heartburn will go away as you decrease coffee, and when you're sleeping better you won't be needing so much aspirin. I'll bet that morning stiffness goes away when you are sleeping better and are off estrogen. Start putting some decaf with the regular coffee after your second cup, Carla, and you'll get used to less caffeine more gradually.

"Now, about your Pap. I'll confess to Dr. Hall that I did it for you. I'll leave it up to you to tell him about your partner."

"Thanks a lot for doing my pelvic and Pap, Dr. Prior," Carla says. "I've known for a while I should have one, but tough old me would rather duck than face it."

"Don't tell anyone else or they'll all be demanding it!" I exclaim. "Most women, I think, would rather have a pelvic exam done by a woman. I remember coming back from my six-weeks check-up after my daughter was born. The gynecologist was patronizing, didn't listen, and literally patted me on the bum. I vowed then that I'd never let a man have anything to do with my female parts. My husband accused me of being sexist! Fancy he'd like a woman urologist poking tubes into him?" We both laugh.

"Ok," I say, "let's get a plan for treatment of those night sweats. I want you to stay on what you're taking right now for the next two weeks while you start your Diary record. That way, we'll get a good sort of baseline. Then I'll prescribe full-dose Prometrium that I want you to take every night before you go to bed. That will treat the night sweats and hot flushes. Plus your breasts will become softer. Progesterone looks like beige, salmon-egg-sized balls and you need to take three at bedtime. Do you have lots of your Premarin pills left?"

Carla shakes her head.

"No? That's good," I say. "I'd like to switch you to a gel form of estrogen called Estragel. Look, here's the estrogen gel—you need to rub it over a large area of skin, anywhere except your face or breasts. It smells like alcohol and evaporates quickly. Alternately, here's an estradiol patch called Estradot that you have to change twice a week. Which would you prefer?" I ask.

"I like the gel—it's clean and tidy," says Carla. "I'd worry about the patch falling off."

"That's fine. As I mentioned earlier, since the results of the Women's Health Initiative (23;27), there is no way I'll prescribe estrogen as pills. It caused a 211 percent increase in the risk for blood clots compared with healthy women on placebo. That's just too risky. Although estrogen itself causes an increased risk for clots, *pill* estrogen is worse because it is absorbed through the intestines, goes to the liver, and instructs the liver to make extra clotting proteins. We don't know for sure, but it looks like estrogen delivered through the skin is less likely to cause blood clots (92).

"You've been to the Centre for Menstrual Cycle and Ovulation Research website, right? Please go back again and look at the 'Stopping Estrogen Therapy' article—it's in the menopause section, I think. A single pump of Estragel each day is about the same dose as your Premarin pill. Follow the instructions on the website about gradually decreasing the amount of estrogen. The idea is that it will take about three or maybe as many as six months to stop estrogen therapy completely. You will be decreasing it by about 10 percent every two weeks."

"What do I do about the little progestin pills?" Carla asks.

"I'd also like you to take two of your medroxyprogesterone pills in the morning every day until they are gone. They will also help with the night sweats." I hold out a lab slip.

"Here's a lab slip," I say. "I've ordered a blood count, a fasting blood sugar, a couple of liver tests and a test for hepatitis. It's important to know what kind of hepatitis you had. Some kinds can continue to be active. I think your stiffness is just perimenopause, poor sleep, and high estrogen levels, but I've also ordered an ESR, which is an old-fashioned test to see whether you have any kind of arthritis."

"Can I get that test now?" Carla asks.

"No, it's better to get it when you're back home," I say. "Besides, you need to go first thing in the morning before breakfast and have had nothing to eat or drink from dinner the night before. I want to make sure that your extra hungriness in the afternoon is not early diabetes. I don't think so. You will get a copy of those test results as will your family doctor. It's also a good idea to go see him in a few weeks and get your blood pressure checked. By then he should have gotten my letter. I'll say that you are in the early phases of perimenopause and have very high estrogen levels. I'm telling him that you have severe night sweats and that you have excess endogenous estrogen because of perimeno-pause plus the estrogen pill therapy. I'll also write that you have severe sleep disturbance, multiple joint and muscle aches, and caffeine excess."

"Whew!" says Carla. "That'll be some letter!"

"Do you have any questions?" I ask. "We're almost finished for today."

"Can I bring Jane next time?" Carla asks. "She's younger than me, and I'd like her to know what's going on. I'm sure she would like to start learning what's ahead."

"That'd be great, Carla. You can support each other. Remember that it may take you many months to successfully stop the estrogen. After that, there will continue to be unexpected perimenopausal changes for a number of years before you're home free."

"I got it," Carla says.

"I'd like to see you in six months," I say. "If, when you're completely off the estrogen, you're still having night sweats, let me know. We can increase the dose of the Prometrium to four or five capsules a night. I'll let Dr. Hall know that also—but he's unlikely to feel comfortable prescribing that high a dose. By the way, I almost forgot to tell you. If you are strapped financially—Prometrium is expensive—a 100-mg capsule costs about seventy cents so the total is over two dollars a day. If you need something cheaper, you could use high dose medroxyprogesterone—that's a white pill—10 mg in the morning and 10 mg at night. I already wrote that as an alternate to Prometrium on your prescription. Just tell your pharmacist which you prefer. Or, there are compounding pharmacists in Victoria that will make a 300-mg capsule of oral micronized progesterone in oil for one dollar a day. Here's a start with a sample of 28 Prometrium pills."

"Thanks, Doc," she says. "I want to ask—are you, yourself, really taking Prometrium?"

"Yes," I reply. "I am a few years after menopause, but still having night sweats and hot flushes. And when they're not controlled, I get migraines again. I know my flushes get worse the more stressed I am, like now when I'm behind! So I still need to take three every night!"

"I've never had a doctor I could talk to and that knew, you know, what I meant. Thanks again."

"You're welcome, Carla," I say. "You've done a lot to help yourself be well. Mine is just a small part. See you in six months!"

A little over six months later, I meet Carla in the waiting room.

"Hi, Carla. How are you?"

"I'm great, Doc. This is my partner, Jane."

"Good to meet you, Jane. I'm glad you came." We settle into our chairs in the small exam room. "Now, Carla, tell me what you've learned."

"I learned that I too can survive perimenopause!" she says, and we all laugh. "And, we just started this website called 'Growing Girls' that has video clips, pictures and written instructions for learning to use the computer. Jane was a fantastic help—with her background in teaching. And we're just getting our computer repair business going."

"You forgot the most important thing—you're no longer a bitch!" Jane says.

"Sounds like you, Carla, and the two of you, are doing great!" I say, grinning at Jane. "When did you finally get off that estrogen, Carla?"

"I decreased the amount of that gel I pumped out until I was on just a sniff," she says. "I guess it's been about two months since I took any."

"I gather that the hot flushes are better, too," I say, and she nods. "You look good on paper, Carla. Your mammogram came back as multinodular and cystic, but that will improve on progesterone. Your fasting blood sugar was quite normal at 4.3, your blood count was great, and your liver tests were fine. It looks as though you probably had Hepatitis A when you were a kid.

That's a kind that spreads through whole communities and doesn't usually cause problems later."

"Great," says Carla. "I feel better than I have for years. I even told Dr. Hall that Jane was my partner. He seemed ok with it, but said he wouldn't put it in my chart, just in case."

"Just in case what? I hope he put Jane as your next of kin."

"I didn't think of that," she says. "I'll be sure he does."

"Let's see what your Diary shows," I say.

"Jane remembered, just before we left early this morning, and printed them out. We had to race to catch the ferry! If you'd like it on diskette, I've got that too."

Carla hands me the papers, and I spread them on the desk so that we can all see them.

"Thanks, yes, I'd be happy to have both," I say. "Looks like the Premarin was just as awful for you as it sounded. Frustration, depression and some anxiety all the time, plus fluid retention, sore breasts and low energy.

"Look, even though you took the Premarin regularly, the Diary shows variability from day to day, suggesting both changes in your stress and the effects of your own variable estrogen production."

"I don't understand—I thought hot flushes meant low estrogen. . ." Jane interrupts.

"Most people, doctors included, explain hot flushes as the perfect example of 'estrogen deficiency.' But it's really clear that hot flushes start in perimenopause in women with regular periods (16) who couldn't possibly have low estrogen levels. In fact about 50-70 percent of perimenopausal women have hot flushes during the last year or two of perimenopause—that's nearly as high a percentage as in menopausal women. That says to me that it can't be low estrogen causing them. After all, men and kids have low estrogen levels and don't get flushes. Right?"

"So what does cause them, Doc?" Carla asks. "I never really thought about it before."

"Hot flushes originate in the deep and essential hypothalamus part of the brain. So if anyone says, 'It's all in your head!' you tell them, 'You're darned tooting it is!' Carla and Jane grin.

"For hot flushes to occur," I continue, "I think that it is necessary that the hypothalamus has gotten used to higher estrogen levels. Then when estrogen levels drop, either to normal or to low levels, the brain reacts. The best thing

I can liken it to is drug withdrawal. The heroin addict who doesn't have a fix gets irritable and anxious. He sweats, feels sick, his heart races. And all of those symptoms are caused by the same set of hormones released when a woman has a hot flush."

## CARLA'S DIARY OF STOPPING ESTROGEN

**Name: CARLA**     Month: _____     Year: _____

| Cycle Day | 1 | 2 | 3 | 4 | 5 | 6 | 7 | 8 | 9 | 10 | 11 | 12 | 13 | 14 | 15 | 16 | 17 | 18 | 19 | 20 | 21 | 22 | 23 | 24 | 25 | 26 | 27 | 28 | 29 | 30 | 31 |
|---|---|---|---|---|---|---|---|---|---|---|---|---|---|---|---|---|---|---|---|---|---|---|---|---|---|---|---|---|---|---|---|
| Date | 11 | 12 | 13 | 14 | 15 | 16 | 17 | 18 | 19 | 20 | 21 | 22 | 23 | 24 | 25 | 26 | 27 | 28 | 29 | 30 | 1 | 2 | 3 | 4 | 5 | 6 | 7 | 8 | 9 | 10 | 11 |
| Tampons/pads/day | hysterectomy---------------------------------------------------------------------------------------------------- | | | | | | | | | | | | | | | | | | | | | | | | | | | | | | |

Record  0 = none, 1 = minimal, 2 = moderate, 3 = moderately intense, 4 = very intense

| | 1 | 2 | 3 | 4 | 5 | 6 | 7 | 8 | 9 | 10 | 11 | 12 | 13 | 14 | 15 | 16 | 17 | 18 | 19 | 20 | 21 | 22 | 23 | 24 | 25 | 26 | 27 | 28 | 29 | 30 | 31 |
|---|---|---|---|---|---|---|---|---|---|---|---|---|---|---|---|---|---|---|---|---|---|---|---|---|---|---|---|---|---|---|---|
| Amount flow | NONE | | | | | | | | | | | | | | | | | | | | | | | | | | | | | | |
| Cramps | NONE | | | | | | | | | | | | | | | | | | | | | | | | | | | | | | |
| Breast Sore: Side | 2 | 2 | 1 | 0 | 0 | 0 | 1 | 0 | 0 | 0 | 0 | 0 | 0 | 0 | 1 | 0 | 1 | 0 | 0 | 0 | 0 | 0 | 0 | 0 | 0 | 0 | 0 | 0 | 0 | 0 | 0 |
| Breast Sore: Front | 3 | 2 | 1 | 1 | 1 | 1 | 1 | 0 | 1 | 1 | 1 | 1 | 1 | 1 | 2 | 1 | 1 | 1 | 2 | 0 | 0 | 0 | 0 | 0 | 0 | 0 | 0 | 0 | 0 | 0 | 0 |
| Fluid Retention | 3 | 2 | 3 | 2 | 2 | 3 | 1 | 1 | 2 | 2 | 3 | 2 | 3 | 2 | 2 | 3 | 2 | 1 | 1 | 1 | 0 | 1 | 1 | 1 | 2 | 1 | 1 | 1 | 1 | 1 | 0 |
| Hot flushes - day | 2 | 2 | 2 | 1 | 2 | 2 | 3 | 2 | 2 | 1 | 1 | 2 | 1 | 3 | 1 | 0 | 0 | 1 | 2 | 0 | 0 | 0 | 1 | 1 | 1 | 0 | 0 | 0 | 0 | 1 | 0 |
| # of flushes - day | 3 | 5 | 2 | 2 | 2 | 3 | 5 | 1 | 4 | 3 | 2 | 3 | 4 | 5 | 1 | 0 | 0 | 1 | 1 | 0 | 0 | 0 | 1 | 2 | 1 | 0 | 0 | 0 | 0 | 1 | 0 |
| Hot flushes - night | 4 | 3 | 2 | 2 | 3 | 2 | 2 | 4 | 2 | 2 | 2 | 3 | 3 | 3 | 2 | 2 | 1 | 0 | 2 | 0 | 2 | 0 | 0 | 0 | 2 | 0 | 0 | 0 | 0 | 0 | 2 |
| # of flushes - night | 1 | 3 | 1 | 2 | 1 | 2 | 3 | 4 | 2 | 3 | 1 | 2 | 5 | 8 | 2 | 1 | 2 | 1 | 0 | 1 | 0 | 1 | 0 | 0 | 0 | 1 | 0 | 0 | 0 | 0 | 1 |
| Mucous Secretion | hysterectomy---------------------------------------------------------------------------------------------------- | | | | | | | | | | | | | | | | | | | | | | | | | | | | | | |
| Constipation | 2 | 1 | 1 | 0 | 1 | 2 | 1 | 1 | 1 | 2 | 2 | 1 | 0 | 0 | 1 | 0 | 0 | 0 | 0 | 2 | 1 | 0 | 0 | 0 | 0 | 0 | 0 | 0 | 0 | 1 | 0 |
| Headache | 2 | 4 | 0 | 0 | 2 | 2 | 1 | 3 | 0 | 0 | 0 | 0 | 0 | 2 | 0 | 1 | 0 | 0 | 0 | 0 | 1 | 0 | 0 | 0 | 0 | 1 | 0 | 0 | 0 | 0 | 1 |
| Sleep Problems | 3 | 3 | 1 | 2 | 2 | 2 | 3 | 4 | 2 | 2 | 1 | 1 | 3 | 4 | 1 | 1 | 2 | 0 | 0 | 0 | 0 | 1 | 0 | 0 | 0 | 0 | 0 | 0 | 0 | 0 | 1 |
| Feeling Frustrated | 3 | 2 | 2 | 1 | 1 | 2 | 1 | 4 | 3 | 2 | 1 | 1 | 3 | 4 | 3 | 2 | 2 | 1 | 0 | 1 | 1 | 0 | 0 | 0 | 2 | 0 | 0 | 1 | 2 | 0 | 0 |
| Feeling Depressed | 1 | 0 | 0 | 0 | 0 | 0 | 0 | 2 | 3 | 0 | 0 | 1 | 2 | 3 | 0 | 0 | 1 | 0 | 0 | 0 | 1 | 0 | 0 | 0 | 1 | 0 | 0 | 0 | 0 | 2 | 0 |
| Feeling Anxious | 0 | 1 | 0 | 0 | 1 | 1 | 1 | 2 | 1 | 2 | 2 | 2 | 1 | 1 | 0 | 0 | 1 | 0 | 0 | 1 | 0 | 0 | 1 | 0 | 0 | 0 | 0 | 0 | 0 | 0 | 1 |

Record  M = much less, L = a little less, U = usual, Y = a little increased, Z = much increased

| | 1 | 2 | 3 | 4 | 5 | 6 | 7 | 8 | 9 | 10 | 11 | 12 | 13 | 14 | 15 | 16 | 17 | 18 | 19 | 20 | 21 | 22 | 23 | 24 | 25 | 26 | 27 | 28 | 29 | 30 | 31 |
|---|---|---|---|---|---|---|---|---|---|---|---|---|---|---|---|---|---|---|---|---|---|---|---|---|---|---|---|---|---|---|---|
| Appetite | Y | Y | Z | U | Y | Y | U | Z | U | U | Y | U | U | Y | Y | U | U | U | U | L | U | U | U | U | U | U | U | U | Y | U | U |
| Breast Size | Y | Y | Y | Y | Z | Y | U | U | Y | Y | Y | Y | Y | U | U | Z | Y | Y | U | U | U | U | Y | Y | Y | U | U | U | U | U | U |
| Interest In Sex | L | U | Y | Y | U | U | U | L | U | U | Y | U | L | L | L | U | U | U | Y | Y | U | U | U | U | Y | U | U | U | Y | U | U |
| Feeling Of Energy | L | U | L | L | U | L | L | L | U | U | L | L | L | L | L | U | U | U | U | U | Y | Y | U | U | U | Y | U | Y | U | U | U |
| Feeling Of Self-Worth | L | L | O | L | U | U | U | U | L | L | M | L | U | U | U | L | U | L | L | L | U | U | Y | Y | U | U | Y | U | L | Y | U |
| Outside Stresses | U | Y | L | L | L | U | U | U | Y | U | U | L | U | Y | Z | U | U | U | L | L | U | U | U | U | U | U | L | L | L | U | L |
| Treatments or Supplement | | | | | | | | | | | | | | | | | | | | | | | | | | | | | | | |
| Premarin 0.625 | √ | √ | √ | √ | √ | √ | √ | √ | √ | √ | √ | √ | √ | √ | 0 | 0 | 0 | 0 | 0 | 0 | 0 | 0 | 0 | 0 | 0 | 0 | 0 | 0 | 0 | 0 | 0 |
| Provera 2.5 | √ | √ | √ | √ | √ | √ | √ | √ | √ | √ | √ | √ | √ | √ | 2 | 2 | 2 | 2 | 2 | 2 | 2 | 2 | 2 | 2 | 2 | 2 | 0 | 0 | 0 | 0 | 0 |
| Estragel pump | NONE | | | | | | | | | | | | | | 1 | 1 | 1 | 1 | 1 | 1 | 1 | 3/4 | 3/4 | 3/4 | 3/4 | 3/4 | 3/4 | 3/4 | 3/4 | | |
| Prometrium | | | | | | | | | | | | | | | 3 | 3 | 3 | 3 | 3 | 3 | 3 | 3 | 3 | 3 | 3 | 3 | 3 | 3 | 3 | 3 | 3 |
| Comments (Temperature Taken Late, Feeling Sick, Poor Sleep, Etc.) | WICKED HEADACHE | | | | | | JANE TICKED | | AWFUL NIGHT | | | | | | | | | | | | | | | | | | | | | | |

"But if estrogen levels are high in perimenopause, why would the hot flushes start then?" asks Carla.

"You see, perimenopausal estrogen levels are variable, unpredictable and erratic," I say. "They average higher than normal, and sometimes double the highest they should ever be during the menstrual cycle. When they drop into the normal range, the hypothalamus interprets that as a big change and voil`a! A hot flush!"

"But I thought," Jane says tentatively, "that estrogen levels dropped in peri-menopause until they got to be really low after menopause."

"You and most of the world thinks that, Jane," I say. "But we now know that's wrong. Estrogen levels are high or normal until at least a year after the last period. I learned that from a study of randomly picked midlife women ages 45–55 from Australia." I pull out a diagram and show them.

ESTROGEN LEVELS IN PERIMENOPAUSE (6)

Menstrual Status Category

"Women in this study," I continue, "had blood drawn three to eight days af-ter the start of flow. That's a time of the cycle when estrogen levels are normally pretty low and just starting to increase. Women were divided up into five groups by their report of flow. Women with no change in how far apart their periods were, or in how much flow, were called group I and considered to be 'pre-menopausal.' Women with periods farther apart or closer together were group

II. Those with flow that was lighter or heavier made up group III. Those with changes in both cycle length and flow were considered to be group IV. Women who had been three but not yet 12 months without a period were group V. Well, between group I and group V, average estrogen levels did drop. But about 20 percent of estrogen levels were high and about 10 percent were *extremely* high in every group, including group V that is almost menopausal (6).

"Estrogen levels are higher the closer to the top of the page they are," I point to the figure."They should all be clustered around this solid line here, which is about the average for days 3-8 of the menstrual cycle. This dashed line is the average highest normal level in the middle of the cycle. Some women, even those who have skipped six months of flow, have very high levels (7)."

"Carla doesn't have a uterus so she can't get flow, but her estrogen levels are still really high and bouncing," Jane says. "Do I understand?"

"That's right," I say. "But when she started to get flushes after her hysterectomy, Dr. Hall figured she was menopausal, so he gave her estrogen treatment."

"I still don't get it," Carla says, thoughtfully. "If estrogen takes away hot flushes after menopause, why didn't it work for me in *perimenopause?*"

"I don't know for sure, Carla. But good population-based studies show perimenopausal women on estrogen treatment have more flushes than do untreated perimenopausal women (93;94).

"I would like to do a study to see whether we could document that the response of hot flushes to estrogen differs before and after menopause. I'm sure it does," I say.

"How did you come up with the idea that progesterone would help?" Carla asks. "It works like a hot damn! I can sleep, I feel more relaxed, and I'm rarely bitchy now."

"Well," I say, "we could have known, based on many early studies, that progestins help hot flushes. But estrogen got all the press. And we didn't have the natural progesterone available until about ten years ago."

"Why was that?" asks Carla. "I thought progesterone was the basic thing that progestins were made from."

"You're quite right," I answer. "Progestins should be synthesized from the basic chemical structure of progesterone. Instead, it's easier to make progestins from testosterone. That's why all the old progestins, except medroxyprogesterone, and most of the ones still used in birth control pills, are derived from testosterone. Very early on, someone—I don't know who—discovered that progesterone by mouth was inactive. Apparently, as a pill, progesterone got digested into bits and no longer acted like a hormone. It wasn't until the 1970s that folks in France learned to micronize it—that means to process the progesterone molecule into very small pieces each surrounded by oil, so that it would stay active when taken by mouth. It took more than 10 years, however, before that bright idea made it across the Atlantic."

"But if hot flushes are caused by dropping brain estrogen levels, how does progesterone treat them?" asks Jane.

"I don't think anyone really understands," I say. "It is probably through some progesterone action in the hypothalamus. We know, for example, that progesterone works in the hypothalamus to increase the body's core temperature (95). That's the higher basal temperature level we see after ovulation (2). Progesterone also works in the brain to increase deep sleep and shorten the time it takes to fall asleep (81). For these and other reasons, I think progesterone acts in the hypothalamus to prevent the drug withdrawal reaction when estrogen levels drop. It may simply stabilize hypothalamic nerve cells."

Carla listens intently. "I was about to start taking an anti-depressant for hot flushes when I first came to see you, Dr. Madrona," she says. "My doctor said, and Jane had read somewhere, that the new serotonin re-uptake inhibitor anti-depressants help hot flushes. What about them?"

"I'm glad you didn't start an SSRI anti-depressant because I think progesterone is more effective and safer," I say. "Progesterone is addressing the primary problem, whereas SSRIs are treating a symptom of the problem. For example, some SSRIs cause sleep *trouble* rather than improving sleep as progesterone does. Also, all of the different SSRI anti-depressants have important side effects—not least of which is that they are hard to stop. SSRIs have only been shown to be effective against hot flushes in short studies, less than two months long, compared with three to 12-month studies of progesterone (96) and progestins (75). Most importantly, SSRIs appear to decrease hot flushes by only about 50-60 percent, which is just slightly better than placebo (97) compared with an 80-95 percent decrease for progestins (74;98). I do think SSRIs help hot flushes, but mainly by treating depression and decreasing stress hormones that are related to depression."

"It sounds like you think that stress hormones from depression are part of the reason for hot flushes," Jane says.

"Good ears! Yes, definitely stress makes hot flushes worse (99). And hot flushes themselves increase brain stress hormones (100). Therefore one of the most important aspects of treating hot flushes is practicing relaxation or meditation (46;101;102). An additional way that progesterone may work to decrease hot flushes is through decreasing anxiety (103)."

"That's interesting," says Carla. "One of the things Jane and I have been doing is practicing yoga breathing for about 15 minutes before bedtime each night. After that, as we quietly get ready for bed, I often think about things, sort things out in my head, and can sometimes understand enough to share important, deep stuff about my day."

"Yes," I say, "that's my experience, too—a little quiet time that looks like doing nothing unlocks key ideas that were there all along."

"That's how we came up with the 'Growing Girls' website! That calm and positive thinking has really guided development of our computer repair business," says Carla.

"I'm very glad you're both doing so well," I say. "But we'd better get busy here. A few quick questions and then I'll examine you again, Carla. You and Jane can decide whether Jane will stay here or go out to the waiting area."

~

I've finished Carla's examination, and we're again sitting around the desk.

"Well, Carla," I say, "You've done a good job decreasing to two or three coffees a day and doing your breast self-examination. Your weight is down a bit to 78.5 kg. I think it helps that you're not eating to try to compensate for low energy and lost sleep!"

Carla smiles broadly.

"Your blood pressure was excellent at 128 over 84," I say. "What I found most remarkable on your exam is that your breasts are much softer. I can still feel evidence of estrogen's action, but it is much less than before."

"I hardly recognize them," she says. "They're softer and healthy feeling!"

"Your breasts definitely feel less risky," I say. "And I'll bet your next mammogram will show it."

"Should I have a mammogram this year?" Carla asks.

"No, you just had one, didn't you?" I reply. "You can go every two years from now on."

"Shall I continue on Prometrium, three each night?" Carla asks.

"Yes," I say, "it's important to continue until the hot flushes go away. Can you afford them?" A glance between the women shows that finances are a concern. "Remember the compounding pharmacy route. A couple of them in Victoria," I say. "will compound progesterone in olive oil at the cost of a dollar for a 300-mg capsule. We helped them with a little experiment about its absorption. So, for the sake of your pocketbook, I'll write that prescription as 'Oral Micronized Progesterone compounded in oil' so you can get it filled there. This prescription is good for 12 months. I don't need to see you again for a year, Carla."

"Great! Now Jane and I have a 'day on the town' in Vancouver! We plan to visit a few computer repair stores here and get some advice. We're also rounding up old computers that we'll scrub clean, check, and re-install software on so that we can give them to older women to use for emails and writing. Let us know if you have any we could take off your hands."

"You bet we do!" I reply. "It's a great help to us for you to take them away. I'll ask Lana to round up the old computer stuff we're no longer using. We've got about half a dozen monitors, keyboards and mainframes hanging around. Because of security and research confidentiality we've already scrubbed the hard drives. See you in a year!"

"Thanks," says Carla. She and Jane wave and walk down the hall, then Carla turns back.

"Oh, Dr. Madrona. I almost forgot! The bunch of us that first met for that group session in the fall about a year and a half ago are going to have a bit of a party soon. Alison said she'd told you about it and would call Lana with the details. Jane and I plan on coming over. Hope you can make it."

"I hope so, too," I say as we again wave goodbye.

# 11

*eva*

## lead legs

"Good afternoon, Eva," I say as I enter the waiting area. "Thanks for mailing me your diaries a few weeks ago. That gave me a chance to have a look at them."

We walk down the hall to my examination room-office.

"What's bothering me most is that I can't seem to train properly," she says as she sits down. "I don't understand it. No one has a clue about female hormones and being athletic—I've done some looking on the Internet and even bugged our local librarian. That's how I found out about some old research on women athletes from this centre. And there's little out there about exercise in perimenopause!"

"I've not actively researched women's cycles and exercise," I say. "However, I'm physically active, I was taught by and worked with Dr. Prior and know her exercise studies (44), and I have friends and colleagues in sports medicine and kinesiology, so I have some hunches. First I need to find out a little more about what you've noticed. Tell me about your running."

"I was not active as a child," she says, "but did have to walk about three miles to school when I lived in northern Manitoba. I finished high school, moved to Regina for university, and found myself on a not-so-special women's track team. That's where I learned that I love to run. Later, when I got premenstrual breast tenderness, bloating, and mood swings in my mid-thirties, I began some jogging to see if that would help. It did. And it felt good. So I started running things like the 10-km Vancouver Sun Run. And I started a training program through one of the running stores. That year I came first in my age category in the 8-km Terry Fox run. I was hooked! Since then, I've joined a running club and am registered as a *master's athlete*. Can you beat that? Women qualify when they are 40! I train for and run several races a year."

"What was your personal best 10-km time, Eva?" I ask.

"My best 10-km was 37 minutes," she says as she pulls a printed spiral-bound runner's record from her metal briefcase. "That was in the spring of 1999. Since then, even though I've been training more consistently, I've never run it under 42."

"You really are a talented runner, Eva. My personal best for a 10-km is 49 minutes, and I usually run it in about an hour. Do you know what the Canadian or world record is for a woman in a 10-km?"

"I don't know," she says. "But I do know that if I could get back to my best, I'd win most races in my age category. In three years, when I'm over 50, I'll be even more likely to win. But to do that I've got to solve my problem."

"How are you training?" I ask.

"I run about 5-8 km on a usual day, taking about 30 minutes. Once a week I do a 12- or 15-km run. On the other days I do sprints, hills and some weight training. If I can manage to finish my run I feel very tired, but also happy. But I'm finding it hard to get myself out there."

"That sounds like a sensible training schedule," I say. "Do you ever take days off?"

"I would, except I feel so fat and sluggish. It's better if I do something every day."

"What do you think is the problem, Eva?"

"I get lead legs," she says, and sighs. "Like it's just *too much work*, especially the hills. I have to walk the ones I used to sprint up."

"If I remember, you said in the group session you aren't anemic—and I have good lab results from your doctor. Have you had your thyroid checked?" I asked.

"I don't know about the thyroid," she says. "I think the problem is that I get so hungry. I work from nine to three, four days a week. I try to do my runs before work, but sometimes when I've had a bad night, I just have to eat some breakfast, and then it's hopeless to try to run. I get off work at three and do my weights or sprints then. But I am so hungry I just have to eat something before I go. Even in the mornings I have to have a yogurt or an energy bar before I can go out. So I'm never really training on an empty stomach. For sure I can't eat something really sweet like a chocolate bar or some candy before I run. Then I really feel I'm dragging."

"So the big problem is that you're overly hungry," I say. "If your insulin levels are high because of eating something sweet, that could make fuel go into fat for storage instead of into muscle to help you run. Perhaps having a little something small, something with complex carbohydrates and protein, won't interfere with your run, Eva. Have you tried that?"

"I've just found I can't eat and run. Period." Eva slumps in her chair.

"What's happened with your weight?" I ask.

"Oh, I'm getting fatter and fatter," she says. "I've dieted so many times, but I always gain it back. I come from European peasant stock, so it's as though my body just wants to get stout. I weighed 57 kg when I ran that personal best. Now I probably weigh over 60. Even though I watch everything I eat. I've just decided to start a low-carb diet. . ."

I lean forward. "It's not a good idea to severely restrict carbohydrates when you're training, Eva. The goal is to have a normal weight. That may be more than you'd like, because muscle weighs more than fat. However, a stable weight is important. More than that, I think that 60 kg is an excellent weight for your height. You are *not* fat!" I say emphatically.

"Well, I *feel* fat. And I am scared I'll gain more."

"Tell me," I say, "how many times have you lost and regained about 5 kg in your lifetime?"

"Let's see," she says, "I went on my first diet when I was in my final year of high school—the prom and all that. I lost 6 kg that time. I had regained it by the time I started university, but then I lost weight because life was stressful, moving away from home and making new friends. I've probably been on a diet at least once or twice a year since then. So about 20 times!"

"That's not good for your metabolism nor for your bones, Eva," I say. "We'll talk more about bones in a minute. For now, I want to ask whether there are any times of your menstrual cycle when your running is better or worse?"

"Yes," she says. "I used to have my best runs at the end of my period. On those days I felt like I could fly. Now, I can't tell. It seems like no days are good days." She thinks for a moment. "I know that if I have very sore breasts in the middle of the month, the next two weeks will be tough. Now I'm not sure what's going to happen. I almost skipped this last period."

"Your Diary shows a lot of stretchy mucus and breast soreness from about Day 16 until flow. It is unusual, in my experience, for a runner to have those high estrogen signs. That tells me you are for sure in perimenopause. Plus it suggests that you aren't ovulating normally, especially when you have mucus just before flow."

"Yeah," she says, "the worst-ever days are any days when my breasts feel swollen and sore. I can only jog slowly, and I usually run on the flat, those days. I figured that out a long time ago, in my mid-thirties. I also learned that I could decrease the bloating, mood swings, and breast tenderness by being more consistent with exercise. I would specifically increase both the intensity and the duration of exercise until things were fine again. But I've not been able to increase my exercise or to help my premenstrual symptoms now, no matter what I do."

"Your last cycle was 41 days long," I say. "Is that the first time you've had some irregularity?"

"Before this funny cycle," she says, "I never skipped a period except once when I had been dieting and was also going through divorce."

"That longer cycle means you are starting Phase C of perimenopause, Eva. And that suggests that soon you will have fewer and fewer days of high estrogen levels and lead legs."

"But I want to do a 20-km run in three weeks. It involves hills, and I'm not ready. To lose will not be any fun."

"I thought you loved running for its own sake, not just for winning, Eva!"

I smile, but Eva doesn't smile back.

"I used to," she says, "but now when I think about running, I think about the problems and not about the fun. That's it—it's just no fun any more! So I'm fighting for something I've lost."

"The good news is that perimenopause doesn't last forever," I say. "I think it will be fun again, Eva. You just have to have patience." I glance briefly at my notes, then look up.

"Are you taking the birth control pill, Eva?" I ask.

"No," she says, looking puzzled. "If I have a relationship, we use condoms. Why?"

"Although you do need effective contraception during all of perimenopause," I say. "I'm glad you're not on the Pill. I believe that it can interfere with exercise performance. A colleague of mine did a randomized, placebo-controlled study of maximal exercise performance. . ."

"You mean $VO_2$ max?" she interrupts.

"That's right. $VO_2$ max was lower while taking the Pill compared to each woman's untreated baseline. But VO$_2$ max didn't change in women on placebo (104)."

"Really?" she says. "I didn't know that. There are only a few women in my running group, but most of them are on the Pill. They told me, when I was complaining about not improving my personal best, that I should start it!"

"When was your last period, Eva?"

"It's due any day now," she replies. "But I'm not sure because the last was about two weeks late. In fact, for the first time, I didn't get sore breasts for about three weeks. I swear I feel engorged now! It will be here soon."

"So, your experience is telling you your period will come soon. Hopefully that predictive sign will continue for the rest of your perimenopause. To see how high your estrogen is, I'll order a blood level now. And I'll also order a progesterone level to see whether you are ovulating. To be complete, I'll order thyroid tests too. Hyperthyroidism, or overactive thyroid problems can definitely interfere with strength and performance. Are you warmer or colder than other people?"

"I tend to be colder, especially my hands and feet. I think it's because I've got less insulation than most of those in my office!"

"Does your whole body feel cold?" I ask.

Eva shakes her head.

"Cold hands and feet *can* be because you are cold," I continue, "but they usually mean you are reacting to stress. Are you ever aware of your heartbeat except when you're running?"

"I feel it sometimes in the night when I wake for no reason. I normally don't have to get up, but if I wake like that, I can't fall asleep until I get up and urinate."

"Have you ever had a running injury that kept you away from exercise for a couple of weeks?" I ask.

"I got a stress fracture of my tibia when I was on the track team in university. I thought it was shin splints, but it would ache especially at the end of and after a run. X-rays were negative, but the coach told me to only bicycle for a month. Because my shin continued to ache, we got another X-ray before I went back to running. It showed a healed fracture."

"There may be some connection between your yo-yo dieting and that fracture, Eva. Stress fractures were more likely, in a study from Australia, in athletic women with worry about what they eat, which is also called eating restraint (105). And a huge study tracking middle-aged Norwegian men and women over many years showed that, in women who lost and regained weight, the hip fracture risk was doubled (106)."

"I don't diet now. I just watch what I eat. And it seems like I'm just watching myself get fat! So I may have to go on a diet as the only way I can keep from becoming a tub!"

"Let's talk about what you normally eat, Eva," I say. "Tell me what you had for breakfast today."

"I had whole wheat nut toast with melted low-fat swiss cheese, a glass of milk, an orange and a cup of coffee."

"That sounds good," I say. "What did you have for lunch and snacks so far today?"

"I ate an energy bar on the way here because I didn't have time for lunch. And I grabbed a mocha latte. I know that's got sugar and more coffee, but at least it's made with milk." She laughs and looks guilty.

"You can do better about lunch than that," I say, "even when you're busy. What did you have for supper last night?"

"I went for my run after work because I had been too tired in the morning. I was starved, so I had a turkey vegetable wrap at my break about two o'clock yesterday. After the run I was tired and didn't feel like cooking, so I grabbed a Greek salad and a muffin from the deli near my place. Because I was still hungry"—she pauses and glances up at me—"I ended up making and eating a bag of microwave popcorn later in the evening."

"I succumb too, Eva!" I say. "So, in that 24-hour day you got only one vegetable and one fruit. You're generally good at avoiding sweets, except for that mocha latte. But you may not be getting enough protein. Also, in spite of your best efforts, there are a lot of hidden fats in your diet, like in that muffin and in the microwave popcorn. I'll bet that bag you ate had 100 calories in it. I know—I was shocked when I looked at the label on a bag of microwave popcorn that I could happily eat after supper. Nowadays I buy plain popcorn and pop it when I feel like munching."

"But that was not a usual day, Dr. Madrona!" Eva protests. "I usually have a yogurt, carrots, an apple and some cheese and rye crackers for lunch. And I often make pasta and salad in the evening. The problem is that when I should feel full, I'm still hungry."

"That sounds better, Eva. I think the key is to increase your protein and probably add some good oils. You seem to be sensitive to carbohydrates. Does anybody in your family have diabetes?"

"Not that I know of," she replies. "I guess I could add some soy nuts as a morning snack. I don't buy much fish or chicken or meat, partly because I haven't liked it much since I started running regularly, and partly because of cost. I'm trying to save to buy a condo—renting where I live in the West End is so expensive. It's like throwing money away. At least I'm near enough to work so I can walk or bicycle. My job is part-time, and I've got almost no benefits. A legal assistant must be well dressed, obedient, fast, and efficient, but doesn't have much to look forward to except being laid off."

"That sounds discouraging, Eva," I say. "No wonder you put your energy and enthusiasm into running."

"And that's also why it's so frustrating to be failing at that," she says.

I nod reassuringly. "You're still more fit than the majority of women! Tell me about your periods," I ask. "What age you were when they first started and how they have been throughout your life?"

"I started when I was almost 14," she says. "I think I skipped a bit in my teens, but then they got regular in university. After my abortion, I started on the Pill for a year or so. But I didn't like it and stopped. I've used a condom plus jelly or foam ever since, without any problem. My periods came regularly but without warning until I started to get that premenstrual mood and bloating stuff in my thirties and began serious running."

"Who's at home with you?" I ask.

"Nobody, now. I've had some roommates in the past, and I've lived with various guys, but somehow things never worked out. Oh, Mabel's at home with me. She's my two-year-old German pointer. She's a great runner—she runs with me most days. She keeps me from feeling lonely. At least I'm not talking to *myself*!"

"I'm glad you've got a pet, Eva. Are you allergic to anything?" I ask.

"Not any foods or medicines that I know of, but I get a really bad rash with tape. The first time I taped a sprain in high school, it looked like a major burn."

"Ouch!" I say. "Now, tell me about your abortion and any other pregnancies."

"I got pregnant once and had an early abortion in my twenties, as I mentioned. I've never really been sick or in the hospital. And I've had no other fractures except that stress one. But I did have some kind of fever the year I was supposed to start school. My knees hurt—they kept me at home in bed. I started school in January, but I caught up with my class quickly. Otherwise I've been well."

"Was that rheumatic fever, Eva?" I ask.

"Yeah, I think so," she says. "I remember a lot of pain, but my mom read to me and dad brought me milk warm from our cow. They said my heart was fine. I had a penicillin shot, I remember that."

"Are there any illnesses that run in your family?"

"My dad is retired from farming now, and they've moved closer to Flin-Flon. Mom still has a huge garden and sells free-range chickens and eggs plus all kinds of vegetables at the Saturday Market. They're both in their late sixties and fine. My older brother, Will, is well and has a family in Winnipeg. My grandparents were in the old country, so I didn't know them. But I think they lived to good old ages except for my grandpa who died in the war."

"That's a healthy family history, Eva," I say. "What supplements, vitamins, or medicines are you regularly taking?"

"I take oil of evening primrose capsules twice a day when I feel PMS, Vitamin E at 400 IU a day, a multivitamin for women, and a 1,000-IU vitamin D pill like your handout suggested. I also take 1,300 mg of calcium and a slow-release 1,000-mg vitamin C."

"That's good," I say. "However, I think we should track your oil of evening primrose. It can act like estrogen. And the latest studies suggest that Vitamin E is not an effective anti-oxidant and may cause harm. How do you get the calcium you mentioned?"

"I just take two 650-mg pills with my other supplements in the morning."

"It would be better to take one pill with a meal at which you're not having a dairy food, like one at dinner. Take the second pill at bedtime, to compensate for no calcium foods in your system overnight. More than 500-600 mg of calcium at a time can't be absorbed from your intestines. Next time you buy calcium pills, get 500-mg ones and take one at lunch, dinner, and bedtime, or three a day. With your yogurt and one milk, that will make 2,000 mg a day of elemental calcium, which is the amount I want you to get."

I wait while Eva jots a few notes on a very small computer she's taken out of her briefcase, then I resume taking her history. "You mentioned coffee in the morning," I say. "Tell me about other caffeine, and about alcohol and cigarettes."

"I only have the one cup of coffee usually," she replies. "I used to drink it at work, but I got quite jittery and had a headache in the afternoons. I rarely drink alcohol because even a little makes my legs feel funny." She laughs as she pats her upper thighs. "They get a weak feeling with any alcohol. I know that's weird! And I've never smoked."

"Do you regularly check your breasts?" I ask.

"Yes, Dr. Gregory showed me how when I first started with her. I do it two weeks after my period every month. She insisted I have a mammogram when I turned 40. My test was fine, but I wasn't—they peeled the skin off my ribs! I've not been back. And she does a Pap every three years. It's always fine."

"I'm glad you're checking your own breasts, Eva, especially because you'd like to avoid a mammogram. But I'd like you to move the time of the cycle when you do your breast exam. It should be at the end of your flow. That's a time of the cycle when estrogen's most likely to be low and when breasts are least likely to be sore or swollen." I pause and then continue. "I've run out of questions. I'd like to examine you, and then we'll get a plan for figuring out what's up with your running. Please take off everything except your pant-ies—you can hang your jacket and skirt on that hook. Put on this gown, lie down there and relax. I'll knock when I come back." I go out, after pulling the curtain shut behind me.

~

After knocking quietly, I enter the examining room, noticing her suit on a hanger behind the door and the carefully folded blouse on top of her bra. "How are you doing?" I ask.

"Good," she says. "It's so relaxing in here. I'm glad you have that smaller light. My eyes are quite sensitive, especially to fluorescent lights. I got premen-strual migraines from my teens until I went off the Pill. Sorry, I forgot to tell you."

"No problem," I say. "I'm glad you remembered to tell me. That's impor-tant to know because it influences how I prescribe progesterone. I'm very glad you're not having migraines in perimenopause. I did, and they were horrid. Now let me check you.

"Your blood pressure is excellent at 112 over 64 with a pulse of 56. Your reflex relaxation is, if anything, slightly slow. That makes it very unlikely that you have an overactive thyroid. And your heart sounds are quite normal with-out any murmur. You do have an easily palpable PMI, meaning the hardest heart thump I can feel on the chest, but that's normal in a thin athlete."

"But I'm not thin," Eva protests. "Just look at my breasts and tummy!"

"Speaking of breasts, yours are full and dense without any masses. They *are* sore aren't they?" Eva nods. "The only part of you that's really thin is your arms. You know, that's common in women who are stressed, especially with the worry, like you have, about becoming overweight. It looks like you have over-pronation, but I can see that you wear orthotics even in your work shoes." I gesture to her stylish pumps beside the exam table. "That's good."

"Yes," she says, "I've been wearing them for years."

"Ok, sit up now so I can check your back. Does that hurt?" I use the side of my fist to tap each of the vertebrae in her spine. "No? Good. Swallow for me. Ok, your thyroid gland is easy to see because it's high in your lean neck. It's symmetrical and normal. All right, come here to the scale. Let's get your height and weight."

"Can I go to washroom first?" she asks.

"You'd have to get dressed to do that since it's out in the corridor past the elevator. Come on. We can take a half-kilogram off if you like. How tall were you at your tallest height?"

"I think I was five foot six."

"Ok, take a deep breath and stand as tall as you can. Your height is 166 cm—hmm, that's about a half inch shorter than you remember. Has Dr. Gregory measured your height before? No? "

"Am I shrinking too?" Eva sounds dismayed.

"Not significantly," I say. "That decrease is within the error of the measurement. Your weight is 62.3 kg. Here, let's measure your waist circumfirence too. It's 69 cm. That is fantastic. Ok, you can take your clothes behind that curtain and get dressed. If you don't mind, I'll sit here and write while you're changing."

When Eva emerges, I begin my review.

"Alright, Eva, I'll summarize what we know so far. You're 47 years old and have just started Phase C of perimenopause with that one late period. You have a history of a stress fracture, perhaps related to over-training and over-pronation, but also possibly to losing and regaining weight over 20 times in your lifetime. You've had some premenstrual symptoms that you formerly controlled with increased exercise. But now you are unable to increase training enough to control breast tenderness and bloating. You're a talented runner who is having trouble improving her personal best. Your physical examination, especially your heart, is normal despite past probable rheumatic fever. Your thyroid is working fine and is unlikely to be an explanation for your exercise problems. Your hands are cool and you have little forearm muscle for the amount of weights you do. Your BMI is 22.6, which is ok but on the low side. Although you've recently gained weight, you've been skinny most of your life."

I stop a minute, looking at Eva, who is sitting quietly and listening intently.

"Am I making sense so far?" I ask. "Now's the hard part. You have what is called cognitive dietary restraint (107)."

"What's that?" she asks.

"It means you are worried, almost to the point of obsession, that the food you eat will cause you to gain weight. In most cases, women with restraint have normal weights and are not too thin."

"I've never been anorexic or weighed too little!" protests Eva.

"I know," I say. "But eating restraint is not about *actually* limiting what you eat. It's more about worry. It's a personal characteristic, a way of being. Restraint means that you constantly worry that what you eat will cause you to gain weight. We've learned a number of things about eating restraint that are relevant for you. First, it is associated with higher levels of the stress hormone, cortisol (108). Although that cortisol level in the women with restraint was just in the high part of the normal range, it may be high enough to interfere with the ability to train and to strengthen muscles. Another thing we've learned is that in premenopausal women, eating restraint is associated with ovulation disturbances like short luteal phase cycles and non-ovulation (109;110). Finally, we know that exercise builds bone in premenopausal women, but with eating restraint that doesn't happen as well (111). Because high cortisol, ovulation disturbances and difficulty building bone with exercise are all reasons for bone loss, you may well be at risk for osteoporosis."

"Why would trouble training and worry about eating become problems for me now?" she asks, looking puzzled.

"I'm not really sure," I reply. "But these are my guesses. In perimenopause, when estrogen levels are high, it is normal for women to gain about 2-5 kg— 5-12 pounds. That's threatening for most of us who care about our looks. But it's very distressing for women who have eating restraint and value thinness. It's also difficult when you're athletic and striving for excellence. In perimenopause, our body's in our face! Weight gain is real, not just a worry any more."

Eva still looks puzzled. "Do you think that explains my trouble training?"

"Partly," I say, "but also, in perimenopause the higher estrogen levels cause us to store energy. Estrogen stores energy as fat. High estrogen also makes insulin resistance that causes increased hunger. The hunger makes it difficult to time exercise so that you have enough fuel, but not so much that you become sluggish. For certain, when you eat anything sweet, your insulin levels soar. The energy is quickly stored, so there is not enough for working muscles. Hence, your lead legs feeling. And your blood sugar levels may well take a nose dive."

"This is starting to make some sense," Eva says thoughtfully. "But what can we do?"

"I'm sure we can figure out something that will give you back the fun of running. I doubt if you'll be able to start winning races again until you're through perimenopause, Eva. But by then you'll be at the top of the podium again. And, given that you've just started Phase C, that should only be about four years away (112)."

"If there's hope, I can hang on," she says.

"Good!" I say. "Now, first I think we could learn more about what's going on by doing a little experiment. I'd like you to run the same distance at the same time of day twice a week for two weeks. That will give us four 'test' runs. Please drink a glass of milk before each run. That will standardize your energy intake—from the milk sugar or lactose—and provide good protein. I'll make you a form on which you can record the time of day, the time you take to run the same distance, and your heart rate after 10 minutes, halfway through, and at the end of the run. I'll ask you to get a blood test for your level of estradiol after work on each day you've had the standardized run. That will give a clue whether I'm right in guessing there are relationships between your exercise performance and your estrogen levels."

"Could I also record how energetic or sluggish I feel?" she asks.

"Great idea! That means you'd also record perceived exertion on a 1 through 4 scale."

I pause and think for a moment. "The therapy part is that, after you've done the test exercises, I'd like you to take progesterone daily. We'll see whether this has any effect."

"Do you think progesterone will help my exercise, Dr. Madrona?"

"I'm not sure about it's effect on training," I answer. "I don't think progesterone either increases or decreases exercise tolerance. A study showed that progestin treatment didn't influence $VO_2$ max (113) but it did increase breathing. My reasons for prescribing progesterone are that your Diary shows you to have high estrogen and probably low progesterone levels based on stretchy mucus and nipple soreness before flow. We don't have any temperature levels to analyze, but we'll know about your progesterone level in this cycle from that blood test. Progesterone treatment is to counterbalance the tissue effects of your high estrogen levels. Another reason for prescribing progesterone is that it helps get rid of water retention. Finally, natural progesterone makes you burn an additional 300 calories or so a day—that's because the body requires that much energy to increase the core temperature after ovulation (114). That should help you feel less worried about your weight and decrease your stress with eating restraint.

"I've prescribed progesterone as Prometrium, which is bio-identical oral micronized progesterone, at bedtime daily. There's a paper called 'Cyclic Progesterone Therapy' on the CeMCOR website. Do you still have the CeMCOR website address?"

"Yes, and I've been to the site many times. I've already got that article in my file." Eva pats her briefcase. "But why did you prescribe it *daily* rather than cyclically?"

"You told me about your past migraine headaches," I say, "so I want to avoid the changes in progesterone levels that cyclic therapy would cause. Women with migraines sometimes react to changes in hormone levels even though progesterone itself doesn't cause migraines."

"Will I still have periods on progesterone?"

"Daily progesterone therapy will let you have regular periods only if you are making high enough estrogen levels to still thicken the endometrium. Meanwhile, keep doing your incredible Diary-keeping and recording your exercise. By the way, would I be able to copy the pages of your exercise log that overlap with your Diary so I can see whether we can observe any patterns already?"

"Sure," Eva says. She fishes in her bag and hands her battered training log to me.

"Finally," I say. "I think you're at high risk for osteoporosis, despite your good exercise. The reasons are your thinness, the up-and-down weight cycling, the eating restraint, probable lack of ovulation, and past stress fracture. All of those are risks even though no one in your family has had fractures.

"We need to address your osteoporosis risk," I continue. "You're doing the right things with the high dose vitamin D totaling 1,400 IU a day. Make sure you get the calcium of 2,000 mg spread across the day, the way we talked about earlier. Keep up your good exercise. The progesterone can start building new bone if decreasing stress, increasing calcium and higher dose vitamin D slow bone loss. Whatever you do, don't go on a diet or try to lose weight. Your weight and BMI are normal now, no matter how fat you feel! And any weight loss will cause bone loss. I'll order a spine and hip bone density scan before your next visit in six months."

We get up and walk down the hall to Lana's desk.

"Lana, Eva has kept an incredibly meticulous exercise record. Could you please copy from November through to the last record? Just have a seat, Eva. When she's done photocopying, Lana will book you a follow-up visit in six months."

I ask Lana to set up a spine and hip bone density test for Eva for next November, with an appointment with me right after that. "Be sure to bring your training logs," I tell Eva. "If you will give Lana your fax number, I'll fax you a form for recording your test runs."

Eva smiles. "I'm not sure this will work, but I have a small glimmer of hope, Dr. Madrona. Thanks so much."

"You're very welcome," I say. "You are doing most of the work yourself. See you in six months!"

About six months later, I see Eva again.

"Eva," I say, "sorry to keep you waiting. I got called to a long distance phone call in the middle of my last consult."

"No worries," she replies. "I've been puzzling over my running records and looking forward to seeing you again."

"Thanks, Eva," I reply. "I feel the same about seeing you again!"

"You know, Dr. Madrona, I've found that your milk-before-a-run trick works! It's enough energy yet I don't get sluggish. I also think that progesterone is helping. I'm sleeping better, and sometimes I get to the end of a meal and realize I've not even worried over what to eat and what not to eat."

"Good for you, Eva. Did you see how I put your test run data together with your estradiol levels?"

Eva groans. "Those bad runs are even worse than I thought. But at least you've discovered a reason. Before, I was blaming *myself* for not training well."

"I think that chart clearly shows that the higher your estrogen levels, the more difficult your run. You go slower, and your pulse is faster. I only wish we had VO$_2$ max values for those!"

## EVA'S RUNNING AND ESTROGEN RECORD

| Date | Time of day | Minutes running | Pulse at 10 minutes | Pulse ½ way thro' run | Pulse end of run | Resting Pulse | Perceived Exertion (1-4) | Estradiol level (pmol/L) |
|---|---|---|---|---|---|---|---|---|
| 07/24 | 0643 | 46 | 174 | 168 | 174 | 52 | 2 | 264 |
| 07/31 | 0650 | 49 | 168 | 180 | 180 | 54 | 4 | 1076 |
| 08/07 | 0645 | 51 | 168 | 186 | 180 | 54 | 4 | 1880 |
| 08/14 | 0633 | 47 | 174 | 174 | 180 | 52 | 3 | 565 |

"You know," interrupts Eva, "things are really looking up for me now. I ran into this woman who works in the same building I do. She's also from the Prairies, and she plays field hockey. She used to be on the Canadian team and went to the Worlds and the Olympics, but now plays just for fun. She invited me to a practice game on Thursday after work, and I really liked it. Plus the gals are a hoot. They have a game against another team each week on a Saturday or a Sunday. She asked me to help out because they were short a couple of players. I went and did a bad job for the first couple of times." She laughs. "But everyone was kind and helpful. Now I'm getting pretty good."

"That's really great, Eva. We humans are social creatures. Your dog Mabel is good—but not sufficient—companionship. One of the things I was worried about when I first saw you was that you were discouraged at work and seemed to be mostly alone."

"Plus," says Eva, " I am having fun now."

"What's happening with your periods?" I ask.

Eva pulls out her Diary sheets, which she's completed with small neat numbers and letters. "Mostly I've been having light flow about every month. I still take progesterone every night."

"It looks like your high estrogen signs are better," I say. "Look, you only had stretchy mucus for a couple of days last month!"

"I certainly know when I'm going to get a period, though. The lead legs come back, my breasts are sore and I feel bloated."

I nod. "You'll probably carry on having hit-or-miss periods for several more years. But it looks as though you're coping well. Not even any hot flushes."

"I think that's because of my exercise," she says.

"I'd like to think so," I say, "but hot flushes are mysterious. There's good evidence that exercise decreases hypothalamic stress hormones, just like re-laxation, does so it *should* help. However, there's really no good evidence yet that exercise prevents hot flushes. All of the studies that have examined the question are biased in one way or another (47;115-117)."

"Well, maybe it's heredity," she says. "My mom didn't have them."

"I'm not sure about that either. It doesn't look like hot flushes run in fami-lies. For example, my mom, my aunt and my older sister got off scot-free of night sweats, but I got them in spades. How's your weight?"

"I've kept my weight steady, as you asked," she replies, "but I'm not happy about it. I feel chunky and I had to get new dress clothes for work."

"You need that weight to fuel your exercise, Eva. You can take your clothes to a store that sells good used clothing on consignment and maybe earn something for your condo fund. Seriously, you need to weigh what you weigh for the sake of your bones. Speaking of bones, let's look at your bone den-sity." I pull out the bone density report and hand it to Eva. "This is for your records." I place the bone density printout on the desk so we both can look at it.

"Here in the four vertebrae in your back, the level is 0.87 g/cm$^2$, which gives a T score of −2.1 or −2.1 standard deviations below young normal values. Do you understand?"

"Kind of," she says. " I assume that a T score of 1 is the average?"

"Not quite," I say, drawing a bell-shaped curve. "Bone densities in all young women put together make a shape like a mountain with most women having an average value"—I mark a 0 in the middle at the peak—"and some normal women have higher and some lower values." I mark on the drawing. "Between −1 and +1 is normal, with 0 being the average for a 20-to 30-year-old woman. We call that peak bone density and use that as the standard because the risk for fractures is the lowest at that age. Women whose bone density is between −1 and −2.5 are said to have osteopenia or low bone density. Those with T scores lower than −2.5 are said to have osteoporosis."

"So where would you put your spine T-score of −2.1 on this curve, Eva?"

"Here." Eva draws an arrow just to the right of the −2.5 line. "And my hip is normal at 0.2, so it goes here, right?" I nod and smile.

## EVA'S BONE DENSITY RESULTS

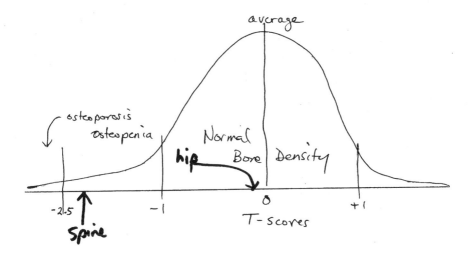

Eva asks, "Why do I almost have osteoporosis in my back and yet my hip is normal?"

"The hip bone we measure is mostly cortical bone that responds, although slowly, to exercise and body weight. Cortical bone is the hard tubular bone like in a drumstick. The spine is mostly made up of cancellous bone that is honey-comb-like and responds quickly to hormonal changes. The pattern you show with low spine density and almost normal hip density is very typical in young women. It's likely that your exercise has protected your hip. But up and down in weight, eating restraint, and not ovulating are hardest on spine bone density."

"Will I always be at risk for fracture, Dr. Madrona?" Eva asks.

"No," I say, "bone is not like concrete. It is a living, remodeling or renovating tissue. It is possible to gain bone between now and menopause. But the other part of your osteoporosis risk picture is that it is normal to lose bone right now. All women start rapidly losing bone at Phase C of perimenopause (118). This loss will continue until you reach menopause and for about three years afterwards (119;120)."

"But Dr. Madrona, I don't want to break any bones—it was awful having that stress fracture!"

"I don't want you to fracture either," I say. "And I don't think you will. I think you'll stay the same or even gain bone density as long as you keep to your current weight and your increased calcium and vitamin D intakes, and continue to find life and eating less stressful. In addition, the progesterone you're taking builds bone in active *premenopausal* women who have mixed-up or no periods (121).

"To be sure you are not losing bone," I continue, "I'll have you do a urine test called deoxypyridinoline or D-Pyr for short. It measures a little cross-linked protein that comes from the protein foundation or matrix of bone. If that is normal, we can be confident you will gain bone. And we'll repeat your bone density again in two years. If you've lost bone, we'll decide then whether you need a non-hormonal therapy that stops bone loss."

"Why don't we start it now?" she asks.

"I'd prefer to see you make the necessary changes so you can gain bone without adding a medicine that hasn't been formally tested in women your age. Have you fallen in the last six months, Eva?"

"Uhh. Yeah. I did," she says. "I tripped on a higher bit of sidewalk and luckily slammed into the tree instead of the cement. Why did you ask?"

"For two reasons. First, because perimenopausal women are reported to fall more frequently than women normally do before their seventies (122). Secondly, because those who fall are more likely to fracture."

"Oh," she says. "I didn't break anything. That's good then."

"Tell me what you are doing now for calcium and vitamin D." I say.

"I have a glass of milk with breakfast and yogurt at lunch. I got some new 500-mg calcium pills like you suggested and am taking three a day."

"What time of day do you take them?"

"I take them at night with the vitamin D and the Prometrium."

"That's the right amount of calcium, and that, plus your food, adds up to about 2,000 mg per day. However, taking 1,500 mg of calcium all at once means you'll only absorb about a third. I suggest that you take one calcium at breakfast, one at dinner and one at bedtime."

Eva is typing on her small computer. "I'm stupid, right? Now I remember your saying to spread them out. All that stuck was that it was important to take calcium at bedtime to prevent the loss of bone that increases during the night when we're not eating."

"Glad you remembered that." I say, "What's your total vitamin D intake?"

"I'm getting some from the milk and sunshine and 1,000 IU in that single pill," she answers.

"I usually don't count the vitamin D either in milk or from sunshine. Milk is supposed to be fortified with vitamin D, but no one checks the levels, so it may have almost none. And, we live in a northern latitude so that from October through March the sun is too low to the horizon. That means sunshine can't effectively make vitamin D in our skin."

"You think I need *more* vitamin D? Couldn't I get too much?"

"You could, but it is safe to take up to 2,000 IU of vitamin D a day. Thought is changing and scientists are pretty sure that even higher doses of vitamin D are likely safe. I'd like you to get 1,400 IU a day. Therefore I suggest you add 400 IU a day from a generic multivitamin to your 1,000-IU vitamin D pill. Given that you're still menstruating and are a runner, find a multivitamin with 4 or 5 mg of iron in it."

"Ok," Eva says, making notes furiously in her small computer.

"You mentioned that you're sleeping better," I say. "How are your bowels?"

"I almost forgot," she says. "I have loose stools, almost like diarrhea, every morning. Since I started the progesterone. Could the diarrhea be caused by that?"

"That's a new one on me," I say. "Did you start anything else around that same time?"

"I'm sure it's the progesterone, Dr. Madrona."

"Ok. We'll do some figuring in a minute. Let's examine you now. Please take off everything from your waist up and lie down there." I gesture to the gown on the exam table and pull the curtain.

"Can I leave my pantyhose on?" Eva asks.

"Sure. I'll be right back after I copy your Diary."

~

"Ok, Eva. You are looking better, more relaxed and comfortable with yourself. Your hands are only a little cool this time. The thing I'm not pleased about is that you did lose some weight—and I measured you with your slacks on! You are now down to 61 kg—that's a loss of 1.3 kg or about three pounds. That makes your BMI just 22. That's not good for your bones."

"That's strange," she says. "I'm eating more regularly and better and not watching what I eat as carefully. Could I be losing weight because of that diarrhea?"

"Yes, that's quite likely. I have a question for you—is there anything besides calcium in the new pills you bought?"

"Sure, I got the ones with magnesium because the pharmacist told me that it helps me to absorb calcium."

"No wonder!" I exclaim. "That magnesium is causing your diarrhea! And you started it at the same time you started progesterone. Makes sense! You've heard of milk of magnesia, haven't you? That's the same stuff in your calcium pills. It's used to clean out the intestines before a bowel X-ray."

"I didn't know that. Why didn't the pharmacist tell me?" she asks.

"Many people think that magnesium supplements are necessary for healthy bones in humans because magnesium has been shown to be important for bone health in studies of rats. Well, the diet for rats is short of magnesium, so they *do* need it to absorb calcium. But you're not a rat! The human diet is rich in magnesium—we get plenty unless we have some bowel disease. The only time I suggest magnesium with calcium is if a woman is having constipation or has had bowel trouble and might not be absorbing adequate amounts."

"It's the same old story, isn't it, Dr. Madrona? Whether true or not, ideas die hard."

"That's right," I say. "So I suggest you substitute one of your old calcium pills without magnesium for one of your three pills a day. And spreading them out will also help. Whatever you do, don't lose more weight. For the sake of your bones, I'd like to see you at 64 kg, which would give you a BMI of 23."

"Ok," says Eva. "I'm beginning to understand that there's more to life than running and lots more to bone health."

"Here's the lab slip for D-pyr every six months for the next two years, and a prescription for progesterone therapy for a year. See you next year!"

"'Bye," she says. "Thanks!"

# 12

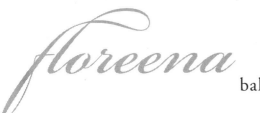 ballistic breasts

"Floreena?"
Floreena stands to greet me. "What a beautiful scarf! I love the interplay of blue and green," I say. "How are you today?"

"I'm fine, thank you." Floreena folds up a small square of what looks like lace. "I came in by train and thought I'd get a lot of tatting done. Instead I just sat back and enjoyed the lovely morning, especially the shades of green from farms, fields and forests up the Valley."

"I've never taken that train," I say. "It starts from Mission, doesn't it? What time did you have to leave?"

"I had to be up at five so my partner could drive me to the station for six o'clock. An early day for me."

I nod as I usher her into the examination room-office, and we each settle down.

"I remember that you spoke about breast lumps in that group session," I begin. "Your doctor has sent the biopsy reports. Have you seen the pathology report from your open breast biopsy?"

"You mean when I had surgery?" At my nod she continues. "I saw it, also the ominous look on my doctor's face," she says. "But I don't really understand what it means."

"Ok, let's see if I can explain," I say. "You have what's called carcinoma in situ. This kind of cancer is midway between actual cancer—by which we mean invasive or spreading cancer—and normal cells. The in situ words mean that the cancer is in one spot and hasn't spread. But the cells themselves look as though they are proliferating, growing too fast, and each has a bigger than normal nucleus. It doesn't look good." I quickly hasten to add, "but I have some ideas. However, first I need to understand a bit more about your breast problems. What can you tell me?"

"Ok," Floreena says. "Where to start? I've always had small breasts. Thankfully they haven't gotten much bigger as you said they usually did in perimenopause. About five years ago, I noticed the first breast lump. I felt it when I was showering. It was very tender, and didn't go away, so my doctor ordered a mammogram. Then I began the usual litany of ultrasounds, more mammograms and eventually had a needle biopsy. It was benign, and I thought that was that. But I've been growing breast lumps consistently since. In fact, it seems that every spring I get a lump and go through the whole scary routine of mammogram, special focused mammogram, ultrasound and then a needle biopsy. It's agonizing waiting for results—I am always *sure* I have cancer. But this last lump was different—it was never tender and from day one it was kind of hard. They said it was suspicious according to the other tests, so I had to have that day surgery."

I nod and she continues. "They told me that there were suspicious cells, but not enough of them to call it cancer. What worries me is that I have increased risks for breast cancer because I've never had children or breast-fed."

"How old are you now, Floreena?"

"I just turned 50," she says. "My menopause seems to be at a normal age."

"Are you still menstruating, Floreena?" I ask. As she nods I say, "You mean *peri*menopause, then, I think."

"Yes, I'm in perimenopause," she corrects herself. "I'm having irregular periods, but haven't started skipping yet. I think the things in my favour with this breast cancer thing are that I've never used alcohol, I don't smoke, and I'm not overweight."

"You've either done a lot of reading or listened well to what doctors have said, Floreena. It turns out that cigarette smoking doesn't relate one way or another to breast cancer (61). But someone who regularly has two or more alcohol drinks a day is about eight percent more likely to get breast cancer (61). I think being overweight and at risk for diabetes are also important risk factors for breast cancer. A colleague of mine showed that women with breast cancer whose waist to hip ratio was greatest at baseline were more likely to die from a breast cancer recurrence over 10 years than those with a slimmer waists (123). In other the words, the apple or round weight-at-the-waist shape that poses a risk for insulin resistance is associated with allowing breast cancer cells to grow."

"What do you mean, 'insulin resistance?'" she asks.

"That means that increasing obesity," I answer, "or inactivity, or heredity cause insulin to not work as well. To be able to do its job, insulin levels must rise. These higher insulin levels seem to stimulate cells to grow—in the breasts, ovary and other parts of the body. They are also related to heart disease."

"Well, I don't know my family so I don't know if I have any genetic risks. I don't even know if anyone had diabetes," Floreena reflects. "But I've never had a thick waist, so I'm probably not at risk for that reason."

"You don't know your family?" I ask.

"I'm adopted," she says flatly.

"I see," I murmur, sensing buried emotion behind her response. "If you would have had any reproductive surgeries such as tubal ligation, hysterectomy by itself, or hysterectomy with removal of your ovaries, your risk for breast cancer could decrease by 13–26 percent (18)."

"Really? I had a tubal ligation two years ago." Floreena pauses for a moment. "We thought it was right at the time. Now I wish we hadn't. I just keep thinking about babies." She pauses again, then resumes. "But I was 40 when we got together, and Sven was already 50. He's got a very busy law practice and just became a partner. So nothing was right for having a family." Another pause. "But it still bothers me."

"I understand, Floreena. There is something very strong and hard to explain about wanting children. Some of us really feel it, especially in perimenopause."

Floreena takes a long slow breath. "I guess you're telling me I should be happy about that tubal ligation," she says, "but I've been wishing I hadn't. I've even thought of adopting, but I don't think Sven would agree." She pauses again, and suddenly asks, "How could tubal ligation decrease the risk for breast cancer?"

"We're not really sure," I reply, "but it looks like any pelvic surgeries interfere with the blood supply to the ovaries. That decreased blood flow causes decreased hormones. What we know is from a study of women in their seventies and eighties. It showed that testosterone levels were lower, but estradiol levels weren't different between women with and without pelvic surgeries (124). The thought is—breast cancer risk is decreased because the lower level of testosterone made by the ovaries after hysterectomy doesn't get converted into as much estrone, the menopausal form of estrogen."

Floreena sits back in her chair. She seems to relax a bit.

"Have you kept any Diaries?" I ask, beginning again.

"I kept them for a couple of months last winter," she says. "And I even remembered to bring those this morning!" she laughs. "I ran back at the last minute and scooped them off the breakfast nook counter." She takes several pages out of her woven African shoulder bag.

I place the pages where we can both see them. "That's good," I say, "you've got a couple of regular cycles, and the last one here was about two weeks late. I see what you mean about breast tenderness before flow. I notice your breasts are most sore in the front, but you're also getting tenderness on the sides."

"I took my temperature," she says, "but I haven't done anything with those numbers. I didn't pick up that sheet you gave—was her name Beverley?—that woman who was trying to get pregnant."

I am scanning the temperatures. "We'll have to analyze the numbers properly to know for sure, but just looking, I don't see an increase suggesting ovulation. Oh—I'll bet you sleep in on weekends, right?"

## FLOREENA'S DIARY

Name: Floreena     Month: _____     Year: _____

| Cycle Day | 1 | 2 | 3 | 4 | 5 | 6 | 7 | 8 | 9 | 10 | 11 | 12 | 13 | 14 | 15 | 16 | 17 | 18 | 19 | 20 | 21 | 22 | 23 | 24 | 25 | 26 | 27 | 28 | 29 | 30 | 31 |
|---|---|---|---|---|---|---|---|---|---|---|---|---|---|---|---|---|---|---|---|---|---|---|---|---|---|---|---|---|---|---|---|
| Date | | | | | | | | | | | | | | | | | | | | | | | | | | | | | | | |
| Tampons/pads/day | | | | | | | | | | | | | | | | | | | | | | | | | | | | | | | |

Record M = much less, L = a little less, U = usual, Y = a little increased, Z = much increased

| | | | | | | | | | | | | | | | | | | | | | | | | | | | | | | | |
|---|---|---|---|---|---|---|---|---|---|---|---|---|---|---|---|---|---|---|---|---|---|---|---|---|---|---|---|---|---|---|---|
| Appetite | L | M | U | U | Y | U | U | U | L | U | U | U | L | L | U | L | C | L | U | L | L | U | U | U | L | U | U | L | U | U | L |
| Breast Size | Y | Y | Y | Y | U | U | Y | Y | Y | Y | Y | Y | X | Y | X | Y | Y | Y | Z | Z | Y | Y | Y | Y | Y | Y | Y | U | U | Y | |
| Interest In Sex | M | M | M | M | L | M | M | L | L | M | M | M | M | L | M | L | M | L | L | M | L | M | M | L | L | L | L | L | L | M | L |
| Feeling Of Energy | U | U | U | Y | U | U | U | U | U | Y | Y | U | U | U | U | U | U | U | L | U | U | U | U | U | U | U | U | U | U | U | U |
| Feeling Of Self-Worth | U | U | U | U | U | U | L | U | U | U | U | U | U | Y | U | U | U | U | Y | Y | U | U | U | U | U | U | Y | U | U | U | Y |
| Outside Stresses | U | Z | Y | U | U | U | U | U | U | L | L | L | U | U | U | Y | L | U | U | U | U | L | L | U | U | U | U | U | U | U | L |
| Basal Temperature | 36.3 | 36.2 | 36.1 | 36.1 | 36.0 | 36.2 | 36.3 | 36.1 | 36.0 | 36.2 | 36.1 | 36.3 | 36.6 | 36.3 | 36.2 | 36.4 | 36.5 | 36.4 | 36.5 | 36.3 | 36.6 | | | | | | | | | | |
| Comments (Temperature Taken Late, Feeling Sick, Poor Sleep, Etc.) | | | | | | | | | | | | | | | | | | | *very sore breasts* | | | | | | | | | | | | |

"Yes, we usually do," she says. "It's the only time Sven relaxes. How did you know?"

"You see, your morning temperature is a little higher for two days every week!" I show her the numbers.

"Amazing," she exclaims. "Staying in bed a little longer makes the temperature higher? I've only got a calendar of periods since then. But it shows that the business with the irregular period has continued. I'll have one that is two weeks apart and then another that takes almost a month and a half to come. I can tell when, though, because I get sore breasts every time."

She puts a hand on her breasts, as though feeling the soreness, then resumes. "And, this spring, I had the worst breast lump and now I have a kind of on-the-spot cancer." She stops, musing. "I want to know how to treat that speck of cancer, and I want to know whether my breast cancer risk is going to get better soon. Can you help me?"

"I'll sure try," I say, making myself sound very confident. "For sure the increased perimenopausal risk for breast cancer should decrease the closer you get to menopause. However, risk of breast cancer continues to increase with increasing age. Even though you are starting to have a few farther-apart cycles, your own estrogen levels haven't decreased to low levels yet, and won't until you are a year past your last flow. You've told me about the usual risks for breast cancer, but I think that there are other factors that are also important, like ovulation and progesterone. So—tell me about your periods, Floreena."

"As I mentioned," she says, "I was 12 for the first one. They came regularly, as far as I remember. I had no trouble with them except I skipped a month or so before my mom died. That was when I was 24. I was very upset after her stroke. She couldn't speak or even swallow properly. It was kind of a relief when she died. She was upset, even though she couldn't talk. I could tell. I lost a lot of weight."

"That kind of fundamental stress and weight loss are common reasons for irregular periods during the premenopausal years, Floreena."

"You see," she says, "they adopted me when they were older. I was really close to them, especially to Mom. I lived at home so I could take care of them. At first they ran a hardware store. I helped out in it from the time I was little. I knew everything there—when to re-order 5-penny nails and wood stain. My dad got so he hadn't a clue what we had and didn't. He relied on me. Which was good. But after Mom died, he changed. I guess it was his way of dealing with grief. He was always telling me that I forgot to do this or that. He was unkind. We ended up having to sell the store. He just suddenly lost touch—he wrecked a dozen pans because he'd leave the burner on, and was always saying that I was not feeding him well because he'd forgotten he just ate."

"That must have been very difficult," I say, reaching out to hold her hand.

"Yes," she says, "I was glad when the pastor and other folks from the church started regularly coming to visit him. Then I could occasionally get out. Finally I organized a home-care worker, and for my sanity worked part-time in a new craft and sewing store that a friend had just opened up in Abbotsford. I got more active in the church, took classes, and then started running a Sunday School class for the young adults. I also took on getting the flowers and decorating the sanctuary. I was eventually elected to the board of deacons. That's where I met Sven. After we got Dad into a nursing home, Sven and I saw more of each other. Eventually I had to sell the old place, and then Sven and I moved in together."

"You've had a lot of responsibility, haven't you?" I say.

She nods. "I still visit my dad once a week at the nursing home. He doesn't recognize me any more. But I still go."

"What do you do for fun?" I ask.

Floreena smiles. "I really like arts and crafts," she says. "I started learning about various hobbies when I worked in my friend's store. Times were tough for her, so she couldn't pay me, but I really enjoy helping out now and then. I found I like pottery, so I took a course at the community centre. I've always done knitting, tatting, crocheting and sewing. Mom taught me those. I give what I make to the church because we always have a Christmas arts and craft sale with the money going to the Mennonite Central Committee. Now I am having a great time making desktop and larger pottery fountains. I learned about wiring the lights and pumps."

"That's great, Floreena.' I point to a turquoise-and-blue fountain on the corner of my desk. "That fountain was made by a patient of mine. I really like it. The sound of running water is soothing."

"I ran out of a market for my little fountains up the Valley, so I've been selling them at the other Christmas craft fairs. In fact, I met Eva, you know, one of the women in the group session we had, also Henrietta at the East Van Christmas fair. We've been planning a party but we haven't got it together yet. When we do, I hope you can come."

"I'd like that if I have time," I reply. "I'm glad you made some connections with the other women. In spite of some rough times, it sounds as though you are being creative and enjoying your life, Floreena."

"Yes, yes, I am," she says. "But I still am looking for something. I guess I need to find some meaning." There is a long pause. "Would it be ok if I asked you something?" she asks.

"Sure," I say, wondering what she seems apprehensive about.

"Is it normal to have no sex drive at all?" she asks. "I've been too shy to talk about it." She pauses. "I wondered if you knew of a reason. I'm just not interested. It has gotten gradually worse over the last two or three years." She stops and begins again. "I actually couldn't care less. But Sven is quite insistent that having sex regularly is what living together is all about. And if I agree, he won't give up until he thinks I'm satisfied. . . It feels like, like work, well, like doing dishes. . ."

Although I find her example quite funny, I manage to be serious. "Did you have a good sex life when you first got together?" I ask.

"Yes, then it was great," she replies.

"And do you care about him and does he for you?"

"Yes, we love each other a lot," she says.

"It's normal," I say, "for sexual interest to decrease in women after about their mid-thirties. We're slower to get lubricated and aroused, and it takes more time to reach orgasm. With a new relationship, sex is usually great. But many, if not most, women go through a spell in perimenopause when they'd rather not bother. Are you having vaginal dryness?"

"No. We use Y-2-K, " she says.

I raise my eyebrows. Then we both begin to laugh.

"I mean K-Y jelly!" she says. I laugh so hard that tears are running down my face.

"I'm glad you realized what you said," I sputter. "I'm not sure I could have managed to keep a straight face!

"Even if you weren't getting irregular periods," I begin more seriously, "not being sexually active for a while can cause a slow start with lubrication. So make sure you have lots of cuddling first, and feel ready for sex. There are many lubricants available besides the one you've been using."

"Are any better than the other?" she asks. "A girlfriend said something about one called Astroslip or something!" She starts to laugh and I join in.

"They are lots—they all have funny names!" I say. "And each is a little different. I'd avoid ones with any alcohol in them—they can be drying. Maybe you can experiment."

"Sven's good and patient and all," Floreena says solemnly. "Just some days I don't want to be touched. Especially on my breasts, I guess because it reminds me of my lumps—I feel afraid."

"That's very natural," I say reassuringly. "You need to tell him I said that it's normal for perimenopausal women to temporarily lose interest in sex. Just keep snuggling and caring for each other. Eventually your interest will return."

Floreena still looks uncomfortable. She leans forward and lowers her voice.

"I was brought up to be honest, you know. But I've gotten so desperate to make Sven happy that I'll sometimes fake a climax."

"That's not good." I say and Floreena nods. "I think many women do that. But what most concerns me is you can't tell him what you're feeling. In some ways, it says you don't trust him. That's not unusual, given your background. But you and he need to work together. For that, openness and honesty are essential." I smile. "In my view, sex is the ultimate team sport!" I pause a moment, wondering how far to go with suggestions. "You know, don't you, that you can always pleasure him in other ways." I try to tell from Floreena's face whether she understands.

"I've never talked with anyone about sex before," she says. "Sven and I have never discussed it. But I know he cares. So I'll tell him what you said." She pauses briefly. "I know! I'll share our Y-2-K joke! See if that helps me tell him what I'm feeling."

"Great idea!" I say. "If you continue to have trouble, I'm sure your pastor would help. The bottom line is that you each care for the other. Sven needs to accept the fact that you're not always ready for intercourse. It's hard for a guy not to think that means you don't love him."

"I guess I thought that it was my responsibility. That if I didn't make him happy, he would leave. We're not married, you know. Sven had a bad first marriage. He doesn't talk about it. He wouldn't consider marrying again. And I don't really care about a ceremony, as long as we are committed to each other and to making a home together."

"I'm glad that you and Sven share your interest and involvement in the church," I say.

"Yes." Floreena relaxes into her chair. "And we have similar values."

I take a deep breath. "Ok, where were we? I still need to know if you have ever been really sick, injured, or hospitalized, or had any operations."

"I had my tonsils out when I was five," she says. "And had an appendectomy at age 11. I don't know anything about my birth or early childhood. I was apparently an out-of-wedlock baby who was given to a children's home.

My foster parents adopted me when I was about two. Otherwise, except for the tubal ligation, and all those breast things, I've had nothing."

"Are you allergic to anything?" I ask.

"Not that I know of."

"Do you regularly exercise?"

"I'm afraid not," she says, smiling ruefully. "Sven and I, occasionally on Saturdays, go to a pick-up volleyball game for the young adult group from the church. I love playing—I've got a great serve. Everyone wants me on their team. We've also taken to having a walk along the Seder Canal some weekend evenings when it's nice, or when he gets home before it's really late."

"You already said you don't drink or smoke. How about coffee?"

"Oh, I like my coffee," she says. "I'll have a couple of good strong cups—teacup size, not mugs—with Sven before he leaves for work, then I drink the rest of a 2-litre pot throughout the day as I'm working on my creations. I can concentrate on designs and things better when I've got something hot to drink."

"So, maybe six or seven cups a day?" She nods. "I'd suggest making regular coffee just enough for a couple of cups for each of you for breakfast. Then make another pot of decaf for you for the rest of the day. I know what you mean about something hot to drink helping you to focus."

"Ok, I'll try that," she says. "What's the matter with too much caffeine, Doctor?"

"It seems to make estrogen have stronger growth-stimulating effects in breast tissue. Plus, caffeine can make anxiety and stress worse and can cause headaches. Finally, you are in the time of perimenopause when *all* women lose bone—and caffeine causes the kidneys to excrete more calcium, which causes bone loss."

"Oh," she says.

"You said you haven't gained any weight. And I'd gather, from what you said about your mom's stroke, that you're one of those people who loses weight with stress. Tell me what you ate yesterday."

"Let's see," she says. "Sven and I, as usual for breakfast, had organic whole-grain porridge cooked with dried cranberries. Milk, and the coffee, as I mentioned. I had a leftover four-bean salad with a scone and local goat cheese for lunch, plus coffee. Then I made a chicken vegetable curry dish and rice for a potluck supper at the church. Of course there I had to taste Monika's lasagna, Mrs. Dirks' deep-dish salmon pie, Isabelle's famous Japanese salad, someone's green gelatin salad, and someone else's lovely Greek salad. Plus a gazillion kinds of desserts." She laughs. "You know, the 'groaning board' where everyone is showing off her best dish."

"You're making me hungry!" I exclaim. "It sounds as though you eat pretty well, but probably skip lunch or just pick at your food if something's upsetting you. I want you to remember that weight loss always increases stress hormones and inevitably causes bone loss"(125). She nods.

"On another note—do you know *anything* about your birth parents?"

"Nothing about my real father," she says. "I think Mom said that my birth mother was from the Prairies and came out here when she knew she was pregnant. But I don't know anything else."

"You know that you can officially find out about the health of your biological parents through the provincial adoption agency? That's a new thing in the last few years. It might be a good idea, given your personal risk for breast cancer, to see if there is any family history for that or for ovarian cancer. There's a hereditary kind of breast cancer that's linked through the family history to ovarian cancer (126). If you want, the agency will provide a name and contact information."

"I didn't know," she says. "I've left all that behind me. But maybe one day I'll get the courage." She pauses. "I'd really like to have my own family."

"You said you've never been pregnant," I say. "Have you ever used the birth control pill?"

"No. I wasn't with anyone until I started going out with Sven. And we used condoms for about eight years until I had my tubes tied."

"Can you tell by the way you feel that your period is coming?" I ask.

"I used to only know by the day of the month," she replies. "Now I know because of sore, swollen and lumpy breasts."

"When you can tell that your period is coming—usually by tenderness high up under the armpit part of the breasts with no other breast soreness, and sometimes also by a little bloating, hunger, or irritability—that's called molimina. When you don't get those signals, and you can only tell by the time of the month, or you have only things our culture tells us to expect, like mood changes, that's strong evidence you didn't ovulate (45)."

"Why do my breasts tell me now?" she asks.

"That front-of-the breast soreness is from high estrogen," I say, "and it doesn't tell us anything about progesterone. How do you sleep?"

"I sleep better cuddled up with Sven. But I've been a poor sleeper all my life. Mom said I'd wake screaming at night when I was a toddler. Before exams in high school, I'd toss and turn. For the last few years I've started to have a different kind of sleep problem. I fall asleep fine, but then wake about two or three. Actually, I know exactly what time it is—I try to not look at the clock. But I always end up looking. It is precisely 2:27 on the dial! It's so strange. Remember Carla in the group said she always woke up at 3:13! Anyway, that'd be ok, but I tend to get to bed late waiting dinner for Sven when he has a deadline or something. And he always is up early. So, after I wake once, I toss and turn until it's time to get up and make his breakfast."

"That's rough, Floreena. Are any other things bothering you—any diarrhea or constipation, skin rashes, joint pains?"

"I tend to get constipation," she says. "It's better now that I make sure to have a fresh fruit, that whole grain porridge and a raw carrot or two every day. Otherwise I'm fine."

"Ok, I've run out of questions, but if I've missed anything, just let me know. I'd like to check you over. But I won't do a pelvic because your doctor said that your Pap test and pelvic exam were normal recently. After that, we'll see what we can do about those breast lumps and your risk for breast cancer. Here's a gown. Put your clothes on that table there, take everything off except your panties and lie down. If I may, I'll go photocopy your Diaries while you're changing."

～

"Knock, knock. It's just me," I say. "You don't look very relaxed," Floreena is lying stiffly on the table. I take her hand and rub it—it is very cold. "Have you ever tried meditating? No? It's important to learn how to meditate. You pray, don't you? Meditation is very much the same as silent prayer. A preacher when I was a kid always used to say, 'Let go and let God.' Meditation or prayer can be very relaxing."

Floreena takes a long breath, and I start the examination.

"Your blood pressure is on the high side at 142 over 92 and your pulse is at 84. I'll repeat these later when you are more relaxed. Your breasts,"—I help Floreena put her arms up over her head—"are not only very small, they've never grown up!"

"What do you mean?" she asks? "They're still a child's?"

"Not those of a kid, but of a young teen. I'll draw the growing-up breast phases for you when you're dressed. I see what you mean about lumpy! Is that place sore now?" I feel her left breast.

"Not bad, just a tiny bit tender," she says. "But there are so many lumpy bits I can't remember them. My doctor kept telling me to check my breasts. But I couldn't remember. Finally I decided to draw the lumpy bits and firm areas on each breast. I have one page for each breast! It's the only way I have a prayer of remembering—they're so fibrous."

"That's a clever idea, Floreena. Not everyone is as good at sketching as you are, but I'll suggest that to other patients who have a difficult time keeping track of lumps. This was where you had your biopsy, right? Because it's still healing, it feels more firm around here than it does in the same area of your opposite breast. I'm always relieved, myself, when I find a lump and then realize it's pretty lumpy in the same area of the opposite breast, too. So another reassurance, besides your drawings, is that your two breasts roughly match.

"I also see that your reflexes are quick, you've very little fat or muscle on your arms or trunk, and your heart sounds fine. Sit up a second. Oh, oh, you need to work on your tummy muscles."

"Why do you say that?" Floreena asks.

"When you sat up, your legs flew off the bed. I have an informal abdominal strength scale I grade as women sit up from lying down. A little leg movement is a 1, about half a foot is a 2, a foot is a 3 and more or hauling yourself up with your hands is a 4. Four is the weakest—I'm afraid that's your score!" I feel the vertebrae in her back from top to bottom and then punch down her back, asking, "Is that tender?"

"No," she says.

"That's good. Turn around this way, hold your chin level and swallow so I can check your thyroid."

Suddenly Floreena grabs my wrists roughly. Her nails are blanched and she looks terrified.

"What's the matter?" I ask. I gently remove my wrists from her clutch. "It's ok, Floreena, you can let go now. It's all right, Floreena." As she releases me I begin rubbing her cold hands. "I won't check your neck and thyroid if it frightens you."

"I'm sorry, Dr. Madrona. I didn't mean to. . ." She stops, looking shaken. "Of course, it's ok. Go ahead and check my thyroid."

"If you're sure." I say. She nods. I keep my left hand on Floreena's shoulder while I gently use my right thumb to feel the right side of her thyroid gland rise as she swallows. Then I trade hands and feel the other thyroid lobe. "Your thyroid is fine. Watch my finger. Focus on the tip." I move my finger in close to her nose.

"Ok, let's get your height and weight and then you can get dressed."

~

When Floreena joins me, I say, "Oh, I forgot to get your blood pressure again. Just ask your family doctor to check next time you're in, Floreena. Your weight is 56.8 kg and your height is 176 cm. That makes you very slim with a BMI of just over 18—that's at the edge of the 'underweight' category for a teenager. Do you know what I mean by BMI?"

"Yes, I do," she answers. "I've read about it. And I know a high BMI is associated with breast cancer."

As we sit again around the corner of the desk, I ask gently, "Do you know why you were frightened, Floreena?"

Floreena shakes her head slowly. She still looks unsteady.

"It's possible," I say, "that something happened when you were little, too young to remember, that seriously hurt or frightened you. That's a huge fear to get over."

"I've always been nervous if someone touches my neck," she says. "I don't know why."

I let a long silence fill the room. "What I do know," Floreena says, changing the subject, "is that I'm not ovulating now—because of perimenopause. But I've had perfectly regular menstrual cycles. What would make you say I've never ovulated?"

"Your breasts told me," I say. "Let's talk about breast stages—they're named after a Doctor Tanner who photographed girls in an orphanage in Britain and recorded breast maturation (127)." I take a pencil, a one-side used piece of scrap paper and a two-dollar coin from my drawer and begin to draw.

"See, let's say this is what your breasts were like when you were a child. This is Tanner Stage I. There's no breast bump at all as you can see in the view from the side, here. As you shot up in height, your breasts probably grew a little bigger and began to stick out a bit. That is Tanner Stage II. Around the time you had your first period, they grew bigger yet to what we call Tanner Stage III. But they haven't matured past that."

"How can you tell?" she asks quizzically.

## TANNER'S BREAST MATURATION STAGES

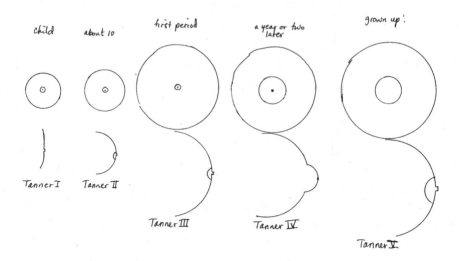

"Tonight when you get ready for bed, look at the size of the darker part of your breast, the areola, surrounding the nipple. It's still small, like a quarter. It should get to be the size of a one-or a two-dollar coin. Maturation beyond Tanner Stage III takes progesterone as well as estrogen. Here in Tanner Stage IV the areola is bigger and puffy but the nipple is still underdeveloped. When women ovulate regularly, breasts mature to Tanner Stage V. What's different about the grown-up breast is that the areola is big and the nipple stands up when you look at it from the side."

"What makes those breast changes?" she asks.

"I'm not absolutely sure, but it looks to me like it's the action of progesterone and estrogen together in Tanner Stages IV and V, but estrogen alone in earlier stages. You're still at Tanner Stage III. That's why I don't think you've ovulated."

"Neat, Dr. Madrona! But why wouldn't I ovulate?" she asks.

"The biggest reason for not ovulating is stress—and you've had plenty in your life. And being skinny. Those two together are plenty to explain your underdeveloped breasts. And I think not ovulating is the biggest reason for your breast lumps and that biopsy showing carcinoma in situ. You have had regular periods, which means normal estrogen levels, most of your life. But regular cycles don't mean regular ovulation."

"I get that, Dr. Madrona. But how does not ovulating relate to breast cancer?"

"Here's the way I understand these hormones and the breast," I reply. "Estrogen's job is to make breast tissue grow or proliferate. Progesterone's job is to counterbalance that growth and to cause differentiation. That means to help tissues become mature, or grow up (128;129). That bigger areola and the standing-up nipple in Tanner Stage V are part of progesterone's work in breast maturation."

"Please remind me," she says, "what you mean by proliferation and differentiation?"

"Sure," I say. "Proliferation means that the cells are growing and dividing. That growth, if unchecked, can lead to cancer. Differentiation means that the cells are becoming more grown-up or mature. Cancer cells are typically growing fast and are very immature."

"So my breasts have been going ballistic with all this estrogen!" she quips. "Only it isn't funny. Does that mean I should take the medicine my cancer doctor suggested that works against estrogen? I think it was called Tamoxifen."

"Tamoxifen *is* probably what your doctor suggested." I agree. "That'd be a great idea if Tamoxifen and others like it were purely estrogen antagonists. But they also work like estrogen. So I don't want you to take Tamoxifen because it not only antagonizes, but also mimics estrogen. Instead, given that you are in perimenopause and already have high estrogen levels, we need to counterbalance those high estrogen effects in your breast. For these reasons I would like you to take a high dose of progesterone every day. The idea is that the progesterone will work to make your breast cells more mature and to prevent your perimenopausal high estrogen levels from causing abnormal growth. You can stop the progesterone and consider Tamoxifen when you have been two full years without flow. How does that sound?"

"I don't know," Floreena looks anxious. "You're the expert."

"Floreena," I say firmly, "this may be difficult for you because you like to do what authorities suggest. What I'm suggesting fits with what I know about perimenopause and how estrogen and progesterone work in breasts. But it will be considered controversial. I expect that your family doctor, and for sure your oncologist, your cancer doctor, will disagree with progesterone therapy. First of all, giving it to you as a treatment is not standard. It is rather like an experiment based on good evidence about how estrogen and progesterone act in breast cells. But that good information about progesterone and breast cells is new, so your doctors may not know about it. Your doctors also were taught, and may believe, that progesterone is one of the causes for breast cancer."

"Why would they think that?" she asks.

"First of all," I say, "it's awfully hard to separate the effects of estrogen from the effects of progesterone. You remember that picture of the normal menstrual cycle I showed you in the group? You have to reach high estrogen levels before you can get ovulation. And most doctors wrongly believe, just as you thought, that regular cycles mean that there are both normal estrogen and normal progesterone levels. Instead, regular cycles, like you've had most of your life, can happen with no ovulating at all. Another reason doctors are worried about progesterone and breast cancer is that some kinds of progestins, when added to breast cancer cells in a laboratory, cause the cancer cells to grow for a few days. Most studies don't continue long enough to see that progesterone later causes differentiation and maturation. The most important recent reason is that the big Women's Health Initiative controlled study of hormone therapy for menopause showed increased breast cancer with estrogen plus progestin (130) and didn't show increased risk with estrogen alone (27;130)."

Floreena looks worried. "But don't the women who've had a hysterectomy and who would have taken estrogen by itself have a lower breast cancer risk?"

"Yes," I say, "but your doctors may not know about the breast cancer-protective effects of pelvic surgery (18). I didn't, myself, until a year or so ago. Let me try to explain why the Women's Health Initiative studies showed the breast cancer results that they did. The estrogen-only study didn't have enough women with a high enough risk to even show breast cancer risk. When the estrogen-only study was planned, they knew they didn't have enough statistical power—or mathematical likelihood of finding something—to show breast cancer risk (131). It's like you wouldn't be able with your eyes to see a dog in a yard a km away. But you could if you looked with binocular that have magnifying power. Plus the study enrolled fewer women than they had planned, women dropped out after the estrogen plus progestin results were announced, and that arm of the study was also stopped a year early. So there are many reasons it didn't show an increased risk for breast cancer."

She nods. "All of the women who got estrogen by itself had hysterectomies, right? And that surgery decreased their breast cancer risk."

"Exactly right!" I say. "In addition, the Women's Health Initiative study was planned before we knew that pelvic surgery decreases the risk for breast cancer (18).

"So, based on what estrogen and progesterone do in breast cells, I think that the risk for breast cancer increases with estrogen primarily when there is not enough progesterone to counterbalance estrogen's breast cell growth effects. There were two randomized controlled experiments, one in premenopausal and one in menopausal women, showing this. All of the women in those two studies were scheduled to have a surgical breast biopsy like you've had. An extra bit of tissue was taken that was far away from the lump that they removed—and all the lumps were benign. The cells of women on progesterone showed decreased proliferation. Proliferation in breast cells is a sign of increased cancer risk" (128;129).

"Do we know what high estrogen did?" she asks.

"Yes," I answer. "Because all of the women in the study were randomized into one of four hormone therapy groups. They had the hormone as a cream that they rubbed onto the breast that was to have surgery. One group rubbed on an inactive cream, another an estrogen cream, another a progesterone cream, and the final group rubbed progesterone plus estrogen cream. All of the hormone doses were natural, and all of the women used the cream for 11 days. The women who were premenopausal rubbed the cream in starting on the first day of the period (128;129)."

"What did the four groups show?" she asks, listening intently.

"At the time of the biopsy," I answer, "those who got estrogen showed increased cellular proliferation and those who got progesterone alone showed decreased proliferation and more mature cells. Those with the combined hormones also had decreased proliferation, especially less than in the estrogen-only group (128;129)."

"But aren't there studies showing that menopausal women on estrogen plus progestin are more likely to get breast cancer than women on dummy pills?" Floreena asks anxiously. "My cancer doctor said that women on just estrogen were less likely to get breast cancer than women on estrogen and progestin."

"Yes," I reply, "because women on estrogen alone all had hysterectomy."

"You are saying that study didn't have enough women to show breast cancer when women with hysterectomies got estrogen by itself, right?"

"That's right," I say. "And I was warning you that your oncologist may strongly disagree with the idea of progesterone treatment."

Floreena sits up straight, leaning forward.

"To help us with this difficult idea about treatment," I say, making my voice strong and reassuring, "let's gather some more information about your present risks. I'll write this lab slip for you to have blood drawn for levels of estrogen, progesterone, testosterone and some stress hormones called cortisol and DHEAS. Have the blood drawn on a day when your breasts are sore and you think your period is coming. I'll write this slip so you can repeat it twice about a month apart. You will get a copy as well as your family doctor and your oncologist. We won't start any treatment until we have those results. In the meantime, I'll write a letter describing your situation to your oncologist and explaining why I want to treat you with high-dose progesterone therapy."

I hand her the lab slip. "Since you're here now, I'll give you the prescription for oral micronized progesterone—it's called Prometrium. Take 400 mg every day at bedtime."

She still looks worried. "You want me to have two blood tests, go see my family doctor and see the cancer specialist before I start this?"

"Yes, I'd like you to," I say. "The final decision about therapy is yours, Floreena. But I want you and all of those caring for you, to understand why I'm making this suggestion. I'll send you and your family doctor copies of my letter to your oncologist, too. I'll explain that we are trying to counterbalance the effects of your body's perimenopausal high estrogen production on your breast cells."

"I don't know what to do, Dr. Madrona! It's all so confusing." Floreena is shaking her head and practically moaning.

"You need to talk about your decision with your doctors and also with Sven," I say.

"What are the side-effects of high-dose progesterone treatment, Dr. Madrona?" she asks.

"The most common one is drowsiness and a deeper sleep (81). Those are good effects because you only take the progesterone on your way to bed at night. Otherwise, you may have fewer periods, lighter flow, and in about a cycle or two your breasts will generally be less sore and lumpy. Progesterone has no serious side-effects like estrogen has. Progesterone doesn't cause blood clots or migraine headaches and may be helpful in preventing heart attacks, although we don't yet have big studies on that (132). In short, I think progesterone is very safe and will be positive for you."

She sighs and nods thoughtfully. "I do trust you, Dr. Madrona. But can I ask you a question? What would you do if you were me?"

"I'd take progesterone, Floreena." I say this very clearly. "But if you decide to follow your oncologist's advice—after all, he is the cancer specialist—and take Tamoxifen, just make sure you understand its risks and benefits, and what evidence there is that it will help with breast cancer in situ."

Still looking worried and unsure, she says, "I just need some time to think it over and make careful decisions. In the meantime, I should work on more exercise, strengthen my stomach muscles and find out about my birth parents' health."

"Those would all be helpful," I say. "Of course you're confused, Floreena. And you have good reason to be frightened of breast cancer. Although breast cancer in situ means the cancer hasn't spread, I'm very concerned, too. I certainly don't want you to take anything that makes you uncomfortable. I can't prove that progesterone will be effective, but I'm sure that a high dose will not increase your risks for breast cancer. You're doing your breast self-examination every month and getting a mammogram every year, right? When are you scheduled to see your oncologist at the Cancer Agency?"

She looks in her date book. "I have an appointment at the Fraser Valley Clinic in August. And yes, I check my breasts monthly and have my mammograms every six or 12 months, whenever I get a reminder letter."

"That's great," I say. "I will write that letter about your situation and my progesterone suggestion tomorrow after I can give it more thought. I'll include the references, especially the new ones about hysterectomy and tubal ligation and the Women's Health Initiative estrogen-only arm's statistical power. You realize, don't you, that I understand progesterone differently than other doctors? That's because I've learned from Dr. Prior and worked with her on some studies. I was sceptical, too, until I read the papers she suggested. Most of what doctors have been taught about women—our menstrual cycles, hormone levels and health risks—is negative for women. Doctors and our society have also believed for decades that estrogen does good things for us. By the same token, we've either blamed anything bad on progesterone or ignored it!

"Meanwhile, Floreena, if you would restart your Diary record and record your basal temperature—at least until you start therapy—that will give us more information. Because of lack of ovulation (133), all the stresses of your life (134), and your leanness, you are also at risk for low bone density. So I'm also going to order a bone density scan as a baseline."

"You think I might have osteoporosis, too, Dr. Madrona?" she asks.

"Yes, I have some bone concerns," I say. "Usually women at risk for breast cancer are heavier, have had more periods and have a low risk for osteoporosis (135). Your history is different, and I think low bone density is a risk for you. At any rate, it will be worth it to take that off your list of worries if it's normal. The good news is that treatment with progestin increases bone density (136;137).

Ask Sven to go to the CeMCOR website—that's www.cemcor.ubc.ca—and download and print out the 'ABCs of Osteoporosis Prevention for Midlife Women' for you. I'd suggest following those practical instructions very closely, Floreena, whether or not your bone density turns out to be normal."

She carefully writes the CeMCOR website address into her book.

A few minutes later, we've finished and are walking down the hall to Lana's desk. I ask Lana to book a bone density scan for Floreena as soon as possible and schedule a six-month follow-up with me.

"How are you doing, Floreena?" Lana asks. "You sounded worried when I spoke with you on the phone to remind you about this visit. Make sure we get copies of all of your lab tests, mammograms, ultrasounds and your oncologist's report, ok?"

"I'll be sure to do that," Floreena answers.

"One more thing, Lana," I say. "Please find Floreena's Cancer Agency number so we that we can send a copy of my consult to her agency chart, as well as my letter to her oncologist."

As Floreena prepares to leave, I give her cool hands a little squeeze. "You are a strong woman, Floreena. You've had a tough go of it so far. Just have faith."

"Thanks, Dr Madrona," she says. "I'll try." She turns away with tears in her eyes.

A few months later, I see Floreena again.

"Hello, Floreena. It doesn't seem that six months have gone by. I guess not quite, because I last saw you in July."

Floreena looks worried. "Actually, Dr Madrona, I called Lana early because I was so confused about what to do. She made this appointment for me when she had a cancellation. I'm so grateful you would see me again."

"I'm happy to see you, too," I say, smiling. "Now tell me what's been going on."

Floreena doesn't return my smile. "I had a set of special mammograms and a bunch of blood tests. My oncologist seemed upset at me and at your letter (see page 214). I didn't know what to do. I talked with women at the Cancer Clinic, with a social worker, with my family doctor and with Sven. I just couldn't decide. And I even got really mad at you for *making* me." She's looking at me intently.

"I'm sorry you feel that way, Floreena. But you're the one with the breast cancer in situ, so *you're* the one who has to decide. I wouldn't want someone making that choice for me. What did you learn about Tamoxifen?"

I glance at some new reports in Floreena's chart.

"Well," she says, "in menopausal women it decreases the risk of recurrent breast cancer by 20 percent (138). But it causes blood clots, can cause cancer of the uterus, and makes some women have horrible hot flushes. Experts don't really have any ideas about how it would work for carcinoma in situ. And no one knows how it would work for someone who's still in perimenopause. I just don't like the sound of Tamoxifen. But everyone I've talked with is very negative about progesterone."

"I tried to warn you, Floreena, about the bad rap progesterone has! Well, so what did you do?"

"I tried Tamoxifen for about ten days," she says. "I felt like I was poisoning myself. So I stopped it."

She pauses and takes a deep breath. "I walk every day now," she continues, "about forty-five minutes or an hour, usually right after Sven goes to work. And he and I talked about—you know—sex and that, and he is now more willing to just touch me or give me a backrub if I say I'm not interested."

"That's really good," I say. "What does he think about your treatment?"

"Sven's a lawyer, right? He read the letter you wrote very carefully—several times. He thinks I could do that experiment you suggested. Did my oncologist call you?"

"No." I reply. "I thought he would, but he didn't."

"Sven came with me to see him and wasn't too impressed. And Sven said the oncologist was not very professional in the way he talked about you and the idea of progesterone treatment. By the way, what did my blood tests show?"

"Yes!" I say. "I wanted to go over those with you. The one in late July was when you were feeling premenstrual, right? It showed a very high estrogen level and a low progesterone level—1733 pmol/L and 7 nmol/L. Clearly you didn't ovulate and your estrogen was *way too high*. The one in August showed an even higher estrogen level at 2076 pmol/L, which is about the highest I've ever seen, and a low normal progesterone level of 19 nmol/L. The testosterone levels were normal at 0.4 and 0.6, but the DHEAS and cortisol were both on the high side of normal."

"Oh—and I have the results of this test. Did you get it?" Floreena pulls a slip from her purse and gives it to me.

"Thank you," I say. "I was wondering whether they got enough tissue to assess breast hormone receptor status. Your breast cancer cells are estrogen receptor positive. That's what I thought they would show.

"I've got some other results, Floreena, like your bone density, that I need to discuss with you. We did that bone density test in August. Did your family doctor talk with you about it? I think I mentioned that your bone density was low in my letter to your oncologist. Anyway, here's the report for your file."

After handing Floreena the report, I spread the printout of the hip and spine density in front of us. "This shows that both your spine and especially your hip are on the low-density side. We use the results of women ages 20–30 as the gold standard and compare you to that using a standard deviation or T-Score. We call a T-Score of +1 to –1 normal. Your spine is –1.8 and your hip is –2.3. Both of these values show low bone density or osteopenia."

"But why?" Floreena asks. "I've walked all my life, I eat well, and I always take calcium. How can I have low bone density when I do everything right?"

"It turns out," I say, "that the important things for bone density in young women are things most people don't know about, like ovulating, and not being too stressed, and having and keeping a normal weight."

"I'm working on some things," she says. "Since we met, I've increased my calcium to 2,000 mg a day from milk and a latte at breakfast, a yogurt at lunch and a decaf latte at supper. Sven bought me an espresso machine for my birthday. It foams milk and makes great coffee—even decaffeinated. And I get 500 mg from a calcium pill at bedtime. Plus I am taking 1,400 IU of vitamin D, just like you said. I've been eating almonds between meals and snacking before bed to increase my weight. Most of all, if something's bothering me, I *make* myself eat. Sven is good at reminding me."

"That's great," I say. "And I gather you've cut down on your coffee."

"Yes, I have decaf coffee after breakfast and limit my breakfast coffee to two or three small cups. Oh, I forgot to tell you—I did call the government adoption agency, and they gave me the name and address of my birth mother. I have only talked with her on the phone, but she doesn't think anyone related to her had breast cancer. We're going to meet at a craft sale in early December. I'm scared, but I also can't wait. She sounded nice. She had been thinking about me and was happy I called."

"Good for you!" I exclaim. "It's hard to get over all the sadness over feeling abandoned, and it's really hard to make those calls. I've known lots of adopted people who found that their birth families sort of set things right for them." Floreena smiles.

"I'd like to examine you now, Floreena," I say. "Before I do that, I think I need to talk with your oncologist. I'll try to call him while you change. Here's the gown. Lie down and relax."

~

Later, I knock and enter the examining room. "I'm sorry I took so long, Floreena. At first Lana couldn't get through the switchboard to get your oncologist's phone extension. Then he was with patients. Anyway he's promised to call me back at 12:30 today when we're both on our lunch break. Lana will take her lunch late to make sure I get through."

"I appreciate what you and Lana do, Dr. Madrona. It's like both of you care. How can you afford to spend so much time with each patient?"

"I can't afford not to," I say. "Otherwise, I don't feel as though I've done a good job, and the patient feels rushed. I have a university salary, so I'm a lucky physician. I take a full hour with every patient."

Floreena nods as she points to an area in the upper outer part of her left breast. "I was checking my breasts while I was waiting—I think I feel a new lump here."

"Let's see," I say. "Well there is a nodular area there, but it matches a similar firmer area on your right breast. The rest of your breast is nodular and more firm than I like to feel, but without any masses.

"Come, let's check your weight and height. Your weight is slightly better at 55.5 kg. That's an increase of 0.7 kg or not quite 2 lb since you were here five months ago. And your height is the same."

After I finish the exam and Floreena is dressed again, I say, "We got through the thyroid exam better this time! It must have helped that I was careful to use one hand at a time and explain everything to you before I did it."

"Yes, thank you," she says. "I took a deep breath and tried to relax."

"Good for us! Ok, you're doing the right things with calcium, vitamin D, weight gain and more exercise to improve your bone density. The only thing I would like to add is progesterone, which will cause you to make more new bone. However, that's still your decision. I guess another possibility is to take Tamoxifen along with progesterone."

"Dr. Madrona, I've thought about it, and I've talked with Sven. I feel ready to make a decision. I'd like to do a trial of progesterone as you suggested in your letter and to just see what the breast biopsy shows. Would you discuss that with my oncologist when you talk with him?"

"Ok," I say. "We need to do the two needle biopsies about a month apart. It's probably best to choose early in your own cycle for the first biopsy. Progesterone in a high dose and taken every day will probably make your period stop. I'll write the laboratory slip for you to get blood hormone levels of estrogen and progesterone in the morning on the same day as each of the two biopsies. You, as well as your doctors, should get copies of those results."

"I've still got that prescription for progesterone, Dr Madrona. But tell me again how I should take it and why."

"I wrote for you to take 400 mg of Prometrium at bedtime daily," I reply. "The reasons are that you are in perimenopause with high estrogen levels that *average* about 30 percent higher than normal (8). I've prescribed progesterone daily and in a dose that is about 30 percent higher than the usual ovulation amount. We want the progesterone to counterbalance the actions of estrogen in your breast cells, to stop proliferation and to cause differentiation. That means to stop the frantic cell growth and instead allow the cells to mature. I think that will take away the abnormal cells that are the breast cancer in situ. We know that kind of cure happens in the uterus with endometrial hyperplasia, and the risk for cancer totally disappears. Also, given your bone density results, we have another reason for progesterone. That's to stimulate new bone to grow so that you won't have any fractures as a result of osteoporosis."

"After the month and the second biopsy on progesterone, shall I stop taking it and wait for the results?" she asks.

"It's up to you," I say. "If you feel good on it and your breasts are feeling softer and less lumpy, then I suggest that you just continue to take it. Several months may pass before we have the biopsy results read and properly compared."

"I'm going to let them go through the regular pathology process in the Valley Cancer Centre," I explain. "But I'll also get the original slides, make sure there's no identification except the dates and your ID, and ask a really skilled pathologist here at the provincial Cancer Agency to look at the two sets. I won't tell her anything except that they are from the same woman and a month apart. I'll ask her to stain them for proliferation and to make comparisons."

"I feel good about this, Dr. Madrona. The information you'll learn here will also help other women, won't it?"

"Yes, I'm sure it will," I say. "Everything I learn I pass on to my patients and students and residents. Life is pretty complex, but as long as we have puzzles to solve, it's also very interesting."

Floreena smiles at me. "I like the way you look at the whole picture—not just my breasts, but my history, and my cycles, and bones, and perimenopause. It feels right to try this. And I'll know from my Diary if the progesterone causes me any problems."

"Speaking of which," I ask, "may I copy your Diary sheets since July? I was so busy trying to make that phone call that I forgot to copy them. Did you write down the days on which you tried Tamoxifen?"

She nods. "I'll see you in six months, Floreena. If anything new comes up in my talk with your oncologist, I'll let you know."

"Thanks again, Dr. Madrona. I'll set up that appointment with Lana."

## Dr. Kailey Madrona, BA, MD, FRCPC
*Centre for Menstrual Cycle and Ovulation Research*

Suite 380 – 575 West 8th Avenue
Vancouver, BC Canada V5Z 1C6
Email: kmadrona@cemcor.ca

July 18, 2004

Dr. Mark Aster
Breast Cancer Programme
c/o Fraser Valley Centre
Cancer Agency of British Columbia

**Re: Floreena van Hoff**
Birth Date June 22, 1953, ID # FV-2002-087-5122

Dear Dr. Mark Aster:

I am writing to you about our mutual patient whom I have just seen for perimenopause and breast tenderness with recurrent breast lumps. I have the results of a couple of mammograms showing increased breast density and numerous nodular and cystic appearing lesions. I also have a copy of the right breast biopsy showing an area of carcinoma *in situ*.

I have suggested that she begin a high dose of oral micronized progesterone. I prescribed Prometrium® 400-mg daily at bedtime. This letter is to explain the reasons I believe progesterone therapy will be both safe and effective for her. I know that the idea of prescribing high dose progesterone for a woman with *in situ* breast cancer will seem a strange and maybe a "crazy" idea to you. However, I want to describe the science behind this suggestion. After reading this letter and having a chance to think about my suggested therapy, I would be happy to discuss this with you if you wish to call. I'll be available except for the last two weeks in August.

As you know, by history Floreena van Hoff is a healthy woman who is 50 years old and has just begun to have irregular menstrual cycles in perimenopause. Her major risk factor for breast cancer is nulliparity plus whatever the influence of increased breast density and the multiple lumps and biopsies she has had in the last few years. She has no other established risk factors. She is lean, has never used alcohol, her menarche was at age 12 and she shows no evidence of anovulatory androgen excess (as I call Polycystic Ovary Syndrome). She has never taken exogenous estrogen or used oral contraceptives. As you also know, she is adopted so we have no knowledge of any genetic risk for breast cancer.

I believe that she has two other major risk factors for breast cancer. These are, first that she has never ovulated despite having regular cycles, and second, that she has been having high levels of estrogen for at least the last three years in perimenopause. She gave a history of always having regular cycles but never any "molimina." Molimina means being able to predict by a set of experiences that a period is going to start. Absence of molimina is a sensitive and specific indicator of anovulation (1). Her recent basal temperature record, quantitatively analysed (2) over four cycles showed no evidence of ovulation. Only the last of these four cycles was irregular—it was 43 days long. The most important evidence for chronic anovulation is that her breasts show Tanner Stage III morphology. That is a sure sign she has never consistently ovulated.

Why do I say that lack of ovulation is a risk factor for breast cancer? I am first basing it on the breast tissue actions of estrogen and progesterone (3) as well as the target tissue actions and receptor interactions of estrogen and progesterone (4). Briefly this basic science work shows that estrogen increases proliferation and progesterone causes differentiation. Cell culture studies that only observe cells for a few days always show that both estrogen and progesterone cause proliferation. However, after a short initial proliferative action progesterone causes differentiation or inhibition of proliferation in breast tissue. The same pattern is true for progesterone's action in other tissues. That is supported by two older cohort control studies showing that women with infertility due to anovulation or with polycystic ovary syndrome had risk ratios of greater than three for breast cancer over controls (5;6). There are also many more epidemiological studies supporting this idea (7;8) I've not cited them here but would be happy to discuss them with you.

The strongest evidence that progesterone would be protective against breast cancer comes from recent *in vivo* human data. Two parallel but independent randomized double blind placebo-controlled studies studied breast proliferation and histology after 11 days of transdermal hormone therapy applied to the biopsied breast. One study was in premenopausal women and the other in menopausal women (9;10), respectively. Each study randomized women to four groups, one on a vehicle cream, one on estrogen cream, one using progesterone cream and the final one using estrogen plus progesterone cream. Each woman applied the cream to the breast scheduled for an open breast biopsy. Both estrogen and progesterone achieved physiological luteal phase levels in the breast tissue. In addition to removing the lump, a biopsy was taken more than a centimetre from the nodule and the tissue was analysed histologically for proliferation using K1a antigen and also for mitoses. Both studies showed that estrogen significantly increased breast proliferation, progesterone significantly decreased it and the combined therapy showed intermediate results most resembling progesterone's effect (9;10).

My best analysis of all of these data is that progesterone acts to oppose the effects of estrogen. Because estrogen is proliferative, progesterone by decreasing proliferation and mitoses acts to decrease the risk for invasive breast cancer.

I know that you will cite the Women's Health Initiative (WHI) estrogen plus progestin results showing an increased RR for breast cancer of 1.26 (11). You will also remind me that the estrogen only arm of the WHI in women with hysterectomy tended to show a decreased risk for breast cancer (12). The implication from these two large randomized controlled trials is that progestin *increases* the breast cancer risk. But that WHI estrogen/placebo study had about 5,000 fewer women in it than the estrogen plus progestin one and all of those enrolled in it had undergone hysterectomy. The WHI estrogen arm also was not powered to show increased risk for breast cancer (13). And that power calculation was done before we knew that women who have had a hysterectomy have a lower risk for breast cancer (14). That data comes from a population-based case control study showing that the *a priori* risk for breast cancer is decreased by 13-26% in women who have had a hysterectomy with or without bilateral ovariectomy (14). Therefore I believe that the WHI estrogen plus progestin study primarily showed the effect of *estrogen* therapy in women who haven't had a hysterectomy. The progestin dose, at 25% of the equivalent estrogen dose, was simply too low to effectively counterbalance the estrogen effect. That over 40% of the women on combined therapy experienced abnormal uterine bleeding sufficiently severe that the code had to be broken, is evidence for the estrogen-progestin dose imbalance in the combined hormone arm of the WHI (15). The WHI estrogen study showed no increased breast cancer risk because it didn't have power to show it (because it was initially underpowered, it didn't take into account the effect of hysterectomy, it had fewer women in it, and it was stopped early).

Because our concept has been that progestin is only given to prevent endometrial cancer during estrogen therapy, women who have had a hysterectomy rarely if ever are treated with progestin. Therefore estrogen treatment alone is given to women who have a *lower intrinsic risk* for breast cancer. Numerous observational epidemiology studies purport to show that progestin with estrogen is more risky than estrogen alone. However the apparent increased risk from combined therapy compared with estrogen is on an order of magnitude consistent with the decreased risk for breast cancer after hysterectomy (16-18). This represents confounding by indication.

Which brings me to a question for you. Our mutual patient is in perimenopause. Average perimenopausal estrogen levels are increased about 30% above premenopausal values from a meta-analysis Dr. Prior published several years ago (19). I have provided evidence that she is not now ovulating and that she hasn't ever consistently ovulated. So here's the question—knowing that she has *breast cancer in situ* are you going to let her continue to be exposed to high levels of estrogen without progesterone?

I guess there are other options to decrease her high estrogen levels. I am not suggesting that she have a bilateral ovariectomy. I am also not suggesting you begin her on gonadotrophin releasing hormone agonist therapy (mostly because she is already at increased risk for osteopenia because of anovulation (20) and cognitive dietary restraint (21)). I don't think that she currently has an indication for chemotherapy or for a selective estrogen receptor modulator therapy such as Tamoxifen or Raloxifene. However, in case you are thinking of any of those therapies, remember that all of them cause hot flushes. Tamoxifen acts a bit like estrogen on bone in menopausal women and prevents loss (22). However, Tamoxifen *causes* bone loss in premenopausal women (23).

I've ordered a baseline bone density test with a copy to you. Dr. Prior earlier showed in a meta-analysis that perimenopausal spinal bone loss at −1.8% on average a year is more rapid than the rate of loss after menopause (19).

Instead of those more dramatic and unproven therapies for breast carcinoma *in situ* I suggest that she take 130% of a full luteal phase equivalent dose of oral micronized progesterone (Prometrium) daily. That should be sufficient to overcome the effects of her increased endogenous estrogen. I also believe Prometrium therapy will decrease her sleep disturbance and in turn decrease the stress hormones related to insomnia and to her intense worry about active breast cancer. The recent aromatase inhibitor data in breast cancer therapy suggest that decreasing high adrenal steroids is a good idea.

If you are still sceptical about progesterone therapy after reading this and looking at the citations, I suggest that we could, if Floreena were willing, perform an experiment of one. We could do a needle aspiration of her breast during the follicular phase now, and measure serum estrogen, DHEAS, testosterone and cortisol levels. We could repeat the blood tests and biopsy after a month of daily progesterone therapy. I trust that the Cancer Agency would analyse the specimens for mitoses and also for K1a antigen—this would need to be done in a blinded fashion. I am reasonably sure that she would agree to this little experiment given that she has had quite a few needle biopsies in her time and is very justifiably worried. Further, I would be happy to come to the Agency's monthly Breast Tumour Rounds and discuss this patient and my suggestion for use of progesterone therapy.

I am looking forward to a discussion with you about this.

Sincerely,

*Kailey Madrona*

Kailey Madrona BA, MD, FRCPC
Clinical Associate Professor of Endocrinology
Scientist, Centre for Menstrual Cycle and Ovulation Research

Cc:  Dr Phelps
     Fraser Valley Cancer Agency
     Floreena van Hoff

* References attached.

**Reference List**

1. Prior JC. Ovulatory disturbances: they do matter. Can.J.Diagnosis 1997;February:64-80.

2. Prior JC, Vigna YM, Schulzer M, Hall JE, Bonen A. Determination of luteal phase length by quantitative basal temperature methods: validation against the midcycle LH peak. Clin.Invest.Med. 1990;13:123-31.

3. Clarke CL, Sutherland RL. Progestin regulation of cellular proliferation. Endocr.Rev. 1990;11:266-301.

4. Graham JD, Clarke CL. Physiological action of progesterone in target tissue. Endocr.Rev. 1997;18:592-19.

5. Coulam CB, Annegers JF, Kranz JS. Chronic anovulation syndrome and associated neoplasia. Obstetrics and Gynecology 1983;61:403-7.

6. Cowan LD, Gordis L, Tonascia JA, Jones GS. Breast cancer incidence in women with a history of progesterone deficiency. Am J Epidemiol. 1981;114(2):209-17.

7. Swain MC, Bulbrook RD, Hayward JL. Ovulatory failure in a normal population and in patients with breast cancer. J.Obstet.Gynaecol.Br.Commonw. 1974;81(8):640-3.

8. Bulbrook RD, Moore JW, Clark GMG, Wang DY, Tang D, Hayward JL. Plasma oestradoil and progesterone levels in women with varying degrees of risk of breast cancer. Eur.J.Cancer. 1978;14:1369-75.

9. Chang KJ, Lee TTY, Linares-Cruz G, Fournier S, de Lignieres B. Influence of percutaneous administration of estradiol and progesterone on human breast epithelial cell cycle in vivo. Fertil.Steril. 1995;63:785-91.

10. Foidart J, Collin C, Denoo X, Desreux J, Belliard A, Fournier S et al. Estradiol and progesterone regulate the proliferation of human breast epithelial cells. Fertil.Steril. 1998;5:963-9.

11. Chlebowski RT, Hendrix SL, Langer RD, Stefanick ML, Gass M, Lane D et al. Influence of estrogen plus progestin on breast cancer and mammography in healthy postmenopausal women: the Women's Health Initiative Randomized Trial. JAMA 2003;289(24):3243-53.

12. Anderson GL, Limacher M, Assaf AR, Bassford T, Beresford SA, Black H et al. Effects of conjugated equine estrogen in postmenopausal women with

hysterectomy: the Women's Health Initiative randomized controlled trial. JAMA 2004;291(14):1701-12.

13. The Women's Health Initiative Study Group. Design of the Women's Health Initiative clinical trial and observational study. Control Clin Trials 1998;19(1):61-109.

14. Kreiger N, Sloan M, Cotterchio M, Kirsh V. The risk of breast cancer following reproductive surgery. Eur.J.Cancer. 1999;35:97-101.

15. Writing Group for the Women's Health Initiative Investigators. Risks and benefits of estrogen plus progestin in health postmenopausal women: principal results from the Women's Health Initiative Randomized Control trial. JAMA 2002;288:321-33.

16. Schairer C, Lubin J, Troisi R, Sturgeon S, Brinton L, Hoover R. Menopausal estrogen and estrogen-progestin replacement therapy and breast cancer risk. JAMA 2000;283:485-91.

17. Bergkvist L, Adami HO, Persson I, Hoover RN, Schairer C. The risk of breast cancer after estrogen and estrogen-progestin replacement. N Engl J Med 1989;321:293-7.

18. Li CI, Malone KE, Porter PL, Weiss NS, Tang MT, Cushing-Haugen KL et al. Relationship between long durations and different regimens of hormone therapy and risk of breast cancer. JAMA 2003;289(24):3254-63.

19. Prior JC. Perimenopause: The complex endocrinology of the menopausal transition. Endocr.Rev. 1998;19:397-428.

20. Prior JC, Vigna YM, Schechter MT, Burgess AE. Spinal bone loss and ovulatory disturbances. N Engl J Med 1990;323:1221-7.

21. McLean JA, Barr SI, Prior JC. Dietary restraint, exercise and bone density in young women: are they relate? Med.Sci.Sports Exerc. 2001;33:1292-6.

22. Love RR, Mazess RB, Tormey DC, Barden HS, Newcomb PA, Jordan VC. Bone mineral density in women with breast cancer treated with adjuvant tamoxifen for at least two years. Br.Can.Res.Treat. 1988;12:297-302.

23. Powles TJ, Hickish JA, Tidy A, Ashley S. Effect of Tamoxifen on bone mineral density measured by dual-energy x-ray absorptiometry in healthy premenopausal and postmenopausal women. J.Clin.Oncol. 1996;14:1,78-84.

# 13

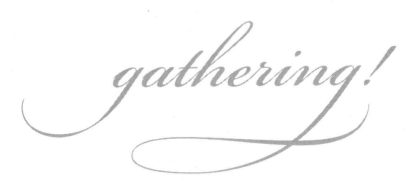

*gathering!*

I walk up the green wooden steps of a stucco-sided, well-kept older home in Kitsilano and ring the doorbell. I wait a few moments, watching a junco flit in the lower branches of an ancient rhododendron just off the porch. I'm just about the ring again when Alison opens the door. "Greetings, Dr. Madrona! I didn't expect to see you so soon."

I see that the folding table and a ping-pong table in the living room are bare, also that Alison's wearing an apron and looking frazzled. "I'm sorry. Looks like I'm early. I had to pick up some music downtown this afternoon and thought coming here afterwards would time it right." I glance at my watch. "Oh, you said six, and it is just five-thirty! That's a guest's unforgivable sin—being early! I can go for a walk, or you can put me to work."

"Don't worry, Dr. Madrona. Just sit here and relax. I'll make you a cup of tea or coffee."

"No, I'm fine, Alison," I protest. "Let me set the tables—just get me the table cloths and point me at the dish cupboards and silverware drawer." Alison hurries out, then returns with ivory tablecloths and shows me to the kitchen.

"Let's see, how many of us are there?" I ask.

"Carla and Jane are coming from the Island. Henrietta doesn't get off until five so she'll be here as soon as she cleans up. That makes six including us. Eva called and said she'd be here a little late because of a game, I think she said hockey. And Jennifer's coming, I think getting a ride with Beverley. I'm not sure about Darlene. I asked Carla to get in touch with her."

"I'd suggest we set it up," I say, "so that we have ten places and we can always take one off if we need to. These tables work just fine," I say as I smooth the cloths."

I've got the table set except for serviettes and glasses when the doorbell rings. Feeling right at home, I answer it. "Welcome, Floreena!" I say. "That's a lovely big spinach salad with—what? Looks like almonds and mandarin oranges." I hand the salad to Alison, who has just joined us.

After setting the salad on the table, Alison takes Floreena's coat. "So," Alison says, looking around at the tables, "you're the artistic one of us. Why don't you fix these on this tray." She hands Floreena a couple of jars of pickles and a plastic ziplocked bag of olives.

"Sure, Alison," says Floreena. "I guess it's good that I got here early. You did too, Dr. Madrona. I wasn't sure of how to find the house, traffic and all, and I didn't want to be late."

"I can always use help. I've shipped my boys and husband off to dinner and a movie so we have the house all to ourselves. I got them to help me haul these tables and chairs in here before they left. We usually eat in the breakfast nook. Somehow we've never gotten a proper dining room set."

"You mentioned Jane," says Floreena. "I don't remember her. Who is she?"

"She's Carla's partner," Alison answers before I have a chance to. "Carla asked if she could bring her. Since it's a girls' party, and she didn't want to come all the way from Victoria by herself, I didn't see why not."

"I'm afraid I don't remember most of the women, since we haven't met as a group before now, even though we all intended to," Floreena remarks. "I did run into Eva and Henrietta at the East Vancouver Christmas Craft Fair this year. I was selling some desktop fountains and things I'd made. I recognized them across the room, but felt kind of shy. Henrietta came right over and greeted me like a long-lost friend."

"It's odd," Alison answers. "From the first, I've felt a bond with the women in that seminar. Like we share something important."

Floreena nods and turns to the table. "Do you have a few place mats or some decoration I could put in the centre?"

"Look in that drawer there. I never know what I have these days. But I used to have some pretty things."

Floreena finds a couple of flower-print placemats and makes a runner out of them in the centre of the two tables. Alison disappears into the kitchen and we drift after her.

"Sorry. I'm busy tending the oven. I've baked a salmon that Walter and the boys caught last fall. And I've got a small turkey that was on sale. I hope I'm timing them right—I think the turkey will take about twice as much time as the salmon, don't you?"

"Probably. Depends how big they are," Floreena says, sniffing with appreciation. "They're both huge. Enough here to feed all of Kitsilano!"

"I've learned that I need more protein and fewer carbohydrates to feel well," Alison says. "Even my migraines are better when I avoid sweets. So I wanted to be sure that we had lots of protein. And some of the women may be avoiding meat, so I wanted the fish."

"Thanks for that choice, Alison," I say. "Lana must have told you that I don't eat anything I couldn't kill."

She nods. "She said you preferred fish."

"By the way, I almost forgot," Floreena says. "I brought some locally pressed organic cider. Maybe others besides me avoid alcohol."

"That's great," says Alison. "Let's see if we can find a spot for it in the fridge. I'll put the other salad with yours on the table. Then there'll be room for the cider."

The doorbell rings and Alison gets there first this time. "Hi Carla! And you must be Jane. Welcome! I've put Floreena and Dr. Madrona to work. Those look like what my kids call 'bird seed buns.' Great! And some local micro-brew beer. You can squeeze those bottles into the fridge. We'll heat the buns after we pull the fish and turkey out of the oven."

"I thought it smelled like Thanksgiving in here!" Carla sniffs appreciatively. "You've got a grand home, Alison."

"We like it! We've been gradually remodelling, but keeping the old look. It was built in the early 1900s and it's solid. Thank god my husband's handy because I'm a slap-dash fixer."

"Can I help with anything, Alison? " asks Jane.

"You could look for salad bowls in that sideboard there, Jane. By the way, Carla, is Darlene coming?"

"I tried and tried her, left quite a few messages. Finally I got through. It turns out that she's just home after having had a hysterectomy with both her ovaries out. She won't be coming."

"That's too bad," Carla murmurs. "I know—that's a horrid surgery, and I kept my ovaries."

Alison pauses, looking at the table. "Well, Dr. Madrona, looks like you can take off one plate. I think everyone else will be here. I'd better check on that turkey." She turns to the kitchen.

Carla is gazing appreciatively at the front yard and then suddenly opens the door. "Hello, Beverley!" Carla says. Beverley looks startled because she didn't even ring the bell. "Hi, Beverley," I say. "It's good to see you."

Jane comes forward, smiling. "Hi, Beverley. I'm Jane—I came with Carla!"

"Come in," Carla steers Beverley into the living room. "Let me hang up your coat. That's a lovely bottle of champagne! Fit for a celebration."

"I don't drink!" says Beverley. "Victor bought for everyone." I see that she whispers something to Alison. Then more loudly Beverley says, "I make these," as she holds out two trays of egg rolls covered with plastic wrap.

"What a great idea!" I exclaim, "I was getting starved smelling the cooking."

"Yes, we could eat them now," Floreena remarks, "before dinner! You set them out on the coffee table there, and I'll go get napkins."

The doorbell rings again and this time Jane is closest. She opens the door to Henrietta who is carrying a huge rectangular glass dish heaping with squares of many kinds. I see a whole pile of Nanaimo bars. "Are we glad to see you, Henrietta!" Carla jokes, ogling the desserts. "Looks like you got carried away with baking!"

"Nope, that's my mom and Aunt Tilly's work," Henrietta says proudly. "My aunt moved from Manitoba to help my mom. She's been a lifesaver to me, too."

As the doorbell rings again, Alison answers it. "Hi Jennifer! Those are lovely!" she exclaims as Jennifer holds out a bouquet of flowers. Alison hands the flowers to Floreena and asks her to arrange them in two vases. Soon twin bouquets are gracing the long table.

"I wasn't sure what to bring," says Jennifer, "so I picked up some light taco chips. I thought they'd be good with my homemade salsa. And I brought this." She unveils a salad bowl filled with shredded cabbage, almonds, and ramen noodles. "Can I help?"

"No, just sit and relax," I reply. "Here's a napkin. You can try those egg rolls that Beverley made."

"That's great, Jennifer. Just what we needed." Alison comes in from the kitchen with an oven mitt on one hand. She sets the newest salad on the table. "I think it's magic the food that appears at potlucks. We always have enough, and usually an amazing variety."

Beverley looks at me, motioning toward one tray. "That one meat." And to the other, "Only vegetables."

I reach out and take one of the vegetable egg rolls.

Looking around, Alison says, "We're only waiting for Eva. Carla, why don't you see what these gals would like to have to drink before dinner? There's skim milk, pop, orange juice, organic cider, beer and white wine in the refrigerator. The salmon and the turkey are almost ready. I don't think I'll bother with potatoes or rice. What do you think?"

"It looks like we've got enough food without them," Jane says. "By the way, thanks for letting me come with Carla—I want to learn more about perimenopause and I've met Dr. Madrona."

At that moment the doorbell rings again. This time Jennifer is closest. Eva stands at the door, brushing back her damp hair and looking flushed. "Come in! We're all here!" Jennifer says.

"This is a rice pilaf, my mom's recipe," says Eva. "It's cooked, but probably needs some warming. I grabbed it on my way home after a great field-hockey game." Eva is glowing with excitement.

"I was just asking everyone whether I should make potatoes or pasta," Alison says. "We've really got our answer now! Our meal is complete! We were just starting to have some egg rolls before dinner. Carla will get you something to drink."

I look around at the women scattered through the cozy living room and think that they are as different as women can be. Then I reach for another egg roll.

After dinner, when the food and dishes are cleared away, we're gathered back on the couches and chairs. Several plates are filled with desserts. A row of plastic wine glasses is standing on the coffee table. "I've made a big pot of decaffeinated coffee and the kettle's on to make tea," Alison sings out from the kitchen.

Then she comes into the living room and holds up the champagne. She passes the chilled bottle of champagne to Beverley. "I think there is something Beverley wants to say."

"You want celebrate with me." Beverley began hesitantly. "I pregnant!"

"That's fantastic," Jennifer says.

"How lovely," murmurs Floreena, the tears welling in her eyes.

"That's really great, Beverley!" I say. "When was your last period?"

"Now three months, almost four ago—wanted be sure."

"I remember when we met, Beverley," Eva says. "You said, 'no more eggs!'"

"How did you get pregnant?" asks Henrietta.

"I make eggs, but not long enough ovulation," Beverley explains.

Several women look toward me questioningly. "She was ovulating," I say, "but had too short luteal phases for egg implantation."

"I take progesterone—make ready for egg," Beverley interjects. "And I not working too hard and not being skinny!"

Everyone laughs appreciatively. "Dr. Madrona was on my case too about being too thin!" Henrietta remarks.

"And me too" says Eva.

Alison turns to Carla. "How are your hot flushes now Carla? I remember that you were miserable and taking Premarin."

"Well, after a big problem with going cold-turkey off the estrogen," Carla laughs ruefully. "Then I finally got with the program! I used the tricks on the CeMCOR website and got myself off estrogen. I'm taking progesterone every day and I never have a hot flush and only rarely feel a night sweat."

"Do you take it every day?" asks Henrietta.

"Yeah, 'cause I had that hysterectomy and don't get periods," replies Carla.

"I wanted to be natural and do everything without pills," Henrietta says. "But I got migraines on cyclic progesterone, then I found I had osteoporosis plus my soaking-the-bed-sweats. I finally gave in and now take progesterone every day. I think I'll survive."

"Your mention of hysterectomy reminds me," Alison interjects, "that Darlene couldn't come because she's just home from the hospital after having a hysterectomy and a total cleanout. Right, Carla?"

"Yeah, she said she gave up on doctors. Her back went out, she was fed up with bleeding, she was depressed, and her gynecologist persuaded her it would be better," Carla says.

"It sounds like you tried to keep her from needing that surgery, Dr. Madrona. What do you think happened?" asks Eva.

"I can't talk about patients," I answer slowly. "Let's just say that she had a hard time taking either advice or medicines."

"I was a pest when I first saw you, too, Dr. Madrona. How do you put up with us?" asks Henrietta.

I look around and smile at them. "Well, it's my job to listen, to try to understand, and to say things in a way that I think will be helpful." I pause. "But I feel very badly that Darlene ended up having ovariectomy and hysterectomy."

"You certainly did good for me!" Jennifer sings out.

"Me too," says Floreena.

"I'd still be a miserable basket case without you," Alison chimes in.

"I have an idea," I say, thinking as I speak. "All of us share the common experience of having a difficult time in perimenopause. Why don't we go around the room and each of us say the main thing that we've learned?"

"Wait a minute!" Alison protests. "Don't get so deadly serious until we've cracked this champagne and toasted Beverley's baby!"

"Anyone besides me who'd like to toast with fresh apple cider?" asks Floreena.

Beverley nods and asks for cider. Soon everyone has a plastic glass filled with some kind of liquid.

"Here's to our perimenopause miracle baby!" shouts Alison. Other happy voices say, "Cheers!" "Congratulations!" "To new life!"

"Here's to surviving perimenopause!" Carla raises her glass and is accompanied by "For surviving!" from many voices.

"Who wants some dessert?" asks Henrietta. "I'll offend my mom and Aunt Tilly if I come home with any!"

"I don't need that," pipes Alison to sympathetic laughter.

Soon all of the women are appreciating the desserts, drinking coffee or tea, and visiting amongst themselves.

"Hey, guys, let's talk about what we've learned," says Carla, calling above the babble of many voices. Jane tings her fork against the side of her china teacup, calling the group to order.

As everyone finds seats and becomes silent, Carla says, "Maybe I'll start. I was brought up to listen to what my mother told me, and to wear clean underwear when seeing the doctor." Several women giggle. Carla grins and then gets serious. "But what I learned in perimenopause is that that, for me, most doctors *suck*!"

"Right! My doctor hadn't a clue why I was sick to my stomach—he said I was 'way too young for menopause," says Jennifer indignantly.

"And mine kept insisting I was depressed," Henrietta adds.

"Doctor made no hope for baby. . ." Beverley murmurs.

"My doctor thought I was having low estrogen because of the night sweats," says Carla, "when really my estrogens were off-the-scale high!"

"My doctor wanted to help with my breast lumps, but didn't know what to do except refer me to other doctors," says Floreena.

Eva, who has been quiet, now says soberly, "I was always worried about what I wore, how I looked, what I ate, and whether I could win that next run. I am learning to accept my body—and it is pretty smart. It has to deal with all the demands *I* make on it as well as to cope with the huge tides of estrogen in perimenopause."

"I'm always critical of my body, too," says Floreena. "I think it's feeling insecure."

"I'm learning to ask for what I need," adds Henrietta thoughtfully. "After we met in that group, my night sweats just got worse and worse. I was working 12 hours a day—remember that I wait tables. Then my mom got sick, didn't take her medicine, and ended up getting burned in a house fire. Oh, yeah, I almost forgot! Around the same time my son, John, whose wife got a job in Cranbrook, asked if he and my seven-year-old grandson could move in with me. I was a wreck! I finally agreed"—she looks at me—"to take progesterone. The flushes and sleep got better, I learned to meditate, and I asked John to help. Then I asked Aunt Tilly out to care for Mom."

"So you stopped trying to do everything by yourself," Jennifer says thoughtfully.

"Wow, you had a rough go there," Jane empathizes. "I know what you mean about getting to the end of your rope. Carla was such a bitch when she was on that horse-piss pill that I almost kicked her out." She pauses. "And the worst is sleeping with a sweaty thrashing machine!"

A huge round of laughter is followed by Alison raising her glass, "Here's to our partners and families who put up with us in perimenopause!" "Cheers for families!" "For partners!" Carla and Jane clink glasses.

Jennifer clears her throat. "I've learned a lot," she starts. "I've had my kids. I don't have anyone to gripe if I'm reading at three in the morning. And I thought I was fine with the idea of menopause—in another ten or 15 years!" Again she stops, collecting her thoughts. "I'm astonished that women have been going through this for eons, yet we know so little. I hadn't a clue that my ovaries would get all riled up, and I'd struggle with sky-high estrogens at my age!"

"I've learned I get breast lumps whenever my estrogen is high," Floreena adds.

"I get nausea," says Jennifer.

"I have migraines up the ying-yang," adds Alison.

"And I can't run worth beans," says Eva.

"I guess what I've really learned," Floreena is speaking thoughtfully again, "is to make up my own mind. I always listened to doctors and did what they said. Then I got breast cancer in situ." Apprehensive sounds sweep across the gathered women. "That means a bit of breast cells are abnormal, but haven't spread. That was bad enough. Then came the arguments. Everything I read, every doctor I saw, everyone I spoke with had a different idea about what I should do. And, of course, no one has studied breast cancer in situ in perimenopause!"

"Just like everything else about perimenopause," Carla mutters.

"Plus I didn't know my family history," Floreena continues. "I'm adopted, you see. I couldn't decide what to do. I lay awake at night agonizing. I was stubborn." She looks over at me. "I didn't take the progesterone Dr. Madrona suggested. I tried Tamoxifen and felt horrid. Finally, I decided we could do a little experiment—we looked at breast cancer cells when my estrogen levels were high and I had low progesterone and then again a month after taking high-dose progesterone. Those tests showed that my own breast cells got less aggressive-looking when I took progesterone. I'm now taking a high dose of progesterone every night. I feel like I did the right thing—I'm also proud because I made up my own mind." There is a murmur of empathy.

"And I contacted my birth mother." Floreena starts again. "I've got no family breast cancer history. My mother is a neat lady—uncanny how much she sounds like me on the telephone!"

"Big changes, Flo," observes Jennifer. "Congratulations to you." She pauses, then asks, "Do your breasts feel any different?"

"Yes! Softer, a lot less sore, and so far I've had no new lumps."

"Me too, since I took progesterone. I don't have my pet rocks anymore!" Alison quips.

"I not so good talking." Beverley starts. Several women say, "It's fine." "It's ok."

"I work too hard, all time. Regular bleeding but no baby. Now I relax!"

"What a good thing to learn, Beverley." Carla muses. "Really to take a few big breaths and feel at home with ourselves is what all of us need to learn."

"I guess I'm last," Alison says. "As each of you was speaking I was thinking how much of what each of you said was true for me too. I'd learned about my body and perimenopause. You know, I had a plan for my life—I was going back to teaching school when my youngest boy got into grade school. Then the migraines made it difficult to cope with just being a mother and at home. I'd be out of commission for three days a week. I tried every herb and vitamin and manipulation and touch therapy and acupuncture. I got told to take this, take that, start hormone replacement." She bit her lower lip, "When anyone has symptoms, that's the bottom line—take estrogen!" There is a skitter of laughter. "I think I've learned that I can cope. I can make plans, but change them if I need to. Most of all, I now have hope that I will survive perimenopause!"

"To surviving perimenopause!" Henrietta raises her empty coffee mug and others follow with glasses and cups clinking and waving in the air.

"Here's to life after perimenopause!" I raise my glass. "Who's going to reach menopause first?"

"I think I am," Henrietta asserts. "I've not had a period for seven months."

"I'm skipping now," says Floreena, "but I'm taking progesterone."

"I went for 16 months without a period," I remember. "I was interviewed and was boasting that I was menopausal. I accidentally noticed very sore breasts again. Then I got another period! At the time I was taking daily progesterone for migraines and hot flushes. So now I say, if you're on daily progesterone, wait two years without a period before you're home free."

"This is a good time, I think." Alison clears her throat. "We wanted to thank you for being such a wise and patient doctor for us, Dr. Madrona. And for sticking your neck out so that eventually our doctors will learn. She points to the flowers on the tables. "These flowers are for you. And, we got you this." She hands me a cheerfully wrapped oblong present. I open it and pull out a unique set of wooden wind chimes. I can feel myself grinning with pleasure as I hold them high for all to see. "It was Carla's idea," Alison continues, "and Floreena got an artisan friend to make them. She did the polishing and finishing herself."

"Thank you." I can't say any more because tears swell my throat. "Thank you for letting me be part of this celebration."

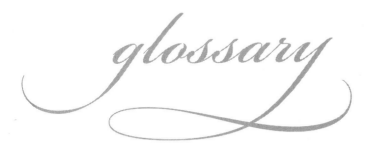

# glossary

Each word is defined. If a word is used that has been defined in another place in the glossary, it looks like _this_.

**24-hour urine sample:** a collection of all the urine passed in one whole day. This is used to assess how well the kidney works, for _cortisol_ and a few other _hormones_.

**5-alpha reductase enzyme:** is a small chemical that helps make _testosterone_ into _dihydrotestosterone_, a hormone that causes male-type hair growth in women, oily skin, and pimples. Progesterone inhibits this enzyme.

**AAE:** or _anovulatory androgen excess._

**Abdominal visceral fat:** a layer of fat surrounding abdominal organs that increases with obesity, especially in those with _insulin resistance_. It is the major contribution to increased _waist circumference._

**Acne:** another name for pimples. It is caused by increased oil formation in hair follicles that plug and cause inflammation. They are especially common on the face and upper back. Acne occurs in the teens _for_ both young women and men but normally goes away after that. It is common in _anovulatory androgen excess._

**Adrenal glands:** small triangular shaped glands that sit on top of the kidneys and make four different kinds of hormones: _cortisol_, _aldosterone_, _androgens_ and _catecholamines_.

**Adrenalin:** a kind of hormone called a _catecholamine_ that is made by nerves and in the centre of the adrenal gland. Adrenalin is released in large amounts with the "fight or flight" response to threat or stress. It causes the heart to beat faster and blood vessels in arms and legs to constrict. It is also called *epinephrine*.

**Aldosterone:** a hormone made in the adrenal glands that causes the kidneys to retain (keep) sodium and water and get rid of *potassium*. High levels can cause *high blood pressure* or hypertension. A medication that can block the effects of aldosterone is called *spironolactone*.

**Alkaline phosphatase:** a chemical made in the bone and liver. Levels will be elevated with some kinds of bone and liver diseases.

**Alopecia:** loss of head hair.

**Alzheimer's:** decreased memory, reasoning and ability to care for ones self that makes a person unable to function. It is a kind of *dementia* that occurs with damage to the brain with aging and with many *strokes*.

**Androgenic alopecia:** male-like head hair loss or thinning starting at the temples and extending back from the forehead. It is related to family inheritance and to higher *androgen* levels.

**Androgenic progestins:** synthetic forms of progesterone that are made from testosterone and act a little like *androgens* as well as like *progesterone*.

**Androgen receptor blocker:** a medicine, like *spironolactone*, that blocks the action of male-type hormones in cells of the body.

**Androgens:** are 'male sex *hormones*', the most important of which is *testosterone*. Androgens are also a normal part of women's reproduction. Besides testosterone, other important androgens are *DHEAS* and *androstenedione*. All androgens increase skin oil production, thicken and darken hair and tend to cause head hair loss in the temple regions. Androgen levels are sometimes high in women with *anovulatory androgen excess*. The term, androgenic, means male hormone-like.

**Androsteinedione:** a kind of *androgen* or male hormone made primarily in the ovary.

**Anemia:** occurs when there are too few red blood cells to carry oxygen to the body. In menstruating women the most common cause for anemia is heavy menstrual flow. This causes iron deficiency and the body cannot make enough iron-carrying red blood cells. By the time anemia develops, the bone marrow no longer has any stores of iron. Low dose daily iron therapy is needed for a full year to rebuild bone marrow reserves. Anemia from inadequate Vitamin $B_{12}$ may occur in vegetarians who are not taking B$_{12}$ supplements or from indaequate *folate* intake in those only eating highly refined grains.

**Anemic:** describes a person with *anemia.*

**Anorexia:** is a severe *eating disorder.* It is associated with a need for control and severe weight loss. The effects of of *undernutrition* include *amenorrhea*, high *cortisol* levels, and bone loss.

**Anorexic:** describes a person with *anorexia*.

**Anovulation:** means a menstrual cycle in which no egg is released and progesterone, which is produced only after ovulation, stays low all the time. May occur in women with regular, normal-length menstrual cycles or those with *oligomenorrhea*. Is variable from cycle to cycle.

**Anovulatory Androgen Excess (AAE):** a more accurate term for what is often called *Polycystic Ovary Syndrome* (PCOS). It is diagnosed when a woman has male-type facial hair growth and acne and evidence of past or present *ovulation disturbances* (*anovulatory* or *short luteal phase* cycles) and often *oligomenorrhea*. It is associated with both *infertility* and risks for *insulin resistance* and *Diabetes Mellitus Type 2*.

**Antihistamine:** a kind of medicine to block the effects of allergy on the body. Older kinds have a useful side-effect to cause drowsiness and are therefore used to help sleep. They may also decrease nausea.

**Anti-prostaglandin:** refers to medicines that block the actions of the small fatty hormones called prostaglandins. They are used to treat menstrual cramps. To be effective they must be taken before symptoms become severe and repeated as soon as the cramps start to return. *Ibuprofen* is one of this group of medicines that also decrease menstrual flow by about twenty-five percent.

**Areola:** the darker and sometimes wrinkly circle in the front of the breast that holds the nipple.

**Aromatase:** an enzyme that helps change male-type hormones into *estrogen*.

**Atypia:** a term used to describe abnormal cells that carry a higher likelihood of becoming cancerous.

**Aura:** sense that something will happen soon. Usually refers to a sense that a migraine, or seizure or hot flush will start.

**Axillary tail of the breast:** the portion of the breast that extends into the armpit. Tenderness here without any other breast soreness indicates ovulation. See *molimina*.

**Basal temperature:** is the lowest temperature the body reaches after falling into a deep sleep—it extends to the person's usual time of getting up in the morning. It is usually measured in the mouth on first awaking. Basal temperature values increase 0.2 to 0.3 degrees Celsius after *ovulation* as evidence of the action of *progesterone* in the *hypothalmus*.

**Bell-shaped curve:** the hill-like shape with valleys on either side. It is a way of sorting things so that the most common size is in the middle with the few extremely small or extremely large sized objects in the valleys on either side.

**Benign:** a term used to mean that something is *not* a cancer.

**Beta-blocker:** a kind of medicine used for *high blood pressure*, *hyperthyroidism*, heart disease, fast heart rates, *migraine* prophylaxis, and performance anxiety that prevents the action of *catecholamines* like *adrenalin* and *noradrenalin*. People with asthma should not take beta-blocker medicines. *Propranolol* is a kind of beta-blocker.

**Bio-identical:** a hormone that is exactly like the one made by the human body. For example, *progesterone* is bio-identical but *medroxyprogesterone* is a synthetic *progestin* and is not.

**Bipolar affective disease:** a mental or emotional illness characterized by extreme mood changes from severe depression to inappropriate hyperactivity and elation. Also called manic-depression. It tends to run in families and is treated differently than other kinds of depression.

**Bisphosphonates:** the general name for a family of bone-seeking medicines that slow the bone loss as well as decreasing the risk for *fracture*. All bisphosphonates must be taken at least an hour away from food and two hours away from *calcium*, *vitamins* and iron intake. Currrently available medicines in the bisphosphonate family include etidronate, clodronate, alendronate, risedronate, zoledronate, pamidronate and ibandronate.

**Black cohosh:** an herb that seems to help with hot flushes and night sweats. It is contained in a medicine called Remifemin®.

**Blood:** the liquid containing red cells, other blood cells and many nutrients, that fills arteries and veins.

**Blood clots:** are clumps formed by certain blood cells. Blood clots stop cuts from continuing to bleed, but are harmful if formed within the _blood stream_ because they can travel to the lungs or block off a blood vessel.

**Blood pressure:** the pressure created by the heart's pumping power and the resisting of blood vessels. When the heart contracts it creates the systolic or top blood pressure number. The diastolic pressure, the bottom blood pressure number, is the resting pressure between heart contractions. The ideal, healthy blood pressure is lower than 135/85. It is written as systolic/diastolic and reported in mm, which is the height of a column of mercury that was originally used for measurement of blood pressure). It is abbreviated as BP.

**Blood stream:** includes all the arteries carrying oxygen-rich blood from the heart to the body, and veins bringing blood without oxygen back to the heart.

**Blood sugar:** the natural energy, also called _glucose_, which is carried in the _blood stream_ and provides energy for the cells of the body. Usually it is measured as _fasting glucose_.

**BMD:** abbreviation for _bone mineral density_.

**Body mass index:** is weight in kilograms divided by height in meters squared (kg/m$^2$). It is used to assess general nutrition. The normal range is 18.5 to 25—lower values mean undernutrition and higher numbers are overweight. It is abbreviated _BMI_.

**Bone resorption:** the process by which old bone tissue is broken down and removed by special cells called _osteoclasts_. Bone resorption is very fast and any one spot takes only about three weeks to be removed. Any weight loss, for reasons that are not clear, causes increased bone loss as does excess stress, caffeine (in women with low calcium intakes) and colas (because the body uses calcium to help excrete the phosphoric acid colas contain). Bone resorption is normally in balance with bone formation. Increased calcium and vitamin D intakes help to keep resorption rates normal.

**Bone marrow:** the collection of cells in the middle of many _cortical_ bones in which new blood cells are made and from which special bone cells are formed. Iron for making hemoglobin is stored here.

**Bone mineral density:** abbreviated _BMD_, is a measure of the amount of bone and its mineral. There are several kinds, but one called _DXA_ uses very low doses of _X-rays_ to make an accurate assessment. The two sites usually measured are in the lower spine and hip. BMD should be repeated in the same season and no more frequently than every two years to obtain an accurate estimate of bone change.

**BMI:** abbreviation for *body mass index*.

**BP pill:** a common way of describing medicines used for *high blood pressure*.

**Breast cancer:** a form of cancer arising in the epithelial or ductal cells of the breast.

**Breast density:** a characteristic on the *mammogram* in which the breast tissue is more closely packed together. Those with the highest breast density have about a five times increased risk for breast cancer. Breast density normally increases with age in *premenopausal* women, is maximal in *perimenopause* and decreases with *menopause*. *Estrogen* therapy increases breast density.

**Breast hormone receptor status:** describes which of the ovarian hormones, *estrogen* or *progesterone*, makes breast cancer cells grow.

**Bulimia:** an eating disorder in which people tend to over-eat (binge) and then vomit or cause diarrhea (purge) to control weight.

**Calcium citrate:** a kind of calcium supplement in which *elemental calcium* is combined with citrate. This is the only kind of calcium a person who has had kidney stones should take.

**Calories:** describes the amount of energy from foods, or energy spent during exercise.

**Cancellous bone:** the kind of bone that has a honey comb-like structure to provide strength without extra weight. It is more responsive to *ovarian hormones* and *cortisol* than to exercise.

**Candidiasis:** infection with a yeast named "Candida"—may be in the vagina, or in the mouth (where it is called thrush).

**Carcinoma in situ:** abnormal cancer cells that are limited to one spot, without any spread.

**Catecholamines:** hypothalamic, nerve and adrenal produced hormones that act on blood vessels and the heart. Catecholamines include *adrenaline* (*epinephrine*) and *noradrenalin* (*norepinephrine*).

**CeMCOR:** abbreviation for the Centre for Menstrual Cycle and Ovulation Research. A virtual research and education centre for women founded in May 2002. The CeMCOR website was launched in October 2003 (www.cemcor.ubc.ca). An international advisory counsel includes women and men from many disciplines and seven countries.

**Cervix:** the mouth or opening of the *uterus* that is situated at the top of the *vagina*.

**Chamomile tea:** an herbal tea from chamomile that is believed to be soothing and assist with a good sleep.

**Chance Health Locus of Control:** see *Health Locus of Control*

**Chest X-ray:** a test using X-rays of the chest to see heart, lung or blood vessel changes.

**Chronic bronchitis:** a form of lung disease in which a person coughs up phlegm for several months every year. It is associated with cigarette abuse.

**Chronic fatigue syndrome:** is the name used for a complex and poorly understood condition that involves low energy, sleep disturbances and often depression.

**Cognitive dietary restraint:** worry that certain foods will cause weight gain. It is also called "eating restraint." It is associated with higher *cortisol* production and *short luteal phase* cycles. It is the mildest kind of *"eating disorder,"* of which *anorexia* is the most severe.

**Complex carbohydrates:** a kind of food in whole grains like rice, wheat, corn and barley.

**Compounding pharmacy:** a store in which medicines are created by a pharmacist rather than a place where manufactured drugs are simply being sold.

**Conjugated equine estrogen:** a pill form of *estrogen* created from the urine of pregnant horses with the brand name *Premarin*®. Contains a mixture of unique horse estrogens and predominately *estrone*, a common type of *estrogen*.

**Cortical bone:** one of the two kinds of bone. It is the very hard outer "shell" of bone, often shaped like a tube or drumstick. Cortical bone responds to exercise, the pull of working muscles and gravity by increasing strength and density.

**Cortisol:** a stress hormone made by the adrenal glands. An essential hormone, it functions to maintain *blood pressure*, assist with fighting infections and preserving health. However, when cortisol levels are too high, as a result of stress, illness, or undernutrition, bone loss results. Cortisol causes increased *bone resorption* and decreased *bone formation*. *Progesterone* competes for the cortisol receptor on the *osteoblast*, possibly preventing cortisol from stopping bone growth.

**Creatinine level:** the concentration of a protein in blood that reflects the health of the kidneys. Often is used to correct urine tests of hormones and *bone resorption* for the person's kidney function.

**Cycle day:** the days of the menstrual cycle counted from the first day of flow, called Day One to the day before the next flow starts.

**Cyclic Etidronate:** (Didrocal®, Didronel®) see *Etidronate*.

**Cystic:** a description of a round, fluid-filled structure commonly seen in the *ovaries*, *thyroid gland* or in *breast* tissue. In only rare cases is a cyst a *cancer*.

**Cysts:** mean round, fluid-filled structures that are common in *ovaries*, *thyroid glands* and *breast* tissue. Only rarely is a cyst caused by cancer.

**Daily Perimenopause Diary©1990:** a daily check-list to help show effects of hormone changes in the menstrual cycle, and experiences like hot flushes and sleep disturbances. It may be used by women for self-learning, by physicians in patient care, and by scientists as a tool in research. It can be printed, free, from the CeMCOR website.

**Dementia:** a decreased ability to remember, to reason or speak, associated with diseases, some medicines and aging. (See *Alzheimer's*).

**Deoxypyridinoline:** a test for *bone resorption* that measures the excretion of this protein from bone in morning urine. It is abbreviated *D-pyr*.

**DHEAS:** an *androgenic* hormone made in both the adrenal glands in response to stress, as well as in the ovary. It is made into *estrogen* especially in *menopause*.

**Diabetes or Diabetes mellitus:** an often-hereditary disease in which the blood sugar becomes abnormally high because the body doesn't make enough *insulin* (Type 1) or the insulin that is made is not effective (Type 2). *Insulin resistance*, being overweight or obese, having *anovulatory androgen excess* and being inactive all predispose to diabetes.

**Diagnostic mammogram:** a more detailed mammogram done to rule out breast cancer—usually when a screening mammogram gives an abnormal result.

**Diaphragm and jelly:** a barrier method of contraception involving a rubber ring with thin rubber in the middle that fits over the *cervix* and blocks sperm. Jelly has a chemical that kills sperm and is most effective if a full applicator is inserted once the diaphragm is in place.

**Diastolic:** the lower *blood pressure* reading.

**Differentiation:** the process by which cells become more mature or grown up. The opposite of the change associated with cancer.

**Digitize:** to convert signals into a computer form. Used for measuring things like _breast density_ and spine _fractures_.

**Dihydrotestosterone:** an _androgenic_ hormone made from testosterone that changes soft silky pale hair on the face and body into coarse dark hair, makes more secretions from oil glands and causes loss of head hair or _alopecia_.

**Dimenhydrinate:** a kind of over-the-counter antihistamine that causes drowsiness and has long-lasting action for allergies. It also helps with nausea.

**Diuretic:** a kind of medicine used for fluid retention, swelling, _edema_ and for high _blood pressure_.

**Dominant follicle:** the large _cyst_ in the _ovary_ during each _menstrual cycle_. An egg is released from the dominant follicle with _ovulation_—it that supplies the majority of the _estrogen_ and all of the _progesterone_ for that particular menstrual cycle.

**Dong quai:** a Chinese herb used to improve energy and help with menopausal symptoms in women—it is still lacking scientific evidence of effectiveness.

**Double blind:** a kind of study in which neither the participants nor the researchers know which treatment each person is on. This is used in _randomized, placebo-controlled trials_.

**D-Pyr:** see _Deoxypyridinoline_.

**Dysmenorrhea:** see _Menstrual Cramps_.

**EEG:** a test that measures brain waves.

**Eating disorder:** means a variety of situations in which a person feels the need to control food intake. This varies from a person who is worried that eating certain foods will cause weight gain (_cognitive dietary restraint_, _eating restraint_) and extends to serious diseases such as _anorexia_ or _bulimia_.

**Eating restraint:** see _Cognitive dietary restraint_.

**Edema:** means swelling of the legs and feet, and occasionally the fingers caused because the body keeps too much salt and water. Often associated with high _blood pressure_. It is treated with a low salt diet or _diuretics_.

**Elemental calcium:** means the weight of the calcium by itself in mg, without the weight of the carbonate or citrate that calcium it must be combined with to be used by the body.

**Emphysema:** a chronic lung disease in which small air sacks become damaged so that the person has difficulty breathing, especially with increased exercise. Emphysema is caused by cigarettes or by poorly treated, long-standing asthma.

**Endocrinology:** a specialty of *internal medicine* in which a doctor focuses on understanding the actions of and diseases of glands and hormones.

**Endogenous:** means from within a person's body—for example in perimenopause a woman can be on the Pill and still have high endogenous *estrogen* levels.

**Endometrial ablation:** a kind of day surgery in which heat, pressure, a sharp instrument or laser is used to destroy the lining of the uterus (*endometrium*). It is used to treat heavy flow (*menorrhagia*), especially in *perimenopause*.

**Endometrial biopsy:** an office procedure in which the *cervix* is made larger and a tool is used to cut out a small piece of the *endometrium*. Is a test used to see whether endometrial cancer is present.

**Endometrial cancer:** a cancer of the *endometrium*. Endometrial cancer is caused by *estrogen* without sufficient *progesterone* which blocks the proliferative action of estrogen in the uterus. Being overweight, having *anovulatory androgen excess* and *diabetes mellitus* are also risk factors. It is usually preceded by persistent endometrial growth and *endometrial hyperplasia* (both of which are reversible with progesterone therapy).

**Endometrial hyperplasia:** an overgrowth of the *endometrium*, which is caused by *estrogen* over-stimulation without sufficient *progesterone*. This can lead to *endometrial cancer*.

**Endometrial thickness:** the thickness or depth of the *endometrium* seen on pelvic or vaginal *ultrasound*.

**Endometrium:** the inner lining of the uterus that is stimulated by *estrogen* to become thicker, and is caused by *progesterone* to become mature and ready to support a fertilized egg.

**Error of measurement:** every test has variability that must be known to accurately interpret the result. This variability adds to the error of measurement.

**ESR:** stands for erythrocyte sedimentation rate. It is a general test used to detect inflammation, or infection, such as arthritis or a bone infection.

**Estradiol:** the most powerful form of bio-identical estrogen. Estradiol is made in the ovaries, the placenta and by conversion in fat and muscle cells from androgens into estrogens. It causes growth or *proliferation* of most cells in the body, especially in the breasts, *uterus* and *vagina*.

**Estradot®:** a form of _bio-identical_ _estradiol_ that is _transdermal_ and delivered as a small patch that has a lower risk for blood clots than oral estrogen.

**Estragel®:** a form of _bio-identical_ _estradiol_ as an alcohol-based gel for rubbing on the skin. This _transdermal_ form of estrogen has decreased risks for _blood clots_ than oral estrogen.

**Estriol:** a weak form of _estrogen_ that is high during pregnancy. It is not effective for treatment of _hot flushes_ or _osteoporosis_ but is effective for "vaginal dryness" or _vaginal atrophy_.

**Estrogen:** the name for a family of hormones including _estradiol_, _estrone_ and _estriol_.

**Estrogen receptor positive:** refers to cells in breast cancer that are stimulated by estrogen to grow and undergo proliferation.

**Estrone:** the common form of _estrogen_ in menopausal women. It can be made from adrenal and ovarian _androgens_.

**External Health Locus of Control:** see _Health Locus of Control_

**Etidronate:** an early bisphosphonate taken for two weeks, every three months. Prevents spine _fractures_ in _randomized placebo-controlled trials_. Does not cause heartburn or esophageal injury. See _Bisphosphonates_.

**Fallopian tubes:** flexible hollow tubes that allow an egg released from the ovary to be delivered to the uterus.

**Fasting glucose:** see _fasting blood sugar_.

**Fasting blood sugar:** a blood test taken before breakfast and after no food for the previous 12 hours. It is used to assess the risk for _diabetes mellitus_ and its control.

**Fasting lipids:** a test taken without eating for 12-16 hours. It measures fats in the blood including total cholesterol, high density lipoprotein and low density lipoprotein cholesterol, and triglycerides.

**Ferritin level:** a blood test that reflects iron stores in the _bone marrow_ and therefore the risk for iron-deficiency or blood loss _anemia_.

**Fibroids:** are benign tumors of fibrous and muscular tissue that grow in the muscle wall of the _uterus_. They increase in midlife women, and decrease in _menopause_. They occur commonly without symptoms but are often discovered on vaginal or pelvic _ultrasound_ because they are associated with heavy menstrual flow (_menorrhagia_).

**Fibromyalgia:** is a condition in which pain at *trigger points* is associated with sleep disturbances and decreased exercise. Helped by improved sleep, increased exercise and often by low dose *tricyclic anti-depressant* medications.

**Fracture:** a break in a bone caused by a force of greater intensity than the bone can withstand. Fractures often occur in the spinal bones in the back (vertebrae) and are often not recognized. They can be diagnosed with an X-ray. Those with vertebral compression fractures often develop a rounded upper back (kyphosis).

**Folate:** a vitamin in the B-vitamin family that helps cells to mature and is needed before and during a pregnancy to prevent birth defects.

**Follicle:** the nest of cells surrounding an egg in the ovary. One follicle becomes the *dominant follicle* each *menstrual cycle* and releases the egg with *ovulation*.

**Follicle Stimulating Hormone:** the pituitary hormone that encourages the follicle to grow and produce estrogen. It is abbreviated *FSH*.

**Follicular phase:** the portion of the *menstrual cycle* from the start of flow until the egg is released with *ovulation*.

**FSH:** abbreviation for *follicle stimulating hormone*.

**Gabapentin:** a medicine used for nerve-type pain or some kinds of seizure, that has recently been shown to help hot flushes and night sweats.

**Gastritis:** irritation of the lining of the stomach causing heartburn.

**Glaucoma:** a disease in which pressure builds inside the eyeball. Glaucoma can cause blindness if not treated.

**Glucose tolerance test:** a test measuring the *blood sugar* after a person is given a test dose of glucose (a form of sugar). It measures the effectiveness of the action of *insulin*—it is rarely used except during pregnancy.

**GnRH:** see *Gonadotrophin Releasing Hormone*

**Goiter:** a swelling or enlargement of the *thyroid gland*.

**Gold standard:** the reference value for a test. Used for validation of a new test.

**Gonadotrophin Releasing Hormone:** also GnRH is the hormone from the hypothalamus that integrates signals from stress hormones, *insulin* and other signals to wisely direct actions of the *pituitary* and the *ovary*.

**GP:** short for physician who is a general practitioner. Now, after a family practice residency, general physicians are usually called family physicians.

**Gynecologist:** a surgical specialist that is an expert in _pelvis_, _uterus_ and _ovary_ surgery and the treatment of _infertility_.

**Gynecology:** the surgical specialty that is expert in _pelvis_, _uterus_ and _ovary_ surgery and the treatment of some forms of _infertility_.

**Health Care Providers:** a general term used for physicians, nurses, emergency medical technicians, ambulance personnel and others in health delivery fields.

**HbA1C:** see _hemoglobin_ A1C.

**Health Locus of Control:** means attitude toward one's health. "External" believes doctors are responsible for health; "Chance" says it is fate or luck; "Internal" says what an individual person does determines his/her health.

**Heart palpitations:** a feeling of fluttering or pounding in the chest that usually means a rapid or irregular heartbeat.

**Head CT scan:** a computed tomography form of _X-ray_ that examines structures within the brain including the pituitary gland.

**Hemoglobin:** the chemical compound that requires _iron_ and becomes part of red blood cells to carry oxygen in the bloodstream.

**Hemoglobin A1C:** a test used to monitor those with _diabetes mellitus_. It that tells the percentage of time in the past three months that the blood sugar level has been abnormally high. A normal Hemoglobin A1C is usually four to six percent. Also _HbA1C_.

**Hepatitis:** an infection of the liver usually caused by one of several viruses.

**Hepatitis tests:** blood tests that measure liver enzyme levels.

**High blood pressure:** when the average pressure is more than 140/90 in young people and more than 145/95 in those over 60. Also called hypertension.

**High bone resorption:** means increased bone loss because _osteoclasts_ are removing bone too quickly.

**High intracranial pressure:** a situation caused by several diseases in which the pressure within the bony skull is high enough to cause symptoms, or disturb brain blood vessels.

**Hirsutism:** the presence of coarse hair occurring in a male-type pattern in women. Hair can grow on the chin and upper lip, as well as the sideburn areas of the face or the inner thigh, up from the pubic hair line toward the navel, and around the nipples. It is normal for hair to be present in these areas but it is usually very fine. This is a sign of high androgen levels or actions.

**Homophobia:** the negative attitude toward women or men who choose partners of the same sex.

**Hot flush:** sometimes called hot flash—a sudden feeling of heat often associated with sweating and accompanied by warm hands, a slightly faster heart rate and higher *blood pressure*. The intensity of hot flushes varies from a mild warm feeling without sweating to "a tropical rain storm." Hot flushes originate in the *hypothalamus* that is exposed to *estrogen* withdrawal after first becoming habituated to high estrogen levels. Hot flushes often begin in *perimenopause* (especially in women who have experienced high estrogen signs such as increased *premenstrual symptoms*). Hot flushes are maximal during the year following the final menstrual period. Men having anti-androgen treatment for prostate cancer may also experience them. Along with *night sweats*, hot flushes are part of a general uncomfortable experience called *vasomotor symptoms*.

**HRT:** an inaccurate term for *estrogen* or *estrogen* plus *progesterone/progestin* therapy for menopausal women. See *OHT* or *Ovarian Hormone Therapy* for a more appropriate term.

**Hyperthyroidism:** the term used for an over-active thyroid gland or caused by taking too much thyroid hormone. The person feels too hot, loses weight despite eating well, develops muscle weakness, trembling hands and a fast heart rate. *TSH* is usually low.

**Hypothalamus:** a small and important organ in the centre of the brain that interprets signals from the environment and controls body temperature, breathing, heart rate and reproduction. Emotional signals are translated into hormonal and brain signals.

**Hypothyroidism:** means when the thyroid gland isn't making enough thyroid hormone. Often there is a feeling of coldness, need to sleep more, and sometimes dry skin and hair. Usually the *TSH* level is increased.

**Hysterectomy:** surgery to remove the *uterus*. This is performed primarily for heavy flow in perimenopausal women whose average age is 42-47. Although *fibroids* are commonly present, the surgery is most often performed because of inadequately treated heavy flow. Hysterectomy is indicated for *endometrial cancer* and invasive cervical cancer. The *ovaries* may or may not be removed (ovariectomy*)*, but evidence suggests that even if they remain, ovarian function decreases after a hysterectomy. Women who have had hysterectomy appear to be at lower risk for *breast cancer*.

**Hysterosalpingogram:** a test in which a substance visible on an X-ray is pushed into the *uterus* and *fallopian tubes* to determine whether eggs can travel to the uterus or not. It is an expensive test that is often painful.

**Ibuprofen:** an over-the-counter kind of *anti-prostaglandin medicine* that is very effective for *menstrual cramps* and *menorrhagia* to decrease heavy flow.

**Immitrex®:** a powerful medicine used to treat an acute migraine attack.

**Incontinence:** difficulty keeping urine in the bladder when the bladder is full or with coughing or sneezing. It often appears in *perimenopause* and improves in *menopause*. It is made worse by *estrogen* or *estrogen* plus *progestin* therapy according to *WHI* results.

**Inhibin:** a family of hormones made by the ovarian follicle and part of the control system for *FSH* levels and hence the menstrual cycle. Inhibin B decreases in the *follicular phase* early in *perimenopause*.

**Infertility:** the inability to become pregnant or bear a child after one or more years of trying.

**In situ:** means that the cells, that contain cancer, are still in one spot and not spreading through the blood vessels or to nearby tissues.

**Insulin:** a hormone made in the beta cells of the pancreas that allows sugar (glucose) to move into cells. Lack of insulin causes Type 1 Diabetes Mellitus.

**Insulin resistance:** occurs when abdominal fat and inactivity plus an inherited risk make insulin less effective. It is diagnosed by a *waist circumference* over 88 cm in women and over 100 cm in men.

**Internal examination:** see *pelvic examination.*

**Internal Health Locus of Control:** see Health Locus of Control.

**Internal Medicine:** the name for a physician specialist who is not a surgeon. This specialty includes endocrinologists, cardiologists, dermatologists, gastroenterologists, neurologists, rheumatologists, and those who run intensive care units and often emergency rooms.

**Invasive:** a kind of test that involves pain, high cost and/or potential risks.

**IUD:** an intrauterine device created for birth control. Women wear a small piece of plastic or metal inside their uterus. It may or may not have a medicine in it (such as the *progestin*-releasing IUD, *Mirena*®). It is inserted through the *cervix* and has a string for its eventual removal. An IUD slightly increases menstrual flow (except for the progestin-releasing one) plus it may cause increased cramps.

**Kinesiology:** the science of exercise, sport and movement.

**Lactose:** a milk sugar that some people with lactose intolerance can't breakdown normally.

**Least squares analysis method:** a quantitative way of figuring out whether or not *basal temperatures* are increased after *ovulation*.

**LH:** see *luteinizing hormone*.

**LH peak:** the high level of *luteinizing hormone* that occurs in response to the *estrogen peak* in the middle of the *menstrual cycle* and which triggers *ovulation*.

**Littermate rats:** a kind of laboratory animal in which all are very closely related, like identical twins.

**Low-trauma fracture:** also called a "fragility fracture." It is defined as a broken bone with a fall with less or equal force as a fall from a standing height. A low trauma fracture is one way of defining *osteoporosis*.

**Lubricants:** over-the-counter preparations to help *vaginal dryness*.

**Luteal phase length:** the portion of the normal menstrual cycle from *ovulation* until the day before the next flow. A normal luteal phase is 10 days or longer (assessed by the *quantitative basal temperature* method) or 12 days or longer from the LH peak at midcycle. The length of the luteal phase is roughly proportional to the amount of *progesterone* produced in the cycle.

**Luteinizing hormone:** a pituitary hormone controlled by gonadotrophin releasing hormone, (*GnRH*) from the *hypothalamus*. It stimulates the ovary's outer cells to make *androgens* that are then converted into *estrone* or *estrogen*.

**Magnesium:** an element found abundantly in human food that is often inadequate in the diet of rats and mice. For this reason these animals, but not humans, need supplements for normal *bone remodeling*.

**Mammogram:** a form of *X-ray* used to detect and screen for breast cancer.

**Manic:** a state of high excitement and activity found in bipolar affective disease and occasionally with other mental illness.

**Maternity vitamin:** a multivitamin that includes enough *folate* for the mother's and the fetus' good health.

**Matrix:** the protein produced by *osteoblasts* that becomes full of *calcium* and other minerals and forms the basic structure for bones.

**Maturation:** the process of becoming more mature or grown up.

**Maximal exercise performance:** sometimes called "*VO$_2$max.*" It means the heart, lungs and muscle are working so hard that no more oxygen can be used or the body is working without oxygen.

**Medical menopause:** an artificial kind of menopause in which the ovary stops producing *estrogen* and *progesterone* because of therapy with *GnRH* or other hormones. This is used sometimes for severe endometriosis or migraine headaches.

**Medroxyprogesterone:** a manufactured kind of *progestin* that fairly closely resembles natural *progesterone*.

**Menarche:** a young woman's first period.

**Menstrual cycle:** the time from the start of menstrual flow until the day before the next flow.

**Menopausal:** the situation of being in *menopause* (one year since the final menstrual flow). This term is preferred over "postmenopausal" which is a duplication of ideas.

**Menopausal Transition:** a term used to describe the period of time from irregular periods until the final menstrual flow in *perimenopause*.

**Menopause:** defined when a year has passed since the final menstrual flow. The average age of menopause in western countries is approximately 51. The average age of menopause is younger in smokers and those who have never had children (nulliparous). Low levels of both *estrogen* and *progesterone* are normal after menopause.

**Menorrhagia:** very heavy menstrual bleeding often with clots and flooding. It is usually caused by high *estrogen* levels and associated with *endometrial hyperplasia* from too little *progesterone*. It commonly occurs in *perimenopause* and may also happen in the teen years.

**Menstrual cramps:** the discomfort caused by contraction of the uterus before and during menstrual flow because of *prostaglandins*. It is also called *dysmenorrhea*. It is treated by *anti-prostaglandin agents* such as *ibuprofen*.

**Metoprolol:** a medicine used for high *blood pressure*—it is from the "beta-blocker family" of medicines that work against *catecholamines.* It slows the heart rate, decreases the force of the heart's contraction and decreases blood pressure.

**Micronize:** means to make into very small or microscopic bits. For *oral micronized progesterone*, each tiny amount of hormone is surrounded by fat. This process allows *progesterone* to be taken by mouth.

**Midcycle estrogen peak:** the highest level of estrogen that occurs in the middle of the *menstrual cycle*. This triggers the *luteinizing hormone peak* that leads to *ovulation*.

**Migraine headache:** a severe kind of headache involving blood vessels in the brain. It is usually associated with nausea and is often preceded by an *aura* that may involve a change in how nerves work. Prevention of migraines involves avoiding triggers (like some wines and cheeses), reduction of emotional stress and not taking estrogen-containing medicines such as *the Pill*, and not starting and stopping any hormones suddenly.

**Milk of magnesia:** an over-the-counter medicine containing *magnesium* that helps with constipation and causes diarrhea.

**MinEstrin®:** a lower dose form of oral contraceptive agent containing 20 μg of ethinyl estradiol and an *androgenic progestin* in the same amount for three weeks with one week off. In a 6-cycle *randomized controlled trial* of perimenopausal women with heavy flow, it was shown to decrease flow slightly, but it did not significantly improve hot flushes or quality of life.

**Mirena®:** the brand name of a powerful *androgenic progestin*-releasing *IUD* used to treat *menorrhagia* in *perimenopause*.

**Miscarriage:** means that a woman was pregnant but that the pregnancy ended early. Usually this occurs before three months of pregnancy because the fetus had an abnormality.

**Molimina:** the set of normal experiences that tells a woman that her period is coming and that she has ovulated. Most specific of these is the development of tenderness in the *axillary tail of the breast* under the armpit at a time when the rest of the breast is not sore. Other experiences include some increase in fluid retention, and perhaps increased appetite, and heightened sensitivity to emotions. It is different from *premenstrual symptoms* because it is less intense, has no front-of-the-breast tenderness and no severe mood symptoms. Lack of molimina indiates that the cycle is not *ovulatory*.

**Multinodular:** a term commonly used for the *breast* and *thyroid gland*s that contain many *cysts*.

**Naproxen:** a kind of *anti-prostaglandin* medicine.

**Natural progesterone:** means *bio-identical* *progesterone*. This term is often used to refer to progesterone creams that, in low doses, are sold without a prescription in the USA.

**Needle biopsy:** a test in which a needle is used to gather cells to decide whether a lump is a cancer or *benign*. Often used for diagnosis in breast and thyroid lumps.

**Neural tube defect:** means a birth or congenital problem often related to inadequate *folate* intake by the mother before and early in pregnancy. The baby's spinal canal doesn't close properly so that muscles and nerves in the feet and legs can't develop normally.

**Neurology specialist:** an *internal medicine* physician who is an expert in problems involving the diagnosis and treatment of brain and nerves.

**Neuropathy:** a problem of nerves causing pain or lack of normal functions. This occurs in those with diabetes that is not well controlled.

**Non-steroidal anti-inflammatory drugs:** these are medications that block *prostaglandin* production and therefore treat *menstrual cramps*. Also called *anti-prostaglandin medicines*. Abbreviated *NSAID*.

**Noradrenalin:** a name for a hormone made in sympathetic nerves and the adrenal gland that makes the heart beat faster and harder, and blood vessels constrict in the hands and feet. Also called *norepinephrine*.

**Norepinephrine:** see *Noradrenalin*.

**Normal luteal phase range:** describes the pattern of expected progesterone levels after ovulation in the normal menstrual cycle. This provides the guide for the amount of progesterone used for treatment of heavy flow, hot flushes and breast tenderness.

**NSAID:** see *Non-steroidal Anti-inflammatory drug*.

**Nucleus:** the special centre part of all cells containing genetic material and receptors that allow hormones to direct the cell.

**Obesity:** being heavier than normal for height—a *BMI* more than 30.

**OHT:** see *Ovarian Hormone Therapy*.

**Oil of evening primrose:** a kind of oil that is used for *premenstrual symptoms* and other of women's symptoms. It has not been shown to be effective.

**Oligomenorrhea:** means menstrual cycles farther apart than 36 days but shorter than 180 days. This may normally occur during early adolescence and in *perimenopause*. It is commonly a protective form of hypothalamic suppression in association with weight loss, inappropriately intense exercise training, emotional stress or undernutrition. In teenagers, it may precede the development of *anovulatory androgen excess*.

**Oncologist:** an *internal medicine* specialist in cancer.

**Open biopsy:** a small surgery to remove a breast lump that might be cancer.

**Ophthalmologist:** a doctor that specializes in diseases and surgery of the eye.

**Oral contraceptives:** commonly called *the Pill*. Contain high doses of a synthetic estrogen and moderate doses of a *progestin*, typically an *androgenic progestin*. "Low dose" (20-30 μg) estrogen-containing kinds still have four to five times more estrogen effect than is normal for the menstrual cycle. The Pill prevents ovarian cancer but increases the risks for *migraine headaches*, *blood clots* and *strokes*. The new ring and patch forms of contraception are less likely to cause *blood clots*.

**Oral micronized progesterone:** a way of preparing *progesterone* so that it can be taken by mouth and remain an active therapy. It improves deep sleep, and is a useful therapy in *perimenopause*.

**Orthotics:** special inner soles for shoes crafted to correct foot problems.

**Osteoblasts:** are cells that lay down the protein *matrix* that becomes bone after mineralization (adding *calcium* and other minerals) under the influence of Vitamin D.

**Osteoblast:** cells that form new bone, a slow but essential process in normal bone renewal. Formation is maximal during growth in adolescence. It also increases under the influence of *progesterone* during the *luteal phase* of the menstrual cycle or from therapy with *progesterone*, most *progestins* or parathyroid hormone.

**Osteoclasts:** cells that remove old bone during *bone remodeling* (called *resorption*). Osteoclastic *bone resorption* is fast and occurs over about three weeks in any spot.

**Osteopenia:** a lower than normal *Bone Mineral Density* with a *T-score* between −1 and −2.5. Suggests an increased risk for fracture.

**Osteoporosis:** a weakness of bone sufficient to cause a *fragility fracture* or very low

*Bone Mineral Density* (lower than a *T-Score* of –2.5). Men and women are both at risk with increasing age—almost 25% of adults over age 50 have had one or more spinal compression fractures.

**Ovarian cysts:** normal developing *follicles* in the ovary that release an egg after *ovulation*.

**Ovarian Hormones:** includes estradiol or estrogen and progesterone that are necessary for women's reproduction and general health.

**Ovarian Hormone Therapy:** therapy with *estrogen* and *progesterone* or *progestin* for specific problems that menopausal women may experience. Ovarian Hormone Therapy (or *OHT*) was formerly wrongly called "hormone replacement therapy." The three appropriate reasons for OHT are: *early menopause*, chronically disturbing *hot flushes/night sweats* or *osteoporosis* in a menopausal woman who also has *hot flushes*.

**Ovarian hyperstimulation:** refers to a kind of *infertility* treatment in which dangerous, extremely high *estrogen* levels sometimes occur. "Endogenous ovarian hyperstimulation" is used to describe the perimenopausal high estrogen levels.

**Ovary:** the two glands in the abdomen of women that contain millions of follicles, each of which includes an egg and cells that can make *ovarian hormones*.

**Overactive thyroid:** see *hyperthyroidism*.

**Over-pronation:** a tendency of the foot to tilt toward the middle of the body—can cause foot and knee pain. Commonly corrected by *orthotics*.

**Ovulated:** means the action of ovulation.

**Ovulatory disturbance:** also called ovulation disturbance. Includes *short luteal phase* and *anovulatory* cycles. Ovulatory disturbance occurs in regular cycles and *oligomenorrhea*.

**Ovulation:** is release of an egg from the ovary. It usually occurs in about the middle of the cycle following an *LH peak*. Only after ovulation are *progesterone* levels high.

**Pap test:** short for the Papanicolaou test for cervical cancer. This is performed during an *internal examination*, or *pelvic examination*.

**PCOS:** see *anovulatory androgen excess*.

**Peak bone density:** the highest *bone mineral density* achieved sometime between the teens and about ages 20-30.

**Pedometer:** a small instrument worn to measure the number of steps or how many km a person has walked.

**Pelvic:** relating to the circle of bones sheltering the uterus, bladder and nerves, muscles, and tendons connecting the trunk to the legs.

**Pelvic examination:** this means examination of the *vagina* and *cervix* using a special tool called a speculum. Also includes feeling the size and shape of the uterus and ovaries with one hand in the vagina and one on the lower abdomen. Commonly called an *internal examination*.

**Perceived exertion:** the feeling an exercising person has of how hard she/he is working.

**Percussing:** a technique of tapping on the outside of the body as a way of learning the position and characteristics of internal organs. Percussing is regularly used for the lungs and to determine the position and size of the liver and spleen.

**Perimenopause:** the period of time before and for a year after the final menstrual period during which time ovarian hormonal patterns, experiences and sociocultural roles change. Irregular cycles develop at approximately age 47. Perimenopause probably begins several years before that, in women with regular cycles, whose *ovaries* are making higher amounts of *estrogen* and tending to make lower amounts of *progesterone*. Like *menopause*, this is a normal part of a woman's life cycle.

**Phytoestrogens:** plant-based molecules that act like estrogen at the same time as they act against estrogens in tissues. Soy foods are high in phytoestrogens.

**Pituitary gland:** a small, complex gland just behind the bridge of the nose that makes many hormones under the direction of the *hypothalamus*. The two pituitary hormones directing the ovary's actions are *LH, Luteinizing Hormone* and *FSH, Follicle Stimulating Hormone*.

**Pituitary hormones:** for the front or anterior part of the pituitary gland these in-clude thyroid stimulating hormone *(TSH)*, *prolactin*, follicle stimulating hormone *(FSH)*, luteinizing hormone *(LH)*, growth hormone and adrenocortical stimulat-ing hormone (ACTH). The back or posterior part of the pituitary gland releases anti-diuretic hormone and oxytocin that are made in the hypothalamus.

**PMI:** point of maximum impulse of the heartbeat that can be seen or felt on the chest wall.

**PMS:** the abbreviation for *premenstrual syndrome* that some experts believe is a mental illness. Also used for *premenstrual symptoms*, a set of physical and emotional changes before menstrual flow that occur when estrogen is too high and progesterone too low.

**Placebo:** an inactive medicine that is used for *double blind, randomized controlled trials*.

**Polycystic Ovary Syndrome:** see *Anovulatory Androgen Excess*.

**Population-based studies:** an accurate kind of epidemiology study that asks a random (by chance) set of people to participate. Ideally over 50% of those invited will join the study.

**Potassium level:** the amount of the small electrically charged molecule in the blood stream. Low potassium levels interfere with the work of the heart and blood vessels and are often caused by *diuretics*.

**Pre-eclampsia:** a serious health problem in pregnancy that results in high *blood pressure*, *edema*, abnormal kidney function and carries risks for the health of the mother and baby.

**Premarin®:** brand name for *conjugated equine estrogen*.

**Premenopause:** the years from the first period until *perimenopause*.

**Premenopausal:** women who are in *premenopause*.

**Premenstrual symptoms:** a set of unwanted experiences such as sore breasts, mood swings, fluid retention and food cravings that occur when, right before flow, estrogen levels are too high and progesterone levels are too low. Also sometimes called *PMS*.

**Progesterone:** a hormone made in small amounts by the liver and adrenal glands in men women and children, and by the *ovary* in high levels after *ovulation*. It is also made by the placenta during pregnancy. Its job is to counterbalance the actions of *estrogen* in all body tissues, and to cause cell *maturation* and *differentiation*.

**Progestin:** a synthetic form of progesterone commonly used in *OHT* and *the Pill*. Most progestins are derived from *testosterone* and are *androgenic progestins—medroxyprogesterone* is one of the few progestins that is not androgenic.

**Prolactin:** a pituitary hormone that, when its levels are very high, can cause *amenorrhea*, *oligomenorrhea* and *ovulation disturbances*.

**Proliferating:** describes cells that are growing rapidly. In general the more rapidly proliferating cells carry a higher cancer risk.

**Proliferation:** a process in which cells grow rapidly, dividing frequently and increasing in number. If proliferation gets out of control, it leads to cancer.

**Prometrium®:** the brand name for *oral micronized progesterone.*

**Prophylactic:** a descriptive word for things that are meant for prevention.

**Prophylaxis:** the process or set of treatments used for prevention of a disease or problem.

**Propranolol:** a kind of medicine that blocks the actions of *adrenalin* and *noradrenalin* thus slowing the heart rate and decreasing the contraction force of the heart. Used in *hyperthyroidism*, high *blood pressure* and for *migraine prophylaxis.*

**Prostaglandins:** hormones made in many tissues that cause pain, increased or decreased blood flow and menstrual cramps.

**Provera®:** the most common brand name for the *progestin*, *medroxyprogesterone* acetate.

**Psychiatrist:** a specialist who deals with emotional problems and mental diseases.

**Pulse:** the heart beat including whether or not it has a regular rhythm and its rate.

**Quantitative Basal Temperature:** means the statistical analysis of the basal temperatures recorded during one menstrual cycle to reliably decide whether *ovulation* has occurred and *luteal phase length.*

**Raloxifene®:** a selective estrogen receptor modulator or SERM that prevents spine but not hip fractures. It causes side effects of *hot flushes*, muscle cramps and *blood clots*.

**Randomized, placebo-controlled study:** a scientifically important way of testing that involves assignment to a group by chance, like a roll of dice. One group gets an inactive intervention or placebo therapy. These are usually *double blind* also.

**Rebound increase in flushes:** the increase in hot flushes that occurs when women with past hot flushes suddenly stop estrogen treatment.

**Remifemin®:** a commercial preparation of the herb, *black cohosh.*

**Remodeling:** a term used for the renovation process, including *bone resorption* and bone *formation* that maintains the strength of bone.

**Retina:** the blood vessel-rich tissue in the back of the eyeball that allows sight.

**Rheumatic fever:** an illness caused by a reaction to the germ causing strep throat. It usually involves a fever and sore joints, and often a skin rash and problems with heart valves.

**Sage tea:** a tea made out of the spice, sage—it is believed to help hot flushes. This treatment has not been scientifically studied.

**Secretory:** a tissue that makes special secretions. For example, under the influence of *progesterone*, the *endometrium* in the *luteal phase* becomes glandular and secretes fluids so that a fertilized egg can implant.

**Selective estrogen receptor modulator:** a kind of created non–hormonal medicine that sometimes acts like and sometimes acts against *estrogen*.

**SERM:** see *selective estrogen receptor modulator*.

**Selective serotonin re-uptake inhibitor (SSRIs):** a newer kind of antidepressant that does not cause drowsiness. Some of this kind of anti-depressants are difficult to stop, cause decreased sexual interest and sleep problems, but also improve *hot flushes*. Abbreviated *SSRI*.

**Serum creatinine:** the blood concentration of a chemical that reflects kidney function.

**Shin splints:** a pain in the front of the lower leg that is caused by not enough blood to the working muscles beside the shinbone. May be confused with a stress fracture of the tibia.

**Short luteal phase:** a type of *ovulatory disturbance* in which the *luteal phase* is shorter than normal and *progesterone* production is less than optimal. Shortening of the luteal phase is a common hypothalamic protective response to weight loss, stress, exercise training that is too intense or *cognitive dietary restraint*. Short luteal phase cycles are associated with *infertility*, bone loss and *osteopenia*.

**Soy-based foods:** food made from soy, a member of the legume or bean family of vegetables. These contain high levels of *phytoestrogens*.

**Sperm count:** is an important *infertility* test for men. The number, movement, shape and health of sperm seen after a man ejaculates.

**Spironolactone:** an anti-*androgen* medication that also is used for high blood pressure. It is very helpful when used with *cyclic progesterone therapy* for the treatment of *anovulatory androgen excess.*

**SSRI:** see *selective estrogen receptor inhibitor* antidepressant.

**Statistical power:** a way using math and the variability of what you are studying, to determine whether, in a scientific study, you could detect a difference if there is one.

**Stress fracture:** a kind of broken bone or *fracture* in which there is disruption of *cortical bone* and pain but no crack going through a bone—often occurs with excess exercise of the same kind, a problem of how the foot and leg line up with exercise (like *over-pronation*), or with compulsive exercise.

**Stroke:** a major brain injury in which a *blood clot* or bleeding in the blood vessels of the brain interfere with the brain's function. Stroke risk is increased by high *blood pressure* and *OHT*, *estrogen* treatment or use of *the Pill*.

**Systolic:** the top reading—see *blood pressure*.

**TB:** or tuberculosis is a bacterial disease that attacks the lungs and can spread to the adrenal glands, kidney and bone. It is worse with overcrowding, poor nutrition and AIDS.

**T Score:** the term used to decide whether *bone mineral density* is normal, low (*osteopenia*) or suggests a strong risk for *fragility fracture*, called *osteoporosis*. Is based on the *bell-shaped* curve distribution of bone density from a random sample of men or women ages 20-30.

**Tamoxifen:** a medicine that was the first *SERM*. It decreases breast cancer recurrence but has side effects of *blood clots*, *hot flushes* and *endometrial cancer.*

**Tanner Stage:** a way of describing the maturation of breasts and pubic hair during women's adolescent reproductive development. It includes five stages from a child's characteristics to those of a mature woman.

**Testosterone:** the major *androgen* or male hormone made by the adrenal glands and the ovaries in women, and primarily by the testicles in men.

**The Pill:** common name for *oral contraceptives*.

**Thyroid:** a small butterfly shaped gland in the front of the neck that produces *thyroid hormone* which is important for energy, temperature and heart rate control.

**Thyroid hormone:** $T_4$ or L-thyroxine is the major hormone released by the thyroid gland under the influence of *TSH*. $T_4$ is made, within body cells, into the active hormone, $T_3$, that is tightly controlled and protectively decreases when a person is undernourished or ill or very stressed.

**Tibia:** the shinbone in the lower leg.

**Transdermal:** means absorbed into the blood stream through the inner layer of skin that is called the dermis.

**Tricyclics:** an older form of medicines for depression that cause drowsiness and are used in lower dose for helping sleep, decreasing pain and treating *fibromyalgia* and *chronic fatigue syndrome*.

**Trigger points:** spots where muscles and tendons join bone that are sore when a person does not obtain sufficient deep and refreshing sleep. People with many sore trigger points are said to have *fibromyalgia*.

**TSH level:** TSH is a common abbreviation for "thyroid stimulating hormone" produced from the pituitary. A high TSH level suggest *hypothyroidism* and a low level indicates *hyperthyroidism* or too high a dose of *thyroid hormone* therapy.

**Tubal ligation:** a surgery in which the fallopian tubes are cut, burned or clamped to prevent pregnancy. Is associated with an earlier perimenopause and a decreased risk for *breast cancer*.

**Tuberculosis:** also called *TB*.

**Type 2 diabetes mellitus:** see *diabetes mellitus*.

**Ultrasound:** a technique for bouncing high frequency sound waves off of tissues or structures. Used for visualizing the gallbladder, uterus, endometrium and ovaries. Also used to detect the amount or strength of *bone mineral*.

**Uterus:** the woman's organ, also called "the womb" that is the size of a fist in *premenopause*. It sits in the *pelvis* and responds every month to *menstrual cycle* hormones with shedding of the *endometrium* and menstrual *flow*. It is the organ in which a baby grows in *pregnancy*. It is removed with *hysterectomy*.

**Vagina:** the passage extending from the *uterus* to the outside skin of the groin in women. The vagina is very rich in *estrogen* and *progesterone receptors*. It takes very low levels of estrogen to maintain the elasticity and moisture of the vagina.

**Vaginal atrophy:** usually called "vaginal dryness"—it is a condition in which the surface of the *vagina* becomes thinned and makes less secretions so that there is discomfort with intercourse. Occurs in about thirty percent of women in menopause. Both *estrogen* and *progesterone* therapy in low doses effectively treat it. The most effective and safe therapy is 0.5 mg of *estriol* made by a *compounding pharmacy* applied to the *vagina* one night a week.

**Vasomotor symptoms:** a way to describe *hot flushes* and *night sweats*. They are experienced briefly or in mild forms by most perimenopausal or menopausal women.

Approximately ten or fifteen percent of perimenopausal women and thirty percent of women in early menopause in the developed world report severe disturbances related to them.

**Vitamin B₆:** a vitamin called "pyridoxine" in the Vitamin B family of water-soluble vitamins. It is used in high doses as a treatment for nausea or for *premenstrual symptoms*.

**VO₂ max:** see *Maximal Exercise Performance*.

**Waist circumference:** measurement of the smallest point in the abdomen near the belly button or umbilicus. Ideal values are less than 88 cm in women and less than 100 cm in men. Larger measurements suggest *insulin resistance*.

**Waist to hip ratio:** the waist circumference divided by the hip circumference. A value lower than 0.8 is normal for women and lower than 1.0 is normal for men.

**WHI:** see *Women's Health Initiative* studies:

**Women's Health Initiative studies:** a series of very large studies on the health of menopausal women. WHI includes randomized double-blind, placebo-controlled trials, as well as observational studies of the effect of a low fat diet on breast cancer risk and *vitamin D* and *calcium* for preventing *osteoporosis*. The trials involve *estrogen* or estrogen plus very low dose *medroxyprogesterone* (*ovarian hormone therapy, OHT*) compared with placebo therapy in healthy menopausal women. Results of the estrogen plus *progestin* arm that was discontinued early in July 2002, and the estrogen in hysterecomized women discontinued in 2004 proved that "*hormone replacement therapy*" is not safe for healthy menopausal women and that "*estrogen deficiency*" is the wrong way to think about *menopause*.

**X-rays:** a kind of beam of radiation used commonly for diagnosis of health problems.

**Yellow jaundice:** the yellow color the skin takes on when a person has *hepatitis*.

# references

1. Hale GE, Hitchcock CL, Williams LA, Vigna YM, Prior JC. Cyclicity of breast tenderness and night-time vasomotor symptoms in mid-life women: information collected using the Daily Perimenopause Diary. Climacteric. 2003;6(2):128-39.

2. Prior JC, Vigna YM, Schulzer M, Hall JE, Bonen A. Determination of luteal phase length by quantitative basal temperature methods: validation against the midcycle LH peak. Clin.Invest.Med. 1990;13:123-31.

3. Shostak M. Nisa: the life and words of a !Kung woman. New York: Vintage Books; 1981.

4. Reitz R. Menopause - a positive approach. Middesex: Penquin Books; 1977.

5. Santoro N, Rosenberg J, Adel T, Skurnick JH. Characterization of reproductive hormonal dynamics in the perimenopause. J Clin Endocrinol Metab 1996;81:4,1495-501.

6. Burger HG, Dudley EC, Hopper JL, Shelley JM, Green A, Smith A et al. The endocrinology of the menopausal transition: a cross-sectional study of a population-based sample. J Clin Endocrinol Metab 1995;80:3537-45.

7. Prior JC, Barr SI, Vigna YM. The controversial endocrinology of the menopausal transition (letter). J Clin Endocrinol Metab 1996;81:3127-8.

8. Prior JC. Perimenopause: The complex endocrinology of the menopausal transition. Endocr.Rev. 1998;19:397-428.

9. Prior JC. The ageing female reproductive axis II: ovulatory changes with perimenopause. In: Chadwick DJ, Goode JA, editors. Endocrine Facets of Ageing. Chichester, UK: John Wiley and Sons Ltd; 2002. p. 172-86.

10. Bonnar J, Sheppard BL. Treatment of menorrhagia during menstruation: randomised controlled trial of ethamsylate, mefenamic acid, and tranexamic acid. BMJ 1996;313(7057):579-82.

11. Morse CA, Dudley E, Guthrie J, Dennerstein L. Relationships between premenstrual complaints and perimenopausal experiences. Journal of Psychosomatic Obstetrics and Gynecology 1989;19:182-91.

12. Gold EB, Sternfeld B, Kelsey JL, Brown C, Mouton C, Reame N et al. Relation of demographic and lifestyle factors to symptoms in a multiracial/ethnic population of women 40-55 years of age. Am.J.Epidemiol. 2000;152:463-73.

13. Stewart A, Cummins C, Gold L, Jordan R, Phillips W. The effectiveness of the levonorgestrel-releasing intrauterine system in menorrhagia: a systematic review. BJOG. 2001;108(1):74-86.

14. Milsom I, Andersson K, Andersch B, Rybo G. A comparison of flurbiprofen, tranexamic acid, and a levonorgestrel-releasing intrauterine contraceptive device in the treatment of idiopathic menorrhagia. Am.J Obstet.Gynecol. 1991;164(3):879-83.

15. Kelsea M. Beyond the stethoscope: a nurse practitioner looks at menopause and midlife. In: Sumrall AC, Taylor D, editors. Women of the 14th Moon: writings on menopause. Freedom, California: The Crossing Press; 1991. p. 268-79.

16. Kaufert PA. The perimenopausal woman and her use of health services. Maturitas 1980;2:191-205.

17. Oldenhave A, Jaszmann JB, Everaerd WT, Haspels AA. Hysterectomized women with ovarian conservation report more severe climacteric complaints than do normal climacteric women of similar age. Am.J.Obstet.Gynecol. 1993;168(3):765-71.

18. Kreiger N, Sloan M, Cotterchio M, Kirsh V. The risk of breast cancer following reproductive surgery. Eur.J.Cancer. 1999;35:97-101.

19. Tuppurainen M, Honkanen R, Kroger H, Saarikoski S, Alhava E. Osteoporosis risk factors, gyneacological history and fractures in perimenopausal women-the results of the baseline postal enquiry of the Kupio osteoporosis risk factor and prevention study. Maturitas 1993;17:89-100.

20. Weel AE, Uitterlinden AG, Westendorp IC, Burger H, Schuit SC, Hofman A et al. Estrogen receptor polymorphism predicts the onset of natural and surgical menopause. J.Clin.Endocrinol.Metab 1999;84(9):3146-50.

21. Maresh MJ, Metcalfe MA, McPherson K, Overton C, Hall V, Hargreaves J et al. The VALUE national hysterectomy study: description of the patients and their surgery. Br J Obstet Gynaecol 2002;109(3):302-12.

22. Moen MH, Kahn H, Bjerve KS, Halvorsen TB. Menometrorrhagia in the perimenopause is associated with increased serum estradiol. Maturitas 2004;47(2):151-5.

23. Writing Group for the Women's Health Initiative Investigators. Risks and benefits of estrogen plus progestin in health postmenopausal women: principal results from the Women's Health Initiative Randomized Control trial. JAMA 2002;288:321-33.

24. Shumaker SA, Legault C, Thal L, Wallace RB, Ockene JK, Hendrix SL et al. Estrogen plus progestin and the incidence of dementia and mild cognitive impairment in postmenopausal women: the Women's Health Initiative Memory Study: a randomized controlled trial. JAMA 2003;289(20):2651-62.

25. Barrett-Connor E. Postmenopausal estrogen and prevention bias. Ann. Int.Med. 1991;115:455-6.

26. Petitti DB. Hormone replacement therapy and heart disease prevention. Experimentation Trumps Observation (editorial). Journal of the American Medical Association 1998;280:650-2.

27. Anderson GL, Limacher M, Assaf AR, Bassford T, Beresford SA, Black H et al. Effects of conjugated equine estrogen in postmenopausal women with hysterectomy: the Women's Health Initiative randomized controlled trial. JAMA 2004;291(14):1701-12.

28. Oudshoorn N. Beyond the Natural Body: an archeology of sex hormones. 1ed. London: Routledge; 1994.

29. Beral V, Banks E, Reeves G. Evidence from randomised trials on the long-term effects of hormone replacement therapy. Lancet 2002;360(9337):942-4.

30. Love S, Lindsey K. Dr Susan Love's Menopause and Hormone Book: making informed choices. 3ed. New York: Three Rivers Press, N.Y.; 2003.

31. Richardson SJ, Senikas V, Nelson JF. Follicular depletion during the menopausal transition: evidence for accelerated loss and ultimate exhaustion. J Clin Endocrinol Metab 1987;65:1231.

32. Nielsen HK, Brixen K, Bouillon R, Mosekilde L. Changes in biochemical markers of osteoblastic activity during the menstrual cycle. J Clin Endocrinol Metab 1990;70:1431-7.

33. Van Look PF, Hunter WM, Fraser IS. Impaired estrogen-induced luteinizing hormone release in young women with anovulatory dysfunctional uterine bleeding. J Clin Endocrinol Metab 1978;46:816-21.

34. Park SJ, Goldsmith LT, Weiss G. Age-related changes in the regulation of luteinizing hormone secretion by estrogen in women. Exp.Biol. Med.(Maywood.) 2002;227(7):455-64.

35. Landgren BH, Unden AL, Diczfalusy E. Hormonal profile of the cycle in 68 normally menstruating women. Acta Endocr.Copenhagen 1980;94:89-98.

36. Soules MR, Sherman S, Parrott E, Rebar R, Santoro N, Utian W et al. Executive summary: stages of reproductive aging workshop (STRAW). Fertil.Steril. 2001;76:874-8.

37. Shideler SE, DeVane GW, Kalra PS, Bernirschke K, Lasley BL. Ovarian-pituitary hormone interactions during the perimenopause. Maturitas 1989;11:331-9.

38. Brambilla DJ, McKinlay SM, Johannes CB, Burger HG, Green A, Hopper J et al. Defining the perimenopause for application in epidemiologic investigations. Am.J.Epidemiol. 1994;140:10:1091-5.

39. Dennerstein L, Dudley EC, Hopper JL, Guthrie JR, Burger HG. A prospective population-based study of menopausal symptoms. Obstet Gynecol 2000;96:351-8.

40. Kaufert PA, Gilbert P, Tate R. Defining menopausal status: the impact of longitudinal data. Maturitas 1987;9:217-26.

41. Page L. Menopause and Emotions: making sense of your feelings when your feelings make no sense. 1ed. Vancouver: Primavera Press; 1994.

42. Prior, J. C. "The Puzzle of Perimenopause - Using the Daily Perimenopause Diary". 1999. Ref Type: Video Recording

43. Hallberg L, Hogdahl AM, Nillson L, Rybo G. Menstrual blood loss - a population study. Acta Obstet.Gynecol.Scand. 1966;45:320-51.

44. Prior JC. Exercise-associated menstrual disturbances. In: Adashi EY, Rock JA, Rosenwaks Z, editors. Reproductive Endocrinology, Surgery and Technology. New York: Raven Press; 1996. p. 1077-91.

45. Prior JC. Ovulatory disturbances: they do matter. Can.J.Diagnosis 1997; February:64-80.

46. Freedman RR, Woodward S. Behavioral treatment of menopausal hot flushes: evaluation by ambulatory monitoring. Am.J.Obstet.Gynecol. 1991; 167:436-9.

47. Hammar M, Berg G, Lindgren R. Does physical exercise influence the frequency of postmenopausal hot flushes? Acta Obstet.Gynecol. 1990;69:409-12.

48. Schiff I, Regestein Q, Tulchinsky D, Ryan KJ. Effects of estrogens on sleep and psychological state of hypogonadal women. Journal of the American Medical Association 1979;242:2405-7.

49. Nichols M, O'Hara J. Mark my words - memoirs of a very political reporter. Vancouver: Douglas & McIntyre; 1992.

50. Burger HG, Dudley EC, Cui J, Dennerstein L, Hopper JL. A prospective longitudinal study of serum testosterone, dehydroepiandrosterone sulfate, and sex hormone-binding globulin levels through the menopause transition. J.Clin.Endocrinol.Metab 2000;85(8):2832-8.

51. Zala L, Swan A, Prior JC. Transitions through the Perimenopausal Years. Victoria: Trafford Publishing; 2004.

52. Hunter M, Battersby R, Whitehead M. Relationships between psychological symptoms, somatic complaints and menopausal status. Maturitas 1986;8(3):217-28.

53. Avis NE, Stellato R, Crawford S, Bromberger J, Ganz P, Cain V et al. Is there a menopausal syndrome? Menopausal status and symptoms across racial/ethnic groups. Soc.Sci.Med. 2001;52(3):345-56.

54. Hunter MS. Physiological and somatic experience of the menopause: a prospective study. Psychomatic Med. 1990;52:357-67.

55. McCann L, Holmes DS. Influence of aerobic exercise on depression. J.Personal.Soc.Psych. 1984;46:1142-7.

56. Farmer ME, Locke BZ, Moscicki EK, Dannenberg AL, Larson DB, Radloff LS. Physical activity and depressive symptoms; the NHANES I epidemiologic follow-up study. Am.J.Epidemiol. 1988;128:1340-50.

57. Van Patten CL, Olivotto IA, Chambers GK, Gelman KA, Hislop TG, Templeton E et al. Effect of soy phytoestrogens on hot flashes in postmenopausal women with breast cancer: a randomized, controlled clinical trial. J.Clin.Oncol. 2002;20:1449-55.

58. Ford DE, Kamerow DB. Epidemiologic study of sleep disturbances and psychiatric disorders. An opportunity for prevention? JAMA 1989; 262(11):1479-84.

59. Gur A, Colpan L, Nas K, Cevir R, Sarac J, Erdogan F et al. The role of trace minerals in the pathogenesis of postmenopausal osteoporosis and a new effect of calcitonin. J Bone Miner Metab 2002;20:39-43.

60. Dawson-Hughes B, Dallal GE, Krall EA, Sadowski L, Sahyoun N, Tannenbaum S. A controlled trial of calcium supplementation on bone density in postmenopausal women. N Engl J Med 1990;323:878-83.

61. Hamajima N, Hirose K, Tajima K, Rohan T, Calle EE, Heath CW, Jr. et al. Alcohol, tobacco and breast cancer--collaborative reanalysis of individual data from 53 epidemiological studies, including 58,515 women with breast cancer and 95,067 women without the disease. Br.J.Cancer 2002;87(11):1234-45.

62. Rich-Edwards JW, Spiegelman D, Garland M, Hertzmark E, Hunter DJ, Colditz GA et al. Physical activity, body mass index, and ovulatory disorder infertility. Epidemiol. 2002;13(2):184-90.

63. Prior JC, Vigna YM, Watson D. Spironolactone with physiological female gonadal steroids in the presurgical therapy of male to female transexuals: a new observation. Arch.Sex.Beh. 1989;18:49-57.

64. Cumming DC, Yang JC, Rebar RW, Yen SSC. Treatment of hirsutism with spironolactone. Journal of the American Medical Association 1982;247:1295-8.

65. Tuomilehto J, Lindstrom J, Eriksson JG, Valle TT, Hamalainen H, Ilanne-Parikka P et al. Prevention of type 2 diabetes mellitus by changes in lifestyle among subjects with impaired glucose tolerance. N.Engl.J Med 2001;344(18):1343-50.

66. Knowler WC, Barrett-Connor E, Fowler SE, Hamman RF, Lachin JM, Walker EA et al. Reduction in the incidence of type 2 diabetes with lifestyle intervention or metformin. N.Engl.J Med 2002;346(6):393-403.

67. Prior JC, Alojado N, McKay DW, Vigna YM. No adverse effects of medroxyprogesterone treatment without estrogen in postmenopausal women: double-blind, placebo-controlled, cross-over trial. Obstetrics and Gynecology 1994;83:24-8.

68. Bruchovsky N, Rennie PS, Batzold FH, Goldenberg SL, Fletcher T, McLoughlin MG. Kinetic parameters of 5 alpha-reductase activity in stroma and epithelium of normal, hyperplastic, and carcinomatous human prostates. J Clin Endocrinol.Metab 1988;67(4):806-16.

69. Irvine GA, Campbell-Brown MB, Lumsden MA, Heikkila A, Walker JJ, Cameron IT. Randomised comparative trial of the levonorgestrel intrauterine system and norethisterone for treatment of idiopathic menorrhagia. Br.J Obstet.Gynaecol. 1998;105(6):592-8.

70. Fraser IS. Treatment of ovulatory and anovulatory dysfunctional uterine bleeding with oral progestogens. Aust.N.Z.J Obstet.Gynaecol. 1990;30(4):353-6.

71. Vollman RF. The menstrual cycle. In: Friedman EA, editor. Major Problems in Obstetrics and Gynecology, Vol 7. 1 ed. Toronto: W.B. Saunders Company; 1977. p. 11-193.

72. Rylance PB, Brincat M, Lafferty K, De Trafford JC, Brincat S, Parsons V et al. Natural progesterone and antihypertensive action. Br.Med.J. 1985;290:13-4.

73. Simon JA, Shangold MM, Andrews MC, Buster JC, Hodgen GD. Micronized progesterone therapy: the importance of route of administration and pharmacokinetics on clinical outcome. J Contracept Fertil Sex 1992;20:13-8.

74. Schiff I, Tulchinsky D, Cramer D, Ryan KJ. Oral medroxyprogesterone in the treatment of postmenopausal symptoms. Journal of the American Medical Association 1980;244:1443-5.

75. Prior, J. C., Alojado, N., Vigna, Y. M., Barr, S. I., and McKay, D. W. Estrogen and progestin are equally effective in symptom control post-ovariectomy--a one-year, double-blind, randomized trial in premenopausal women.

Program of the 76th Annual Meeting of the Endocrine Society, Anaheim, Ca. Abstract 12H, 411. 1994. Ref Type: Abstract

76. Roopnarinesingh S. Evaluation of progestational agents from postmeno-pausal hot flushes. Int.J.Gynecol.Obstet. 1982;20:133-5.

77. Lobo RA, McCormick W, Singer F, Roy S. Depo-medroxyprogesterone acetate compared with conjugated estrogens for the treatment of postmeno-pausal women. Obstet.Gynecol. 1984;63(1):1-5.

78. Prior JC, Ho Yeun B, Clement P, Bowie L, Thomas J. Reversible luteal phase changes and infertility associated with marathon training. Lancet 1982;1:269-70.

79. Ferin M. Clinical review 105: Stress and the reproductive cycle. J.Clin. Endocrinol.Metab 1999;84(6):1768-74.

80. Stachenfeld NS, Silva C, Keefe DL. Estrogen modifies the temperature effects of progesterone. J Appl.Physiol 2000;88(5):1643-9.

81. Friess E, Tagaya H, Trachsel L, Holsboer F, Rupprecht R. Progesterone-induced changes in sleep in male subjects. Am.J.Physiol. 1997;272:E885-E891.

82. Kalish GM, Barrett-Connor E, Laughlin GA, Gulanski BI. Association of endogenous sex hormones and insulin resistance among postmenopausal women: results from the Postmenopausal Estrogen/Progestin Intervention Trial. J Clin Endocrinol.Metab 2003;88(4):1646-52.

83. Boyd NF, Byng JW, Jong RA, Fishell EK, Little LE, Miller AB et al. Quantitative classification of mammographic densities and breast cancer risks: results from the Canadian National Breast Screening Study. J.Nation. Can.Inst. 1995;87:670-5.

84. Guttuso T, Jr., Kurlan R, McDermott MP, Kieburtz K. Gabapentin's effects on hot flashes in postmenopausal women: a randomized controlled trial. Obstet.Gynecol. 2003;101(2):337-45.

85. Paul SM, Purdy RH. Neuroactive steroids. FASEB J 1992;6(6):2311-22.

86. Wallston KA, Wallston BS, DeVellis R. Development of the Multidimen-sional health locus of control (MHLC) scales. Health.Educat.Monograph. 1978;6:160-70.

87. Reynolds FA. Perceived control over menopausal hot flushes: exploring the correlates of a standardised measure. Maturitas 1997;27(3):215-21.

88. Rapp SR, Espeland MA, Shumaker SA, Henderson VW, Brunner RL, Manson JE et al. Effect of estrogen plus progestin on global cognitive function in postmenopausal women: the Women's Health Initiative Memory Study: a randomized controlled trial. JAMA 2003;289(20):2663-72.

89. Loprinzi CL, Michalak JC, Quella SK, O'Fallan JR, Hatfield AK, Nelimark RA et al. Megesterol acetate for the prevention of hot flashes. N Engl J Med 1994;331:347-52.

90. Hitchcock CL, Prior JC. Evidence about extending the duration of oral contraceptive use to suppress menstruation. Women's Health Issues 2004;14(6):201-11.

91. Kirschbaum C, Schommer N, Federenko I, Gaab J, Neumann O, Oellers M et al. Short-term estradiol treatment enhances pituitary-adrenal axis and sympathetic responses to psyhosocial stress in healthy young men. J Clin Endocrinol Metab 1996;81:3639-43.

92. Scarabin PY, Oger E, Plu-Bureau. Differential association of oral and transdermal oestrogen-replacement therapy with venous thromboembolism risk. Lancet 2003;362(9382):428-32.

93. Collins A, Landgren B. Reproductive health, use of estrogen and experience of symptoms in perimenopausal women: a population-based study. Maturitas 1995;20:101-11.

94. Guthrie JR, Dennerstein L, Hopper JL, Burger HG. Hot flushes, menstrual status, and hormone levels in a population-based sample of midlife women. Obstetrics and Gynecology 1996;88(3):437-42.

95. Prior JC, Alojado N, McKay DW, Vigna YM. Medroxyprogesterone increases basal temperature: a placebo-controlled crossover trial in postmenopausal women. Fertil.Steril. 1995;63:1222-6.

96. Leonetti HB, Longo S, Anasti JN. Transdermal progesterone cream for vasomotor symptoms and postmenopausal bone loss. Obstetrics and Gynecology 1999;94:225-8.

97. Stearns V, Beebe KL, Iyengar M, Dube E. Paroxetine controlled release in the treatment of menopausal hot flashes: a randomized controlled trial. JAMA 2003;289(21):2827-34.

98. Albrecht BH, Schiff I, Tulchinsky D, Ryan KJ. Objective evidence that placebo and oral medroxyprogesterone acetate therapy diminish menopausal vasomotor flushes. Am.J.Obstet.Gynecol. 1981;139:631-5.

99. Swartzman LC, Edelberg R, Kemmann E. Impact of stress on objectively recorded menopausal hot flushes and on flush report bias. Health Psychology 1990;9:529-45.

100. Freedman RR. Biochemical, metabolic, and vascular mechanisms in menopausal hot flashes. Fertil.Steril. 1998;70(2):332-7.

101. Ganz PA, Greendale GA, Petersen L, Zibecchi L, Kahn B, Belin TR. Managing menopausal symptoms in breast cancer survivors: results of a randomized controlled trial. J Natl.Cancer Inst. 2000;92(13):1054-64.

102. Wijma K, Melin A, Nedstrand E, Hammar M. Treatment of menopausal symptoms with applied relaxation: a pilot study. J.Behav.Ther.Exp.Psychiatry 1997;28(4):251-61.

103. Rodriguez-Sierra JF, Hagley MT, Hendricks SE. Anxiolytic effects of progesterone are sexually dimorphic. Life Sci. 1986;38(20):1841-5.

104. Lebrun CM, Petit MA, McKenzie DC, Taunton JE, Prior JC. Decreased maximal aerobic capacity with use of a triphasic oral contraceptive in highly active women: a randomised controlled trial. Br.J.Sports Med. 2003;37(4):315-20.

105. Bennett KL, Malcolm SA, Thomas SA, Ebeling PR, McCrory PR, Wark JD et al. Risk factors for stress fractures in female track-and-field athletes: a retrospective analysis. Clin.J.Sport.Med. 1995;5:229-35.

106. Meyer HE, Tverdal A, Faich JA. Changes in body weight and incidence of hip fracture among middle aged Norwegians. Br.Med.J. 1995;311:91-2.

107. Schweiger U, Tuschl RJ, Platte P, Broocks A, Laessle RG, Pirke KM. Everyday eating behavior and menstrual function in young women. Fertil. Steril. 1992;57:771-5.

108. McLean JA, Barr SI, Prior JC. Cognitive dietary restraint is associated with higher urinary cortisol excretion in healthy premenopausal women. Am.J.Clin.Nutr. 2001;73:7-12.

109. Barr SI, Janelle KC, Prior JC. Vegetarian versus nonvegetarian diets, dietary restraint, and subclinical ovulatory disturbances: prospective six month study. Am.J.Clin.Nutr. 1994;60:887-94.

110. Barr SI, Prior JC, Vigna YM. Restrained eating and ovulatory disturbances: possible implications for bone health. Am.J.Clin.Nutr. 1994;59:92-7.

111. McLean JA, Barr SI, Prior JC. Dietary restraint, exercise and bone density in young women: are they related? Med.Sci.Sports Exerc. 2001;33:1292-6.

112. McKinlay SM, Brambilla DJ, Posner JG. The normal menopause transition. Maturitas 1992;14:103-15.

113. Collop NA. Medroxyprogesterone acetate and ethanol-induced exacerbation of obstructive sleep apnea. Chest 1994;106:792-9.

114. Barr SI, Janelle KC, Prior JC. Energy intakes are higher during the luteal phase of ovulatory menstrual cycles. Am.J.Clin.Nutr. 1995;61:39-43.

115. Hammar M, Hammar-Henriksson MB, Frisk J, Rickenlund A, Wyon YAM. Few oligo-amenorrheic athletes have vasomotor symptoms. Maturitas 2000;34:219-25.

116. Ivarsson T, Spetz A, Hammar M. Physical exercise and vasomotor symptoms in postmenopausal women. Maturitas 1998;29:139-46.

117. Lindh-Astrand L, Nedstrand E, Wyon Y, Hammar M. Vasomotor symptoms and quality of life in previously sedentary postmenopausal women randomised to physical activity or estrogen therapy. Maturitas 2004;48(2):97-105.

118. Guthrie JR, Ebeling PR, Hopper JL, Barrett-Connor E, Dennerstein L, Dudley EC et al. A prospective study of bone loss in menopausal Australian-born women. Osteoporos.Int. 1998;8:282-90.

119. Okano H, Mizunuma H, Soda M, Kagami I, Miyamoto S, Ohsawa M et al. The long-term effect of menopause on postmenopausal bone loss in Japanese women: results from a prospective study. J.Bone Min.Res. 1998;13(2):303-9.

120. Recker R, Lappe J, Davies K, Heaney R. Characterization of perimenopausal bone loss: a prospective study. J.Bone Min.Res. 2000;15(10):1965-73.

121. Prior JC, Vigna YM, Barr SI, Rexworthy C, Lentle BC. Cyclic medroxyprogesterone treatment increases bone density: a controlled trial in active women with menstrual cycle disturbances. Am.J.Med. 1994;96:521-30.

122. Torgerson DJ, Garton MJ, Reid DM. Falling and perimenopausal women. Age and Ageing 1993;22:59-64.

123. Borugian MJ, Sheps SB, Kim-Sing C, Olivotto IA, Van Patten C, Dunn BP et al. Waist-to-hip ratio and breast cancer mortality. Am J Epidemiol. 2003;158(10):963-8.

124. Laughlin GA, Barrett-Connor E, Kritz-Silverstein D, von Muhlen D. Hysterectomy, oophorectomy, and endogenous sex hormone levels in older women: the Rancho Bernardo Study. J Clin Endocrinol Metab 2000;85:645-51.

125. Pritchard JE, Nowson C, Wark JD. Bone loss accompanying diet-induced or exercise-induced weight loss: a randomised controlled study. Int.J.Obesity 1996;20:513-20.

126. Tavani A, Ricci E, La Vecchia C, Surace M, Benzi G, Parazzini F et al. Influence of menstrual and reproductive factors on ovarian cancer risk in women with and without family history of breast or ovarian cancer. Int. J.Epidemiol. 2000;29(5):799-802.

127. Marshall WA, Tanner JM. Variations in pattern of pubertal changes in girls. Arch.Dis.Child. 1969;44:291-303.

128. Chang KJ, Lee TTY, Linares-Cruz G, Fournier S, de Lignieres B. Influence of percutaneous administration of estradiol and progesterone on human breast epithelial cell cycle in vivo. Fertil.Steril. 1995;63:785-91.

129. Foidart J, Collin C, Denoo X, Desreux J, Belliard A, Fournier S et al. Estradiol and progesterone regulate the proliferation of human breast epithelial cells. Fertil.Steril. 1998;5:963-9.

130. Chlebowski RT, Hendrix SL, Langer RD, Stefanick ML, Gass M, Lane D et al. Influence of estrogen plus progestin on breast cancer and mammography in healthy postmenopausal women: the Women's Health Initiative Randomized Trial. JAMA 2003;289(24):3243-53.

131. The Women's Health Initiative Study Group. Design of the Women's Health Initiative clinical trial and observational study. Control Clin Trials 1998;19(1):61-109.

132. Mather KJ, Norman EG, Prior JC, Elliott TG. Preserved forearm endothelial responses with acute exposure to progesterone: a randomized cross-over trial of 17-b estradiol, progesterone, and 17-b estradiol with progesterone in healthy menopausal women. J Clin Endocrinol Metab 2000;85:4644-9.

133. Prior JC, Vigna YM, Schechter MT, Burgess AE. Spinal bone loss and ovulatory disturbances. N Engl J Med 1990;323:1221-7.

134. Prior JC. The cultural causes of osteoporosis for women. In: Kahn SE,

editor. Women, Stress and Coping: An interdisciplinary research workshop. Vancouver, B.C.: University of British Columbia; 1989. p. 13-22.

135. Cauley JA, Lucas FL, Kuller LH, Vogt TM, Browner WS, Cummings SR. Bone mineral density and risk of breast cancer in older women. Journal of the American Medical Association 1996;276(17):1404-8.

136. Lindsay R, Gallagher JC, Kleerekoper M, Pickar JH. Effect of lower doses of conjugated equine estrogens with and without medroxyprogesterone acetate on bone in early postmenopausal women. JAMA 2002;287:2668-76.

137. Grey A, Cundy T, Evans M, Reid I. Medroxyprogesterone acetate enhances the spinal bone density response to estrogen in late post-menopausal women. Clin.Endocr. 1996;44:293-6.

138. Early Breast Cancer Trialists' Collaborative Group. Systemic disease of early breast cancer by hormonal cytotoxic or immune therapy - 133 randomized trials involving 31,000 recurrences and 24,000 deaths among 75,000 women. Lancet 1992;339:1-15,-71-85.

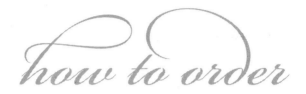

how to order

Available through your local bookstore and from our webpage at:

**www.cemcor.ubc.ca**

Distributed by:

**Sandhill Book Marketing Ltd.**
Distribution for Small Press & Independent Publishers
#99 – 1270 Ellis Street
Cannery Row Building
Kelowna, BC Canada V1Y 1Z4
Tel: 250-763-1406
Fax: 250-763-4051
Website: www.sandhillbooks.com

# *about the author*

Dr. Jerilynn C. Prior grew up in a remote Alaskan fishing village as one of five children. She worked her way through university and medical school with the aid of scholarships and by digging ditches, being a deckhand, and being a fire warden on a lookout tower. She moved to Vancouver, Canada, with her family in 1976. She finished her training in endocrinology at the University of British Columbia and became a full professor in 1994.

As a young faculty member in 1980, Dr. Prior performed the first of many studies of the menstrual cycle. She continues to research the experiences and health issues that are important for women. In 2002, she founded the Centre for Menstrual Cycle and Ovulation Research (www.cemcor.ubc.ca).

Dr. Prior is known internationally for controversial research showing that regular ovulation is needed for optimal health, that progesterone increases bone formation, and that perimenopause is symptomatic because of higher estrogen levels—not lower, as is commonly thought. She has received scientific recognition and many honours, and is a widely sought-after physician, teacher, and mentor. She is invited around the world to address academic and general audiences.